T0073796

The Stigma of Mental Illness

The Stigma of Mental Illness

Models and Methods of Stigma Reduction

Edited by

Keith S. Dobson

Professor of Clinical Psychology
Department of Psychology, University of Calgary, Canada

Heather Stuart

Professor and Bell Canada Mental Health and Anti-stigma Research Chair

Departments of Community Health Sciences, Psychiatry, and School of Rehabilitation Therapy, Queen's University, Kingston, Ontario, Canada

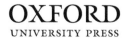

OXFORD
UNIVERSITY PRESS

OXFORD
UNIVERSITY PRESS

Oxford University Press is a department of the University of Oxford. It furthers
the University's objective of excellence in research, scholarship, and education
by publishing worldwide. Oxford is a registered trade mark of Oxford University
Press in the UK and certain other countries.

Published in the United States of America by Oxford University Press
198 Madison Avenue, New York, NY 10016, United States of America.

© Oxford University Press 2021

All rights reserved. No part of this publication may be reproduced, stored in a retrieval system, or transmitted, in any
form or by any means, without the prior permission in writing of Oxford University Press, or as expres sly permitted
by law, by license, or under terms agreed with the appropriate reproduction rights organization. Inquiries concerning
reproduction outside the scope of the above should be sent to the Rights Department, Oxford University Press, at the
address above.

You must not circulate this work in any other form
and you must impose this same condition on any acquirer.

Library of Congress Cataloging-in-Publication Data
Names: Dobson, Keith S., editor. | Stuart, Heather L., editor.
Title: The stigma of mental illness : models and methods of stigma reduction /
[edited by] Keith Dobson, Heather Stuart.
Description: New York, NY : Oxford University Press, [2021] |
Includes bibliographical references and index. |
Identifiers: LCCN 2021017049 (print) | LCCN 2021017050 (ebook) |
ISBN 9780197572597 (hardback) | ISBN 9780197572610 (epub) |
ISBN 9780197572627 (other)
Subjects: MESH: Mental Disorders | Social Stigma | Social Discrimination—prevention & control |
Prejudice | Mental Health Services Classification: LCC RC454 (print) |
LCC RC454 (ebook) | NLM WM 140 | DDC 616.89—dc23
LC record available at https://lccn.loc.gov/2021017049
LC ebook record available at https://lccn.loc.gov/2021017050

This material is not intended to be, and should not be considered, a substitute for medical or other professional advice.
Treatment for the conditions described in this material is highly dependent on the individual circumstances. And,
while this material is designed to offer accurate information with respect to the subject matter covered and to be current
as of the time it was written, research and knowledge about medical and health issues is constantly evolving and dose
schedules for medications are being revised continually, with new side effects recognized and accounted for regularly.
Readers must therefore always check the product information and clinical procedures with the most up-to-date
published product information and data sheets provided by the manufacturers and the most recent codes of conduct and
safety regulation. The publisher and the authors make no representations or warranties to readers, express or implied, as
to the accuracy or completeness of this material. Without limiting the foregoing, the publisher and the authors make no
representations or warranties as to the accuracy or efficacy of the drug dosages mentioned in the material. The authors
and the publisher do not accept, and expressly disclaim, any responsibility for any liability, loss, or risk that may be
claimed or incurred as a consequence of the use and/or application of any of the contents of this material.

DOI: 10.1093/med/9780197572597.001.0001

Contents

Preface

The World Health Organization defines health as "a state of complete physical, mental and social well-being and not merely the absence of disease or infirmity" (see https://www.who.int/about/who-we-are/constitution), and it further states that the "enjoyment of the highest attainable standard of health is one of the fundamental rights of every human being." The incorporation of mental well-being as a critical feature of fundamental human rights underscores the importance of this area of functioning and the need to address the impediments to the attainment of this right. Declining or poor mental health is associated with a multitude of other personal and social problems, including worse physical health, reduced employment opportunities and socioeconomic status, limitations to participation in society, and potentially forced hospitalization and/or treatment.

A recognized corollary of mental health problems or mental illness is the risk of stigma. Stigma can be demonstrated in a variety of forms, including social or public stigma (negative attributes, emotions, and behaviors toward others with mental illness), self-stigma (internalized negative ideas toward and feelings about the self, possible self-limitation or self-handicapping behavior), and structural stigma (organizational policies, procedures, and systems that reduce the rights and opportunities for individuals with mental illness). The range of these varied forms of stigma continues to be exposed, even as their deleterious effects both on people with mental illness and on those who care for and love them are documented.

This volume represents the distillation of years of effort to understand, measure, and reduce the stigma of mental illness. Much of the work represented in this volume is the direct result of work from the Mental Health Commission of Canada, but its scope is global in nature. The Mental Health Commission of Canada was inaugurated in 2007, with an initial 10-year mandate (since renewed) to examine issues related to mental health promotion and the care of people with mental illness in Canada. One aspect of the commission's work is the Opening Minds program (see https://www.mentalhealthcommission.ca/English/opening-minds), which has an explicit focus on understanding the role of stigma related to mental illness and the development and delivery of evidence-based programs to reduce stigma and its consequences. The Opening Minds researchers have adopted a somewhat unique approach to the topic of stigma, including work on assessment tools and multifaceted programs that utilize the emerging science of validated methods to undermine stigma in focused areas. Thus, the program has eschewed the more common strategy of public information and marketing related to mental illness and instead selected domains where stigma has been recognized and where focused work could have an impact. In particular, these areas focus on youth, healthcare, the workplace, and media.

The chapters in this volume are organized into several sections. Introductory chapters define the scope of stigma and conceptual issues in the field. One chapter focuses on the topic of structural stigma because this is a relatively recent construct in the field of stigma, and the exposition of its nature and processes is an important contribution to the field. After presenting the concepts and structures related to stigma, the volume shifts its focus to assessment. Many stigma measures exist, but the vast majority are in the domain of public stigma toward people with mental illness, and most would be relatively unserviceable to evaluate the outcomes of targeted programs. As such, several novel measures are introduced so that the reader can understand the approach taken to measurement and see the resultant measures. Indeed, one of the explicit hopes of this volume is that readers will take the materials presented and, with appropriate modifications or restandardization, utilize them and help to build the empirical literature in this field.

The third section of this volume presents descriptions of and reports from a series of novel intervention programs in the areas of youth, healthcare, the workplace, and media. The reports document the models that were used, the incorporation of validated strategies such as contact-based education, and the outcomes associated with these various interventions. The overall result of this work is a series of documented programs that can be freely shared in other contexts or adapted for use in novel ways or with new populations, languages, cultures, or target groups. A latter chapter explicitly discusses the importance of knowledge dissemination and the methods of implementation science as valuable ways to consider program adaptation and validation. A final chapter discusses the place at which the field of stigma for mental illness has arrived and potential directions for the future evolution of the field.

Chapter authors were encouraged in the writing of this book to provide both scholarly and practical conclusions from their work. In this regard, every chapter concludes with a set of key recommendations or directions for work within the scope of that chapter. We have also purposefully created a set of materials in the appendices that can be borrowed, adapted, and utilized by the reader. In fact, one of the goals in the production of this volume was that others who work in this area will take the practical ideas and materials and continue to develop and evaluate them in ways that we cannot perhaps even imagine.

We must recognize the pivotal importance of the Mental Health Commission of Canada in the funding of and support for much of the work represented in this book. The board of directors has supported the Opening Minds program since the inception of the commission and that support is duly acknowledged. The director of the Opening Minds program, Micheal Pietrus, deserves particular mention because he has been with the commission since it opened, and he has fully supported the work of researchers and clinicians to develop and validate the measures and programs within Opening Minds. We also wish to acknowledge the many other groups within Canada that have been working to reduce the stigma of mental illness. Bell Canada has for many years conducted the "Let's Talk" initiative, which is a strategy to encourage people with mental illness to bring their conditions into the daylight and to force a dialogue about issues related to mental illness. Bell Canada has supported one of us (Dr. Stuart) through a funded chair at Queen's University.

We also wish to take this opportunity to thank the acquisitions editors at Oxford University Press for their willingness to continue to publish in the area of the stigma of mental illness. Stigma is a global problem, and the endorsement of a major publishing firm to undertake this volume should be understood as part of a global response. As coeditors, we have both worked in the field of mental health for many years, and while we have seen considerable developments and improvements, much remains to be done. The recognition of and meaningful response to the stigma of mental illness remains one of the most important set of activities in the field of mental health and illness. It is our fervent hope that readers will take what is presented in this volume and advance this work in multiple directions.

Keith S. Dobson, PhD
University of Calgary, Alberta, Canada
Heather Stuart, PhD
Queen's University, Ontario, Canada
January 2021

Contributors

Shu-Ping Chen, University of Alberta, Edmonton

Keith S. Dobson, University of Calgary, Calgary

Bonnie Kirsh, University of Toronto, Toronto

Stephanie Knaak, University of Calgary, Calgary

Michelle Koller, Queen's University, Kingston

Bianca Lauria-Horner, Dalhousie University, Halifax

Brittany L. Lindsay, University of Calgary, Calgary

Dorothy Luong, University Health Network, Toronto

Beth Milliard, York Regional Police, Toronto

Scott Patten, University of Calgary, Calgary

Heather Stuart, Queen's University, Kingston

Andrew C. H. Szeto, University of Calgary, Calgary

Thomas Ungar, St. Michael's Hospital, Unity Health & University of Toronto, Toronto

Rob Whitley, McGill University and the Douglas Research Centre, Montreal

1

Prejudice and Discrimination Related to Mental Illnesses

Keith S. Dobson and Heather Stuart

According to the *Oxford English Dictionary* (2020), the word *stigma* is derived from the Greek στίγμα, which reflects a mark or brand made by a pointed instrument, termed a *stig* (Arboleda-Flórez & Stuart, 2012). In modern English, however, there are no fewer than seven potential definitions of the word. Several definitions of stigma refer to horticultural or biological phenomena, usually small openings or pores. In the context of mental illness, however, the *Oxford English Dictionary* provides a figurative definition for the word stigma as follows: "A mark of disgrace or infamy; a sign of severe censure or condemnation, regarded as impressed on a person or thing; a 'brand'" (see Figure 1.1). Historians of the stigma concept will also know that it has been applied to the wounds of Jesus suffered during the crucifixion or to stigmata (bleeding hands) experienced by saints and holy men. In this latter meaning, spontaneous openings or bleeding have been associated with a blessed state or affinity with God or a higher being (Simon, 1992). For example, St. Francis of Assisi was reported to have bled spontaneously from the palms of his hands, which was taken as a clear sign of his devotion. Thus, the term *stigma* has been used both as a mark of grace and as a mark of disgrace.

The bulk of stigma research has examined the experiences of people with a mental illness and, to a lesser extent, substance use disorder. However, it is important to note that a wide variety of illnesses and disabilities have been stigmatized, including intellectual disabilities, physical and sensory disabilities, HIV/AIDS, infectious diseases such as leprosy, cancer, obesity, and Alzheimer's disease. Although stereotypes differ among illnesses and disabilities, many of the same underlying mechanisms (such as public fear and intolerance) and impacts (such as social segregation and inequity) likely are at play (Corrigan, 2014).

The use of the term stigma in the field of mental health and illness is typically attributed to the work of Erving Goffman. In 1961, he published the volume *Asylums*, which was a critical analysis of psychiatric facilities and their punitive effect on the mental well-being of the patients they held. This book was followed in 1963 by *Stigma: Notes on the Management of Spoiled Identity*. Goffman argued that the natural consequence of being treated as a psychiatric patient in an asylum was what he termed "spoiled identity" and that this process was enabled by stigma, through which

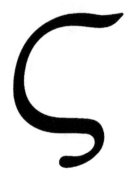

Figure 1.1 The Greek Symbol for Stigma

patients were demeaned, labeled, and entered into what was essentially a negative and self-reinforcing system that was difficult, if not impossible, to escape. One of the principal heritages of these books is that the concept of labeling and diagnosis is often now considered to be perforce stigmatizing and that diagnostic labels have a strong potential within psychiatric settings to become equivalent to enduring, if not permanent, "marks" or "brands."

As a sociologist, Goffman viewed stigma as a relational construct—something conferred by the social group. However, his definition has been criticized for overemphasizing the attributes of the individual patient and the various effects that labeling had on the individual, rather than the power relationships that underlie the creation and maintenance of social inequities. In contrast, Link and Phelan (2001) further contributed to the development of the stigma concept when they identified several important social and structural aspects of the stigmatization process. Included in these aspects was the fact that labeling is done in a social context, typically as a method to differentiate between "normal" and "abnormal" individuals, "us" and "them." They also noted that diagnostic labels most often had negative social connotations and that these negative social connotations usually were associated with discriminatory behavior and reduced social status. Further, there was an inherent social structure and set of authorities involved in the process of labeling and stigmatization, such that the affected individuals were labeled as "patients" and, through this identity, were disadvantaged socially, economically, and politically. Stigmatization occurs in the context of power. Only powerful groups have the ability to create and maintain stigma.

Contemporary models of stigma often distinguish among three related features. Two of these features can be traced to the earlier developments described in the previous paragraphs. Thus, there is both the concept of public (sometimes called social) stigma and the concept of self-stigma. Public stigma refers to the differentiation between us and them in the process of labeling and diagnosis, the identification of an individual as a "patient" who requires treatment or hospitalization, the potential overidentification of the individual with their diagnosis, the risk of self-confirming biases in the way that an individual with a diagnosis is seen and treated, and the pejorative labels that are used ubiquitously in society to refer to disparaged individuals as "crazy," "insane," or other punitive labels. In like manner, self-stigma refers to the ways in which an individual who faces mental health problems can self-handicap, self-label, limit their own development, attribute failure to their diagnosis, and essentially act in a manner that internalizes public biases and turns them against themselves (Corrigan et al., 2016).

More recently, the concept of structural stigma has gained increasing attention (Pincus, 1999). Structural stigma is again a sociological concept that identifies the inherent and intentional effects that derive from social power dynamics and the policies and practices of institutions to restrict the autonomy of people with a mental illness. For example, the practice of involuntary hospitalization has been argued to be a de facto diminishment of the legal rights of people who may consider self-injury. Other forms of structural stigma include the ability of insurance companies to deny payment to families in instances of suicide, the restriction on individuals with a history of a mental illness to be precluded from certain occupations, or the practice on some credit card applications that requires the declaration of psychiatric diagnoses that can preclude entry into some countries. Structural stigma is multifaceted and widely expressed in social groups, making it challenging to address in a comprehensive way. However, there is growing recognition that structural stigma creates and nurtures stigma within and across generations. Thus, it is receiving growing scientific and policy interest.

In addition to the current distinction between public, self, and structural stigma, the critical features of the stigma concept have been elaborated. Whereas earlier concepts of stigma emphasized negative attitudes and beliefs about individuals with a mental illness, contemporary models typically elucidate three features that function under the larger umbrella concept of stigma. These three features include negative attitudes or beliefs, as have been associated with stigma over time, but also negative or pejorative affect and discriminatory behavior at both the individual and the organizational level. The primary affect associated with social stigma is fear. Many depictions of individuals with mental illnesses show them to be unpredictable, unreliable, and potentially dangerous (Goodwin, 2014). Not surprisingly, many aspects of public stigma reinforce the need to isolate people who are mentally ill and to protect society from individuals who have these attributes. In contrast, self-stigma is more associated with feelings of shame, embarrassment, self-hatred, and diminishment. Structural stigma is more associated with concepts related to paternalism and social inequity, but is also infused with the protection of society from someone who can be viewed as potentially unpredictable and dangerous (Livingston, 2020).

Arguably, one of the most important developments within the broader conceptualization of stigma is the awareness that it is also associated with negative behaviors toward individuals with mental illnesses. Discriminatory behaviors can take a number of explicit and subtle forms. In public stigma, discriminatory behaviors can include social isolation and shunning, gossiping about an individual, refusing to promote someone at the workplace because of concerns about reliability, and much

Table 1.1 *Matrix Model of Stigma*

		Type of stigma		
		Public	Self	Structural
Features of stigma	Attitudes, beliefs	Unpredictable Unreliable Dangerousness	Damaged Weak Vulnerable	Unpredictable Unreliable Dangerousness
	Affect	Fear	Embarrassment Self-hatred Diminishment	Fear Parentalism
	Discriminatory behaviors	Social isolation Shunning Limited opportunity	Isolation Self-limitation	Restricted freedoms Limited opportunity

more. Individuals who struggle with mental health challenges can also adopt self-stigmatizing beliefs and act in ways that discriminate against themselves, such as purposefully dressing in a way to be less visible in society, not speaking up for themselves in social situations, or not seeking positions or promotions even if they are fully qualified. Corrigan and colleagues refer to this as the "why try" effect (Corrigan et al., 2009). Structural stigma can also be enacted in different ways, such as policies that prohibit insurance claims based on death by suicide, screening for mental fitness for certain social roles even if the linkage to the role is tenuous, or restricted healthcare for people who have a mental illness. Table 1.1 provides a conceptual overview of the three forms of stigma (public, self, and structural) and the three features of stigma (beliefs, affect, and behaviors) that can be exhibited within these forms.

The Development and Maintenance of Stigma

One of the underexplored issues in the field of stigma is how it develops or is maintained. Multiple overlapping processes can eventuate in stigmatizing attitudes, feelings, or behaviors. Part of the process is likely the inherent way in which humans differentiate or categorize objects and circumstances. From an early age, children look for patterns and apply labels to physical objects and groups. As life continues, this categorization process is extended to social constructs, and it is further attached to emotional valences. Thus, humans learn to like "happy people," to fear "odd behavior," and to seek out, identify, and befriend others who generally agree with their values and perspectives. The specific attributes of people we either seek out or wish to avoid will vary somewhat from culture to culture, and these attributes are also heavily influenced by socialization. Strong social influences that help individuals define what is "normal" and "abnormal" include parents, friends, family, various forms of media, popular film, and literature. In some cases, personal experiences with others who are viewed as odd, eccentric, or abnormal can also influence ideas, affect, and behavior. The formal healthcare system, including the diagnostic system for mental illnesses, also represents an institutionalized and structural system to label and potentially stigmatize individuals.

Once established, mental sets and biases are difficult to change. Humans naturally employ a series of cognitive heuristics and systems to simplify our world and to make sense of our experience. For example, we selectively attend to and recall information that is consistent with our beliefs, while selectively disattending to, minimizing, or forgetting inconsistent information (Kahneman, 2011). Humans have cognitive systems that "think fast" to process information that conforms to existing biases, whereas changing these biases requires effort and "thinking slow." Notably, one feature of the process of thinking fast is loss aversion, in which humans naturally attend to perceived threats more quickly and efficiently. In this regard, the fact that individuals with mental health problems are often portrayed as erratic or dangerous in media and the entertainment industry reinforces the rapid stigmatization and social rejection of such individuals. Labeling and pejorative language help to cement the stereotypical views held toward people with a mental illness.

A Social Justice Perspective

Although the prior discussion frames the manners in which stigma can be experienced and expressed and helps to understand the genesis and maintenance of stigma, it fails to consider the fact that many aspects of stigma exist as self-perpetuating beliefs and biases. Further, it fails to address the need to identify and minimize systems of social control and potential victimization for individuals who experience mental health challenges. In this latter regard, there is a strong need for the perspective of social justice, to ensure that rights, freedoms, abilities, and potentialities are maximized.

Within the Canadian context, it has been recognized for some time that the mental health system can hinder as well as help people who struggle with mental illnesses and that stigma toward mental illnesses often perpetuates the problems faced by people with mental health challenges (Arboleda-Flórez & Sartorius, 2008; Corrigan, 2014; Hinshaw & Stier, 2008). For this reason, the Senate Committee on Social Affairs, Science and Technology explored these issues and released a wide-ranging report (Kirby & Keon, 2006) that included a large number of social policy, legal, educational, media, reporting, workplace, and health service delivery recommendations. One of the most tangible outcomes of the *Out of the Shadows* report was the creation of the Mental Health Commission of Canada (MHCC) in March 2007, funded through and reporting to Health Canada, but operating as a separate not-for-profit organization. Its early goals included the development of a mental health strategy for Canada, a demonstration project in mental health and homelessness, a focus on reduction of prejudice and discrimination, knowledge exchange, and developing partnerships.

The Mental Health Strategy for Canada (MHCC, 2012) reinforced the multipronged and progressive agenda set by the MHCC in its earlier releases.

One of the initiatives of the MHCC and the one that is directly connected to the current volume was Opening Minds (see https://www.mentalhealthcommission.ca/English/opening-minds). Opening Minds, the antistigma agency within the MHCC, was created in 2009 to identify issues related to stigma and to try to reduce stigma as a barrier to care. Opening Minds initially addressed stigma within four target groups: healthcare providers, youth, the workforce, and the media. Large social marketing campaigns were deemed to be inadequate to change behaviors and cost-ineffective. Even by the time of its first report (Pietrus, 2013), it was clear that the Opening Minds teams were active in all of these areas, conducting literature reviews, developing and validating novel assessment tools, developing and evaluating intervention programs related to stigma, and advancing the understanding of the logic behind and strategies to optimize stigma reduction in various domains. Another part of the Opening Minds team was evaluating the manner in which mental health was portrayed in Canadian television and print media (Whitley & Wang, 2017a, 2017b). Even more, a process model was developed to assist with the different phases of design, development, evaluation, and dissemination (see Figure 1.2).

One of the principal features of the work of the Opening Minds program was its reliance on the best possible evidence (Stuart et al., 2014). As different areas of work were initiated, a literature review was typically conducted (Malachowski & Kirsch, 2013; Patten et al., 2012; Szeto et al., 2013; Szeto & Dobson, 2010; Whitley & Berry, 2013) to determine the state of theory and research. In some cases, it was recognized that the measures or metrics needed to properly evaluate work did not exist, and novel measures were created and validated (Kassam et al., 2012; Modgill et al., 2014;

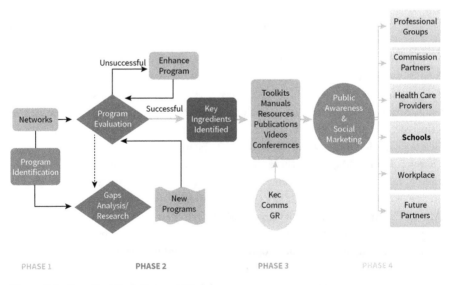

Figure 1.2 Opening Minds Process Model

Szeto & Dobson, 2010). Thereafter, trials were conducted of the many programs that were developed, modified, and put into broad use (cf., Dobson et al., 2019; MHCC, 2016; Papish et al., 2013; Szeto et al., 2019). As can be discerned from the above set of published articles, although the work typically resulted in internal technical reports, web-based announcements, and professional conference presentations, the work was also of such a caliber that it typically emerged in peer-reviewed academic journals.

The current volume is a testament to the widespread activities of the Opening Minds program and the researchers and practitioners who were part of the effort. The reduction of stigma has been recognized as a critical issue for the defensible and just treatment of people who experience mental health challenges (Corrigan, 2018; Stuart et al., 2012), and so this work forms an essential part of that international effort. The book is organized into four sections that address conceptual issues in the field, meas- urement, stigma reduction programs, and future directions for the field. Throughout, an effort has been made to provide clear and succinct messages, coupled with prac- tical tools for researchers and clinicians, so that they are able to take the ideas pre- sented here and apply them in diverse contexts. With this goal in mind, the book includes sets of appendices with copies of reprinted measures and programs. There is also discussion of the process of dissemination and how to adapt what is offered here to other diverse settings, whether this be unique population targets within a given country or diverse global settings.

References

Arboleda-Flórez, J., & Sartorius, N. (Eds.). (2008). *Understanding the stigma of mental ill- ness: Theory and interventions.* J. Wiley & Sons.

Corrigan, P. W. (Ed.). (2014). *Stigma of disease and disability: Understanding causes and over- coming prejudices.* American Psychological Association Press.

Corrigan, P. W. (2018). *The stigma effect: Unintended consequences of mental health campaigns.* Columbia University Press.

Corrigan, P. W., Bink, A. B., Schmidt, A., Jones, N., & Rüsch, N. (2016). What is the impact of self-stigma? Loss of self-respect and the "why try" effect. *Journal of Mental Health, 25*(1), 10–15.

Corrigan, P. W., Larson, J. E., & Rüsch, N. (2009). Self-stigma and the "why try" effect: Impact on life goals and evidence-based practices. *World Psychiatry, 8*(2), 75–81.

Dobson, K. S., Szeto, A. C. H., & Knaak, S. (2019). The Working Mind: A meta-analysis of a workplace mental health and stigma reduction program. *Canadian Journal of Psychiatry. Revue Canadienne de psychiatrie, 64*(1 Suppl.), 39S–47S. https://doi.org/10.1177/ 0706743719842559

Goffman, E. (1961). *Asylums: Essays on the social situation of mental patients and other inmates.* Anchor Books.

Goffman, E. (1963). *Stigma: Notes on the management of spoiled identity.* Prentice Hall.

Goodwin, J. (2014). The horror of stigma: Psychosis and mental health care environments in twenty-first-century horror film (Part I). *Perspectives in Psychiatric Care, 50*(3), 201–209.

Hinshaw, S. P., & Stier, A. (2008). Stigma as related to mental disorders. *Annual Review of Clinical Psychology, 4*, 367–393.

Kahneman, D. (2011). *Thinking, fast and slow*. Farrar, Straus and Giroux.

Kassam, A., Papish, A., Modgill, G., & Patten, S. (2012). The development and psychometric properties of a new scale to measure mental illness related stigma by health care providers: The Opening Minds Scale for Health Care Providers (OMS-HC). *BMC Psychiatry, 12*, 62. https://doi.org/10.1186/1471-244X-12-62

Kirby, M. J., & Keon, W. J. (2006). *Out of the shadows at last: Transforming mental health, mental illness and addiction services in Canada*. Standing Senate Committee on Social Affairs, Science and Technology.

Link, B. G., & Phelan, J. C. (2001). Conceptualizing stigma. *Annual Review of Sociology, 27*, 363–385.

Livingston, J. (2020). *Structural stigma in health-care contexts for people with mental health and substance use issues: A literature review*. Mental Health Commission of Canada.

Malachowski, C., & Kirsh, B. (2013). Workplace anti stigma initiatives: A scoping study. *Psychiatric Services, 64*(7), 694–702. https://doi.org/10.1176/appi. Ps.201200409

Mental Health Commission of Canada. (2012). *Changing directions, changing lives: The Mental Health Strategy for Canada*.

Mental Health Commission of Canada. (2016). *The Mental Health Commission of Canada's HEADSTRONG Youth Anti-Stigma Initiative 2014–2015*. Final Report.

Modgill, G., Patten, S. B., Knaak, S., Kassam, A., & Szeto, A. C. H. (2014). Opening Minds stigma scale for health care providers (OMS-HC): Examination of psychometric properties and responsiveness. *BMC Psychiatry, 14*(1), 120.

Oxford English Dictionary. (2020). Stigma. In *OED.com dictionary*. Retrieved September 9, 2020, from https://www.oed.com/view/Entry/190242

Papish, A., Kassam, A., Modgill, G., Vaz, G., Zanussi, L., & Patten, S. (2013). Reducing the stigma of mental illness in undergraduate medical education: A randomized controlled trial. *BMC Medical Education, 13*, 141 https://doi.org/10.1186/1472-6920-13-141

Patten, S. B., Remillard, A., Phillips, L., Modgill, G., Szeto, A. C. H., Kassam, A., & Gardner, D. M. (2012). Effectiveness of contact-based education for reducing mental illness-related stigma in pharmacy students. *BMC Medical Education, 12*, 120. https://doi.org/10.1186/1472-6920-12-120

Pietrus, M. (2013). *Opening Minds interim report*. Mental Health Commission of Canada. https://www.mentalhealthcommission.ca/English/document/17491/opening-minds-interim-report

Pincus, F. L. (1999). From individual to structural discrimination. In F. L. Pincus & H. J. Ehrlich (Eds.), *Race and ethnic conflict: Contending views on prejudice, this culmination, and ethnoviolence* (pp. 120–124). Westview Press.

Simon, B. (1992). Shame, stigma, and mental illness in ancient Greece. In P. Fink & A. Tasman (Eds.), *Stigma and mental illness*. American Psychiatric Press.

Stuart, H., Arboleda-Flórez, J., & Sartorius, N. (Eds.). (2012). *Paradigms lost: Fighting stigma and the lessons learned*. Oxford University Press.

Stuart, H., Chen, S-P., Christie, R., Dobson, K. S., Kirsh, B., Knaak, S., Koller, M., Krupa, T., Lauria-Horner, B., Luong, D., Modgill, G., Patten, S. B., Pietrus, M., Szeto, A. C. H., & Whitley, R. (2014). Opening Minds in Canada: Targeting change. *Canadian Journal of Psychiatry. Revue canadienne de psychiatrie, 59*(10, Suppl. 1), S13.

Szeto, A. C. H., & Dobson, K. S. (2010). Reducing the stigma of mental disorders at work: A review of current workplace anti-stigma intervention programs. *Applied and Preventive Psychology, 14*, 41–56. https://doi.org/10.1016/j.appsy.2011.11.002

Szeto, A. C. H., Dobson, K. S., & Knaak, S. (2019). The Road to Mental Readiness for first responders: A meta-analysis of program outcomes. *Canadian Journal of Psychiatry. Revue canadienne de psychiatrie, 64*(1 Suppl.):18S–29S. https://doi.org/10.1177/0706743719842562

Szeto, A. C. H., Luong, D., & Dobson, K. S. (2013). Does labeling matter? An examination of attitudes and perceptions of labels for mental disorders. *Social Psychiatry and Psychiatric Epidemiology, 48.* https://doi.org/10-1007/s00127-012-0532-7

Whitley, R., & Berry, S. (2013). Analyzing media representations of mental illness: Lessons learnt from a national project. *Journal of Mental Health, 22*(3), 246–253. https://doi.org/10.3109/09638237.2012.745188

Whitley, R., & Wang J. W. (2017a). Good news? A longitudinal analysis of newspaper portrayals of mental illness in Canada 2005–2015. *Canadian Journal of Psychiatry, 62*(4), 278–285.

Whitley, R., & Wang, J. W. (2017b). Television coverage of mental illness in Canada: 2013–2015. *Social Psychiatry and Psychiatric Epidemiology, 52*(2), 241–244.

2

Prejudice and Discrimination Related to Substance Use Problems

Shu-Ping Chen and Heather Stuart

Background

Stereotypes, prejudice, and discrimination associated with substance use disorders (SUD) are complex psychological, social, and cultural phenomena in which individuals with SUD are devalued and excluded because of societal perspectives concerning the use of substances and the socially discredited condition of addiction. In particular, stigmatizing attitudes regarding illegal substance use are socially endorsed and enshrined in policy. The stigma associated with SUD comes from many sources, including the general public, family members, friends, coworkers, employers, and healthcare providers, and can be manifested at the self, social, and structural levels (Earnshaw et al., 2013). Stigmas at these levels interact and reflect a consensus that the society devalues people with SUD and legitimizes collective actions to penalize them (Smith et al., 2016). Such discriminatory actions not only reinforce the social, economic, and health inequities in substance users, but also devastate their self-perception and discourage them in addressing their substance misuse issues.

Social stigma occurs when the general public projects stereotypes and prejudices onto individuals living with SUD, which may result in discriminatory behavior. A variety of determinants contribute to stigmas related to substance use, including the type of substance, the drug's legal status, the route of entry, and its association with delinquency and crime. Figure 2.1 depicts a conceptual framework of the social stigma mechanisms involving stereotyping, prejudice, and discrimination and the extent to which individuals with SUD have experienced stigma in its various forms and outcomes.

The stigmas associated with SUD are pervasive in society, and over 70% of the general public hold negative and stereotypic views and social distancing toward people with substance use problems (Barry et al., 2014; Crisp et al., 2000; Stuart, 2019). People with a history of substance addiction may continue to be stigmatized even when they have stopped using the substances (Link et al., 1997). For example, people with former SUD have reported job loss as a result of their history (Baldwin et al., 2010).

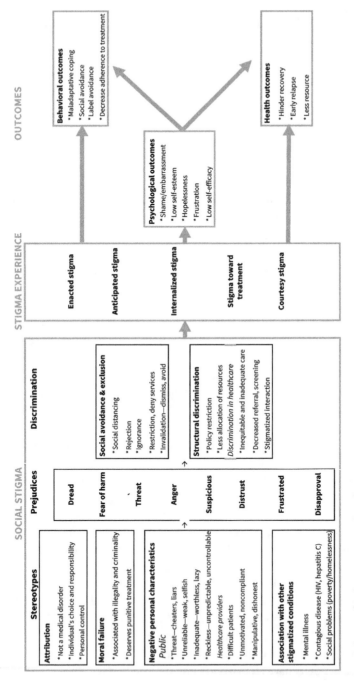

Figure 2.1 Stigma of Substance Use Disorders

Stereotypes and Misperceptions Associated With Substance Use Problems

Stereotypes are harmful and disrespectful beliefs about substance users. They are widely endorsed in society. We discuss the public stereotypes and misperceptions about SUD from four perspectives: attribution, moral failure, negative personal characteristics, and negative associations with other stigmatized conditions.

Attribution

The attribution of personal responsibility for addiction is high in the general public (Schomerus et al., 2011; Yang et al., 2017). Individuals with SUD are believed to have personal control over their use of substances. The perceived degree of intentionality is high, because the public holds the view that the use of substances is under conscious control. Solving the problem of SUD is thus believed to be simply a personal willingness and choice to abstain, and recovery is perceived as dependent on users' personal willpower (Brezing & Marcovitz, 2016). As a result, the individual is held to blame for their use of substances and therefore held responsible for their condition. Based on this notion, treatments such as maintenance therapy, which uses a medication like methadone as a substitute for illicit drugs, are highly misperceived to be a personal weakness of not having the willpower to simply abstain (Stuart, 2019). The internal attribution of control is also associated with the belief that people need to be "totally" sober or achieve "drug-free" status to demonstrate their self-discipline. Compared to abstinence-oriented approaches, harm reduction approaches to therapy are more stigmatized by healthcare professionals and society. People believe that the programs to reduce harm merely replace one addictive drug with another rather than see them as a treatment (Smye et al., 2011). Under these assumptions, substance addiction and abuse is considered a nonhealth issue that is outside the realm of a medical disorder but within the realm of choice (Rasinski et al., 2005).

Moral Failure

Substance use disorder is frequently treated as a moral and criminal issue, especially when the substance being used is illegal (Livingston et al., 2012). The public may perceive a person's criminality based on the legality of the drugs being used. As one user shared, "The stigma comes . . . if it's seen as illegal" (Nieweglowski et al., 2018, p. 325). Indeed, the moralization of substance use is common across many societies (Room, 2006). The perceived moral failure leads to a belief that people who use substances deserve punitive treatment, such as criminal sanctions. The criminalization of substance use exacerbates the stigmatization of SUD. Drug dealing is also associated with violent crime (Rasinski et al., 2005). Such perceptions of dangerousness can further be associated with the moral failure associated with criminal behaviors, such as the notion that "addicts steal" (Nieweglowski et al., 2018, p. 325).

Negative Personal Characteristics

People with SUD may have negative personal characteristics assigned to them, such as being a threat (cheaters and liars), reckless (unpredictable and uncontrollable), un-reliable (weak and selfish), and inadequate (worthless and lazy) (Nieweglowski et al., 2018; Schomerus et al., 2011; Yang et al., 2017). Among these stereotypes, being a threat and being reckless are endorsed more strongly by the general public. People with SUD are thought to be unable to control the things they do. They are viewed as dangerous because of their unpredictable or impulsive behaviors, which can lead to a life of criminality (Nieweglowski et al., 2019). Unusual behaviors (such as smoking crack) being witnessed by the public may also reinforce the perception of these individuals as dangerous (Nieweglowski et al., 2018).

People with SUD are perceived as being in denial, weak, and selfish because of their substance use. The general public considers them lazy, so they are to blame for their own problem. They are seen as not being capable of changing their behaviors and not being able to manage their lives, keep a job, or take care of themselves and finally recover. Eventually, they are assumed to have relapsed, even when they are seeking treatment. Based on this belief, the public views people with SUD as uneducated and irresponsible and, in a paradoxical sense, unable to take responsibility for their actions.

Healthcare professional stigma, which is a type of social stigma, has been elicited from primary care providers, psychiatrists, physicians, and nurses in other specialties, as well as by pharmacists and healthcare students (Brezing & Marcovitz, 2016). People with SUD are seen as noncompliant, out of control, untrustworthy, dishonest, and unwilling to change their risk behaviors in healthcare settings (Earnshaw et al., 2013; Livingston et al., 2012). For example, healthcare providers often think that people with SUD are lying to them to obtain pain medications. People with SUD are also thought to be manipulative and to overuse system resources, and they are often labeled as "demanding," "difficult patients," and "undeserving" of help.

Negative Association With Other Stigmatized Conditions

Substance misuse is often linked symbolically to other stigmatized conditions, such as mental illness, contagious diseases (e.g., HIV/AIDS or hepatitis C virus), unsafe behaviors (e.g., being unhygienic or taking part in impaired driving), and social problems (e.g., poverty, homelessness, family strife, significant legal problems, or unemployment)

(Livingston et al., 2012). People who use intravenous drugs are especially highly associated with infection with HIV/AIDS and risk behaviors such as sharing needles. Indeed, research has suggested that people who use intravenous drugs are the most stigmatized by the general public and healthcare providers (Decety et al., 2009; Luoma et al., 2007). If two stigmatizing conditions co-occur, the chance of stigmatization and the potential for opportunity loss are magnified (Rasinski et al., 2005). These negative associations make the stigmatization of SUD particularly strong.

Prejudice and Discrimination Toward Substance Use Problems

Prejudices are emotional responses and evaluative consequences, typically ones that concord with stereotypes (Corrigan et al., 2017). Stereotypes and misperceptions lead to feelings of dread, threat, anger, suspicion, and distrust (Yang et al., 2017). In particular, the widespread perception of violence and criminality evokes a fear of personal harm. The public may be more wary when people with SUD are around, and such fears may turn into anger or resentment if the general public perceives that people with SUD are in denial, make unrealistic promises, or act in inappropriate ways (Nieweglowski et al., 2019). In a U.S. study, over 70% of participants agreed that injection drug users were "disgusting and a threat to society" (Capitanio & Herek, 1999).

The sense of devaluation and discredit regarding addiction surfaces frequently in the form of "looking down on" or despising people with SUD. People show low expectations and increased embarrassment among both individuals with SUD and their family members. Such prejudices result in restricting opportunities to and unfair treatment of individuals with SUD. Discrimination toward people with SUD can be observed at two levels: (a) social avoidance and exclusion and (b) structural discrimination.

Social Avoidance and Exclusion

Discrimination toward people with SUD includes social distancing, rejection, ignorance, restriction, and the denial of services. The desire to maintain social distance was found to be strong toward substance-dependent people (Schomerus et al., 2011; Yang et al., 2017). The public may act suspicious and watch people with SUD more closely than others, but at the same time dismiss and avoid them. As an example, the general public has opposed locating methadone maintenance therapy clinics in their neighborhoods. Social distancing behaviors also include unwillingness to have a person with SUD work with them or marry into their family, as well as decreased intention to help. Individuals with SUD can be denied services that would improve their life and health, such as renting an apartment, especially when they are viewed as criminals (Nieweglowski et al., 2019).

Most people with SUD feel that others look down on them after they disclose their history of addiction. They may be viewed as poor parents, irresponsible workers, or otherwise at high risk of doing harm to others. For instance, some have been told that they are not trusted to be alone with children or to teach young children. Difficulty in obtaining employment, reduced access to housing, and difficulties with social adjustment are often reported by people with SUD (Luoma et al., 2007). They have frequently heard others say unfavorable or offensive things about them and have experienced various forms of rejection. Past experiences may influence their expectation of future stigma as well. Experiences of stigma can continue even after a person no longer actively uses drugs.

Individuals with SUD who are looking for a job fear that they would not be hired once employers discover their history of addiction or run criminal background checks on them. Those who are employed may worry that their employers or coworkers will discover their history and view them as untrustworthy, show prejudice, and treat them with discrimination. Thus, some individuals with SUD try to avoid this stigma experience by concealing their treatments (Earnshaw et al., 2013). Indeed, some workers in the workplace automatically assume that people with a history of SUD are not reliable. Such beliefs may lead to their being denied important work responsibilities, being denied promotions, or shortening their job tenure.

In addition to social rejection from the public, the close family members or friends of people with SUD may be unsupportive, reject requests for help, or ignore the individuals because of resentment resulting from their past behaviors. Such resentment may lead to more suspicious behaviors in the future. A common experience of stigma among people with SUD is that their family "did not understand or did not care to understand" their addiction (Earnshaw et al., 2013, p. 115). Some people with SUD perceived that they had lost their family's trust as a result of past behaviors, such as stealing or hurting someone when they were using drugs; however, others felt that they had done nothing wrong, but were viewed as untrustworthy only because of their drug addiction (Earnshaw et al., 2013). Some even felt that their family "gave up" on them (Luoma et al., 2007) and that they were not given opportunities to prove themselves reliable. Such experiences of rejection make it difficult for people with SUD to build social networks. Family members' perceptions of untrustworthiness and irresponsibility may lead to discriminatory behavior, like rejection within the family. As a result, people with SUD lose their sense of belonging in the family. Some might react with anger and avoid their family, while others might regret their past and seek to repair their relationships.

Structural Discrimination

Structural discrimination refers to the rules, policies, and procedures of institutions that restrict rights and opportunities for individuals with SUD. Structural discrimination can include the inequitable distribution of resources, the withholding of services, and the fragmentation and poor quality of care (Knaak et al., 2020).

On the one hand, negative perceptions toward SUD are correlated with lower support for policies designed to benefit this population (Kennedy-Hendricks et al., 2017). Policy makers may reduce their willingness to allocate resources to this population. Research showed that increasing government spending on treatment for SUD, such as expanding access to naloxone, was supported by fewer than 50% of Americans (Barry et al., 2014, 2016). On the other hand, stigma is associated with support for punitive policies, such as the arrest and prosecution of individuals who obtain multiple opioid prescriptions from different doctors (Kennedy-Hendricks et al., 2017). Another example of structural discrimination toward people with SUD is restricted coverage of addiction treatment by health insurance. For example, some U.S. health insurance policies require greater deductibles from people receiving substance-related treatment and provide lower annual expenditure limits. Some state Medicaid programs do not include certain critical SUD treatment options in their benefit packages (e.g., methadone) or have restricted the doses or length of treatment (Substance Abuse and Mental Health Services Administration, 2016). Consequently, addiction treatment has suffered losses in funding and reimbursement, with resulting reductions in service availability.

Discrimination in Healthcare

Healthcare providers' negative perceptions toward people with SUD affect access to treatment and can contribute to the inequitable and inadequate provision of care (van Boekel et al., 2013). In particular, individuals with SUD reported denial of adequate treatment and rude treatment after providers learned of their history of addiction. For example, lack of care was reported in one medication maintenance therapy program where staff were described as "ignorant, condescending, patronizing, arrogant, and ingenuine" (Stuart, 2019). Healthcare providers who viewed drug use as "controllable" had prejudicial attitudes toward people who use injection drugs (Brener, von Hippel, Kippax et al., 2010). Providers who endorse negative stereotypes worry that people who use injection drugs may misbehave in treatment settings. The most popular discrimination is denying pain medication based on the assumption that people with SUD overstate their pain to receive painkillers, or "pill shop."

Perceived or actual lack of knowledge and skills in the treatment of addiction leads to unwillingness among healthcare providers to treat people with SUD or the provision of biased and non-evidence-based care. Prejudiced providers may decrease referrals for treatment, refuse to screen for and address substance use problems, or have a zero-tolerance policy regarding substance use or relapse. Stigma also shapes the delivery of care; for example, an emergency room physician with limited awareness of their stereotypes toward SUD may discharge a patient with a drug overdose during a busy shift without considering the need for other services (Brezing & Marcovitz, 2016). Such unawareness can result in reduced opportunity for intervention and referral and overall reduced quality of care.

Structural discrimination in healthcare also significantly restricts access to resources and care. People living with SUD reported being unable to find family doctors who would support them during methadone therapy, as well as difficulties changing prescriptions between geographic locations. These structural barriers make people with SUD less likely to utilize services or to succeed in treatment, both of which can adversely affect their well-being.

Discrimination toward people with SUD can be present not only in general healthcare settings but also in SUD treatment sites. For example, some mutual help groups and recovery programs do not allow participants to be on medication maintenance therapy. On the one hand, providers may become frustrated with people with SUD because of "repeated relapses/admissions." Therefore, individuals with SUD who have more frequent relapses have experienced higher stigma-related rejection and more stigmatized interaction with providers (Brezing & Marcovitz, 2016). Receiving unfair or inadequate treatment makes people feel frustrated with their options for SUD treatment. On the other hand, some people with SUD appear to have negative perceptions toward the treatment of SUD, especially when that treatment is ineffective or punitive. Their concerns, such as restricted choice, loss of freedom, and potential physical harm, contribute to the belief that treatment is a form of punishment (Myers et al., 2009). This perception definitely restricts help-seeking behaviors. For example, negative experiences when receiving methadone maintenance therapy, such as restrictive dispensing schedules and lack of privacy, contribute to overall negative views of replacement therapy that in turn lead to the decision to discontinue treatment (Brezing & Marcovitz, 2016; Crapanzano et al., 2019; Stuart, 2019). People often feel disempowered in methadone clinics because of policies such as required daily visits, frequent and unannounced urinalyses, and termination of treatment for using other drugs (Smye et al., 2011; Stuart, 2019). Perceived stigma within SUD treatment and mutual help settings also appears to be a barrier for people with SUD to access care. For instance, many people with alcohol misuse disorder have negative perceptions toward the 12-step Alcoholics Anonymous group therapy, because they think that the intervention only caters to those with severe alcoholism or significant legal or family issues.

In summary, structural discrimination in healthcare makes it more difficult for people with SUD to engage and thus makes it more difficult for them to continue in a treatment program (Crapanzano et al., 2019). Fear of stigma is a major reason for avoiding treatment (Luoma et al., 2007). As a result, the perceived structural discrimination in healthcare is highly associated with a decreased intention to seek therapy, lower compliance with therapeutic intervention, lower treatment adherence, and a lower quality of life (Brener, von Hippel, von Hippel et al., 2010; Can & Tanriverdi, 2015; Luoma et al., 2007).

Internalized Stigma and Label Avoidance

Given the stigma toward addiction in society, people with SUD often learn to adopt the same stigmatizing attitudes and then internalize this socially conferred stigma after the onset of SUD. Their environments tend to validate these stigmatizing thoughts because they commonly endorse their experiences of rejection. Past experience is also often associated with perceived stigma and internalized shame (Luoma et al., 2007). Internalized stigma can damage people's self-esteem, self-identity, self-efficacy, and self-confidence, leading to feelings of shame, unworthiness, guilt, anxiety, depression, and hopelessness (Can & Tanriverdi, 2015; Corrigan et al., 2017; Crapanzano et al., 2019; Rasinski et al., 2005).

Shame appears to be a core component of the self-devaluation found in self-stigma regarding substance use. Shame is a negative affect and cognition that people have about their personal attributes and personal characteristics (Gilbert, 2000). People with SUD tend to feel ashamed of themselves for their substance use difficulties (Luoma et al., 2013). The sense of belonging to the category of "addiction" leads to a devalued social identity, low self-esteem, and self-perceptions of inferiority to others. Such an experience is associated with poor mental status, depression, anxiety, and sleep disturbances (Birtel et al., 2017). Furthermore, it can negatively affect their interpersonal relationships. Even people who successfully recover from SUD may suffer the psychological effects of social and internalized stigma. They still report experiencing shame and embarrassment regarding other people's attitudes (Link et al., 1997).

Internalized shame tends to infringe on people's personal and social worth and cause them to feel alienated and isolated from others, resulting in their marginalization to the periphery of the society. Such internal perception of stigma has been associated with deterioration in social functioning (Can & Tanriverdi, 2015). As a result of social withdrawal, decreased interpersonal relationships and access to social activities, the ability to maintain social functioning is thus compromised. It is possible that the relationship is mutual, forming a vicious cycle between perceived stigma and its impact on social functioning, the loss of status, and marginalization.

The fear of being labeled and looked down on almost certainly hinders people's social participation and the act of seeking help. Secrecy and social withdrawal are common coping strategies adopted by those with SUD, in part to avoid rejection from others. Secrecy is common in situations where one is likely to be stigmatized, such as job interviews (Luoma et al., 2007). People with SUD tend to cope with the fear of stigma by disengaging from important life events and responsibilities, such as employment. Such avoidant behaviors can interfere with their ability to pursue valued life goals.

Label avoidance is another common behavioral outcome of stigma. Individuals living with SUD who perceive high levels of prejudice and discrimination may choose to hide their problems and avoid entering treatment because it confirms their membership in a stigmatized addiction group. In some cases, they may even forgo treatment to avoid a diagnostic label.

Courtesy Stigma

Families that support an adult member with SUD often report adverse effects on family functioning. Some family members struggle with embarrassment and shame for their family, and such internalized stigma hinders families from seeking help for their family members (Myers et al., 2009). Family members perceive a lack of knowledge and empathy and judgmental attitudes from others, and they fear judgment from others. These experiences further reinforce secrecy, reduced contact with others, and restricted access to potential support (McCann & Lubman, 2018). However, over time, some family members are able to moderate the effect of stigma by challenging others' misperceptions about SUD. They are more "open" to speaking out about their experiences and the need for support.

Key Considerations and Recommendations for Implementation

People who suffer from SUD experience a type of double jeopardy in society. Not only must they manage the symptoms of addiction, but also they face severe stigma attached to their conditions, which negatively impacts their lives. We present several key considerations and recommendations that emerge from this chapter:

- The high level of social stigma endorsement by the general population shapes the lives of individuals with SUD and leads to adverse psychological, behavioral, and health outcomes. The prejudice and discrimination about substance use problems, include social distancing and rejection, result in reduced opportunities in education, employment, housing, relationships, healthcare, public services, and social engagement. Because stigma is often used as a tool with which to marginalize individuals who suffer from SUD, efforts to create social acceptance could fundamentally improve their quality of life. People with SUD should be empowered to be actively involved in planning and implementing solutions to combat stigma.
- Policy and legislative reform designed to prohibit discrimination and improve protections and accommodations for those suffering from a mental illness and addiction in areas such as employment, education, and housing has been successfully used to combat stigma (Arboleda-Flórez & Stuart, 2012). It is critical to advocate for the adoption of a public health approach that promotes prevention, harm reduction, and recovery from SUD.

- Healthcare providers' negative attitudes act as powerful deterrents to entry into treatment, treatment retention, and treatment compliance. These factors may result in early relapse and reduced recovery (Keyes et al., 2010). Stigma in healthcare can result in restricted resources and decreased access to healthcare, fostering health inequities among people with SUD. Comprehensive strategies are needed to solve the structural levels of stigma, including strengthening the integration and coordination of care, achieving equity in resource distribution, expanding access to evidence-based treatment, fostering clients' active and meaningful involvement in the treatment process, and enhancing human rights protections (Knaak et al., 2020).

- People who live with SUD and who experience internalized stigma show low self-esteem and reduced help seeking and treatment compliance. The emotional and instrumental support provided by family members and friends can shield the harmful impact of stress on the experience of rejection and lessen the effects of internalized shame. Based on recovery philosophy, stigma self-management approaches that empower people to overcome their illness identities and move beyond the illness experience to find new meanings in their lives would be a promising way to reduce the impacts of self-stigma (Arboleda-Flórez & Stuart, 2012). It would be a social benefit to empower people to reintegrate into social networks, to buffer against the negative effects of stigma, and to reduce stigma-related burdens.

- Although the stigma of substance use problems is prevalent in society, contact-based interventions, empowerment and recovery approaches, and social support are promising strategies to reduce such public and internalized stigma. Future research should focus on the evaluation of these interventions.

References

Arboleda-Flórez, J., & Stuart, H. (2012). From sin to science: Fighting the stigmatization of mental illnesses. *Canadian Journal of Psychiatry, 57*(8), 457–463.

Baldwin, M., L., Marcus, S. C., & De Simone, J. (2010). Job loss discrimination and former substance use disorders. *Drug and Alcohol Dependence, 110*(1–2), 1–7.

Barry, C. L., Kennedy-Hendricks, A., Gollust, S. E., Niederdeppe, J., Bachhuber, M. A., Webster, D. W., & McGinty, E. E. (2016). Understanding Americans' views on opioid pain reliever abuse. Addiction, *111*, 85–93.

Barry, C. L., McGinty, E. E., Pescosolido, B. A., & Goldman, H. H. (2014). Stigma, discrimination, treatment effectiveness, and policy: Public views about drug addiction and mental illness. *Psychiatric Services, 65*, 1269–1272.

Birtel, M. D., Wood, L., & Kempa, N. J. (2017). Stigma and social support in substance abuse: Implications for mental health and well-being. *Psychiatry Research, 252*, 1–8.

Brener, L., von Hippel, W., Kippax, S., & Preacher, K. J. (2010). The role of physician and nurse attitudes in the health care of injecting drug users. *Substance Use & Misuse, 45*(7–8), 1007–1018.

Brener, L., von Hippel, W., von Hippel, C., Resnick, L., & Treloar, C. (2010). Perceptions of discriminatory treatment by staff as predictors of drug treatment completion: Utility of a mixed methods approach. *Drug and Alcohol Review, 29*(5), 491–497.

Brezing, C., & Marcovitz, D. (2016). Stigma and persons with substance use disorders. In R. Parekh & E. Childs (Eds.), *Stigma and prejudice: Touchstones in understanding diversity in healthcare* (pp. 113–132). Springer International.

Can, G., & Tanriverdi, D. (2015). Social functioning and internalized stigma in individuals diagnosed with substance use disorder. *Archives of Psychiatric Nursing, 29*, 441–446.

Capitanio, J. P., & Herek, G. M. (1999). AIDS-related stigma and attitudes toward injecting drug users among Black and White Americans. *American Behavioral Scientist, 42*, 1148–1161.

Corrigan, P., Schomerus, G., Shuman, V., Kraus, D., Perlick, D., Harnish, A., Kulesza, M., Kane-Willis, K., Qin, S., & Smelson, D. (2017). Developing a research agenda for understanding the stigma of addictions. Part I: Lessons from the mental health stigma literature. *The American Journal of Addiction, 26*, 59–66.

Crapanzano, K. A., Hammarlund, R., Ahmad, B., Hunsinger, N., & Kullar, R. (2019). The association between perceived stigma and substance use disorder treatment outcomes: A review. *Substance Abuse and Rehabilitation, 10*, 1–12.

Crisp, A. H., Gelder, M. G., Rix, S., Meltzer, H. I., & Rowlands, O. J. (2000). Stigmatisation of people with mental illnesses. *British Journal of Psychiatry, 177*, 4–7.

Decety, J., Echols, S., & Correll, J. (2009). The blame game: The effect of responsibility and social stigma on empathy for pain. *Journal of Cognitive Neuroscience, 22*, 985–997.

Earnshaw, V., Smith, L., & Copenhaver, M. (2013). Drug addiction stigma in the context of methadone maintenance therapy: An investigation into understudied sources of stigma. *International Journal of Mental Health and Addiction, 11*, 110–122. https://doi.org/10.1007/s11469-012-9402-5

Gilbert, P. (2000). The relationship of shame, social depression and anxiety: The role of the evaluation of social rank. *Clinical Psychology & Psychotherapy, 7*, 174–189.

Kennedy-Hendricks, A., Barry, C., Gollust, S. E., Ensminger, M. E., Chisolm, M. S., & McGinty, E. E. (2017). Social stigma toward persons with prescription opioid use disorder: Associations with public support for punitive and public health–oriented policies. *Psychiatric Services, 68*, 462–469.

Keyes, K. M., Hatzenbuehler, M. L., McLaughlin, K. A., Link, B., Olfson, M., Grant, B. F., & Hasin, D. (2010). Stigma and treatment for alcohol disorders in the United States. *American Journal of Epidemiology, 172*(12), 1364–1372.

Knaak, S., Livingston, J., Stuart, H., & Ungar, T. (2020). *Combating mental illness- and substance use-related structural stigma in health care.* Mental Health Commission of Canada.

Link, B. G., Stuening, E. L., Rahav, M., Phelan, J. C., & Nuttbrock, L. (1997). On stigma and its consequences: Evidence from a longitudinal study of men with dual diagnoses of mental illness and substance abuse. *Journal of Health and Social Behavior, 38*, 177–190.

Livingston, J. D., Milne, T., Fang, M. L., & Amari, E. (2012). The effectiveness of interventions for reducing stigma related to substance use disorders: A systematic review. *Addiction, 107*, 39–50.

Luoma, J. B., Nobles, R. H., Drake, C. E., Hayes, S. C., O'Hair, A., Fletcher, L., & Kohlenberg, B. S. (2013). Self-stigma in substance abuse: Development of a new measure. *Journal of Psychopathology and Behavioral Assessment, 35*, 223–234. https://doi.org/10.1007/s10862-012-9323-4

Luoma, J. B., Twohig, M. P., Waltz, T., Hayes, S. C., Roget, N., Padilla, M., & Fisher, G. (2007). An investigation of stigma in individuals receiving treatment for substance abuse. *Addictive Behaviors, 32*, 1331–1346.

McCann, T. V., & Lubman, D. I. (2018). Stigma experience of families supporting an adult member with substance misuse. *International Journal of Mental Health Nursing, 27*, 693–701.

Myers, B., Fakier, N., & Louw, J. (2009). Stigma, treatment beliefs, and substance abuse treatment use in historically disadvantaged communities. *African Journal of Psychiatry, 12,* 218–222.

Nieweglowski, K., Corrigan, P., Tyas, T., Tooley, A., Dubke, R., Lara, J., Washington, L., Sayer, J., Sheehan, L., & the Addiction Stigma Research Team. (2018). Exploring the public stigma of substance use disorder through community-based participatory research. *Addiction Research and Theory, 26*(4), 323–329. https://doi.org/10.1080/16066359.2017.1409890

Nieweglowski, K., Dubke, R., Mulfinger, N., Sheehan, L., & Corrigan, P. W. (2019). Understanding the factor structure of the public stigma of substance use disorder. *Addiction Research and Theory, 27*(2), 156–161. https://doi.org/10.1080/16066359.2018.1474205

Rasinski, K. A., Woll, P., & Cooke, A. (2005). Stigma and substance use disorders. In P. W. Corrigan (Ed.), *The stigma of mental illness: Practical strategies for research and social change* (pp. 219–236). American Psychological Association.

Room, R. (2006). Taking account of cultural and societal influences on substance use diagnoses and criteria. *Addiction, 101,* 31–39.

Schomerus, G., Lucht, M., Holzinger, A., Matschinger, H., Carta, M. G., & Angermeyer, M. C. (2011). The stigma of alcohol dependence compared with other mental disorders: A review of population studies. *Alcohol and Alcoholism, 46*(2), 105–112.

Smith, L. R., Earnshaw, V. A., Copenhaver, M. M., & Cunningham, C. O. (2016). Substance use stigma: Reliability and validity of a theory-based scale for substance-using populations. *Drug and Alcohol Dependence, 162,* 34–43.

Smye, V., Browne, A. J., Varcoe, C., & Josewski, V. (2011). Harm reduction, methadone maintenance treatment and the root causes of health and social inequities: An intersectional lens in the Canadian context. *Harm Reduction Journal, 8,* 17.

Stuart, H. (2019). Managing the stigma of opioid use. *Healthcare Management Forum, 32*(2), 78–83.

Substance Abuse and Mental Health Services Administration, Office of the Surgeon General. (2016). Health care system and substance use disorders. In *Facing addiction in America: The Surgeon General's report on alcohol, drugs, and health*. U.S. Department of Health and Human Services. Retrieved August 26, 2020, from https://www.ncbi.nlm.nih.gov/books/NBK424848/

van Boekel, L. C., Brouwers, E. P. M., van Weeghel, J., & Garretsen, H. F. L. (2013). Stigma among health professionals towards patients with substance use disorders and its consequences for healthcare delivery: Systematic review. *Drug and Alcohol Dependence, 131,* 23–35.

Yang, L., Wong, L. Y., Grivel, M. M., & Hasin, D. S. (2017). Stigma and substance use disorders: An international phenomenon. *Current Opinion in Psychiatry, 30*(5), 378–388.

3

Best and Promising Practices in Stigma Reduction

Heather Stuart

Introduction

As discussed elsewhere in this volume, stigma can occur at the individual level (self-stigma), the interpersonal level (public stigma), and the structural level (structural or institutional stigma) (see Chapter 1). Antistigma programming also occurs at any of these levels, individually or simultaneously. Because intervention programs are seldom evaluated, it has been difficult to build a comprehensive evidence base supporting best practices in stigma reduction. In medical research, the gold standard to determine whether an intervention works is a meta-analysis of a large number of high-quality randomized controlled trials. Few randomized trials have been conducted in the antistigma field, so much of our knowledge comes from study designs that would be considered less than ideal by conventional evidence-based standards.

Notwithstanding the limited number of trials that have examined antistigma programs, it may be argued that randomized controlled trials are inappropriate for population-based antistigma initiatives (Stuart, 2016b). Thus, to discuss "best and promising" practices in antistigma programming, it is necessary to adopt a broader and more pragmatic view of evidence. This chapter examines six approaches to antistigma programming, moving from broad structural interventions to individual-level interventions. Three of these approaches (education, contact, and protest) have been widely discussed in the antistigma literature (Corrigan et al., 2012). In addition, this chapter examines legislative reform, advocacy, and stigma self-management strategies (Arboleda-Flórez & Stuart, 2012).

Ways to Disrupt Stigma

Figure 3.1 summarizes six approaches that have been used widely to disrupt the process of stigmatization. Each is discussed in more detail below.

Strategy	Mechanism	Targets	Desired Outcome
Legislative reform	Development and enactment of protective legislations; removal of discriminatory legislation	Legal system, legislators	Improved protections for rights and freedoms; improved access to social entitlements; reduced social inequities
Advocacy	Use of multiple approaches to increase priority of mental health on agendas of decision makers	Politicians, policy makers, decision makers, funders	Greater policy recognition; policy reform; improved services; reduced social inequities; improved avenues of redress
Protest	Formal (often written) objection to negative representations	Opinion leaders or stigmatizers (e.g.: politicians, journalists, manufacturers)	Suppress negative attitudes; remove negative representations and content
Contact-based education	Contact with people who are successfully managing a mental illness usually including opportunities for active discussion and learning	General public or selected sub-groups, such as students, healthcare providers, or police	Reduce stereotypes; improved attitudes; greater empathy; reduce desire for interpersonal distance
Education	Replace myths and misinformation with accurate information	General public or selected sub-groups	Improved knowledge; improved mental health literacy; better recognition of symptoms; promotion of early help-seeking
Stigma self-management & peer support	Peer-led self-learning and peer support workers work within or alongside traditional mental health programs	People who have a mental illness or family members	Reduced personal impact of stigmatization; reduced self-stigma; improved self-esteem;

Figure 3.1 Six Approaches That Disrupt the Process of Stigmatization
Adapted from Arboleda-Flórez and Stuart (2012).

Legislative Reform

Public health researchers and practitioners recognize the importance of legislative reform to promote population health goals because it exerts its effects at the broadest structural levels. Though most would agree that legislation is not enough (there also needs to be monitoring and enforcement), legislative action is indispensable in changing social structures and individual behaviors. Laws can govern actions even when they cannot change attitudes (Callard et al., 2012).

Mental health advocates such as Sayce (2003) have noted that it hardly matters what people think about individuals with mental or substance use disorders, so long as these persons are treated fairly and justly and have an equal opportunity as others to engage in social and occupational spheres. Legislative reform, such as seat belt legislation, smoking restrictions, or speed limits, has been essential to promoting healthy behaviors, even when public attitudes were oppositional (Stuart, 2016b).

Laws can prohibit discriminatory practices and provide the legal basis for advocacy efforts and mechanisms for redress. Laws can also impose duties on sectors and organizations to promote equal opportunities and eliminate discrimination and harassment, such as in workplace settings. Laws shift the emphasis from the attitudes and behaviors of individuals and place the responsibility on broader social structures (Callard et al., 2012). Therefore, legislation is one component of a larger regulatory framework focused on nondiscrimination (Stuart, 2007).

Advocacy

Legislative change and strong advocacy go hand in hand. To be fully effective, laws must be bolstered by social and political activities that reduce or eliminate marginalization and exclusion. Advocacy movements have emerged in recent decades in response to the recognition that people with mental illnesses are particularly vulnerable to human and civil rights violations, including involuntary long-term detention and treatment in large psychiatric institutions (Funk et al., 2006).

The World Health Organization defines advocacy as a broad range of activities that may be undertaken by a variety of players, which are designed to promote the human rights of people with mental disorders under current laws and ensure that mental health is on the agenda of policy makers and funders. Activities that come under the broad umbrella of advocacy include awareness-raising, knowledge exchange, education, training, mutual help, counseling, mediating, defending, and denouncing. The goal of advocacy is to change structures that act as barriers to the full and effective participation of people with mental disorders and to promote greater mental health. Although systematic research quantifying the full effects of advocacy is lacking, the World Health Organization has noted positive outcomes, including improvements in the policies and practices of governments and institutions, changes to laws and regulations, improvements in services, and better human rights protections (World Health Organization, 2003). The core of advocacy activities is giving meaningful voice to people who have a mental disorder to ensure their priorities are known and their needs are met. Service users must be empowered and enabled to speak on their own behalf and to take a leadership role in the healthcare processes that affect them (Varghese, 2015).

Although it would be ideal if advocacy efforts were based on the best available evidence, many are not. For example, biological models that depict mental illnesses as brain disorders (widely used in advocacy efforts) have inadvertently conveyed the message that mental illnesses are genetically determined and have minimal possibilities for recovery (Corrigan & Kosyluk, 2013). Research partnerships are salient for all approaches to stigma reduction, and it is particularly important to have research partners within advocacy efforts (Corrigan & Kosyluk, 2013). One major challenge in uniting advocates (who are often from grass-roots communities) with researchers is that they have different cultures of knowledge, different views of what constitutes evidence, and different time frames for results. Scientific knowledge is slow to materialize, objective, decontextualized, and often of little interest to advocacy groups who desire decision-oriented, pragmatic, and more immediate information. Nevertheless, several large, national antistigma programs (e.g., Time to Change, United Kingdom; Like Minds Like Mine, New Zealand; Opening Minds, Canada) have affiliated with university researchers to conduct formal evaluations of antistigma interventions (Stuart, 2016a). Such partnerships form the nexus for knowledge exchange and provide important insights contributing to the development of better practices in stigma reduction.

Policy reform is a common target for advocates. Rather than trying to change attitudes one person at a time, policy reform can modify the behavior of large groups of people. The person-first language movement is an example of how policies can alter stigmatizing representations and behaviors. This movement began over 2 decades ago based on the idea that labels can denigrate and marginalize. Putting the person first was intended to ensure that people were not dehumanized, such that their most important characteristic was reduced to their diagnosis, and it was viewed as a means to change attitudes, reduce stigma, and ultimately improve lives. This movement has been highly successful on a global scale and requirements for person-first language can now be found in government documents, scientific journals, day-to-day speech, therapeutic interactions, and a host of other situations (Collier, 2012).

Research has shown that a counselor's use of inclusive or exclusive language affects a client's perceptions. Clients expressed greater willingness to see a counselor who used inclusive language (Johnson & Dowling-Guyer, 1996). Other research has shown that the use of pejorative terms such as "substance abuser" compared to "having a substance use disorder" is associated with public perceptions that the individual engages in willful misconduct, is a greater social threat, and is more deserving of punishment. Despite evidence showing potentially positive effects of person-first language, not all members of the wider disability community agree with its use. For example, person-first language can create heated debates among disability communities related to autism, diabetes, or blindness (Collier, 2012). Despite some disagreement, person-first policies can improve the tenor of therapeutic encounters and require a conscious effort on the part of others to recognize and avoid potentially stigmatizing representations.

Protest

Advocates have used protest as a strategy to suppress or eliminate negative representations of people with a mental illness and to change selected organizational policies or practices. Protest often involves open objection to situations and lobbying to modify or eliminate negative images or offensive products (e.g., television shows, video games). Protest efforts are often focused on structural factors, such as organizational policies, that create barriers for people with mental illnesses. This strategy has also been used effectively by advocacy groups in media watch programs and letter-writing campaigns (Arboleda-Flórez & Stuart, 2012). For example, the StigmaWatch program operated since 1999 by SANE Australia is a good example of a grass-roots, protest-based activity (http://www.sane.org). People with a mental illness, friends, and supporters identify stigmatizing images presented in the media and submit a complaint to SANE. The submission is reviewed using the national guidelines for media conduct and, if the media representation is deemed to be inappropriate, StigmaWatch informs the media (or business) about the complaint and encourages an amendment. According to SANE, the majority of recipients are embarrassed, apologize for any offense, respond positively, and promise to think twice in the future.

The book *From Psychiatric Patient to Citizen* (Sayce, 2000) provides a number of advocacy success stories, even while it recognizes that results can be mixed. For example, the American National Stigma Clearinghouse successfully diverted scriptwriters from having Superman killed by a "superlunatic" from an interplanetary insane asylum. When advertisements for the film *Crazy People* appeared with the slogan "Warning: crazy people are coming" and "Warning: crazy people are here," advocates picketed the cinema and local newspaper, which offered free tickets to people who could prove they were crazy. The advertisements were discontinued and the newspaper offered a written apology. A number of local and national newspaper articles highlighted the story and the role of the advocacy organizations to remove the offensive advertisements.

Many protests focus on a specific instance, such as an infringement of someone's legal rights (where a legal protest may be mounted) or, as the previous examples illustrate, an offensive advertisement or product. Consequently, it is never clear how far-reaching the effects of protest have been. The service user movement is a recent example of how people who had been former patients in psychiatric facilities mounted a broad concerted front to protest their treatment and fight for their rights. They became vocal critics, denouncing the medical model that had been used to force hospitalization and involuntary treatment. Along with the antipsychiatry and civil rights movements, these protests have had wide-reaching effects culminating in broad social changes such as deinstitutionalization, the community mental health movement, and the recovery movement (Moncrieff & Steingard, 2019).

Contact-Based Education

Based on the contact hypothesis, many antistigma programs use personal contact as part of an educational intervention to replace negative stereotypes with positive images of recovery and reduce fear and the desire for social distance. In these interventions, people who have lived experience with a mental or substance use disorder tell their personal recovery stories and provide an opportunity for recipients to ask questions and interact. In some cases, contact is indirect through videos of people with a mental illness or actors who are portraying people with a mental illness (Stuart, 2016b).

Ideally, contact-based education provides an opportunity for transformative learning. In addition to being provided to undifferentiated groups, such as students, contact-based education can be directed to specific subgroups that have particular influence in the lives of people with a mental illness, such as healthcare providers (Knaak et al., 2014) or police (Henderson, 2020). In a large meta-analysis of 72 outcome studies, Corrigan and colleagues (2012) found that contact-based educational approaches were superior to more traditional educational approaches, particularly in changing attitudes. Behavioral intentions were more difficult to change, but contact-based approaches were still superior to traditional approaches. One difficulty with meta-analyses is the heterogeneity of contact-based approaches that may be used and differing methods and measures of assessing outcomes. A more detailed analysis of contact-based approaches that were evaluated under the auspices of the Opening Minds initiative of the Mental Health Commission of Canada appears in this book.

Jorm (2020) has argued that the literature supporting contact-based education is relatively weak, with a large number of observational studies, only a few high-quality clinical trials, and a lack of standardization of measures to assess behavioral change. He also noted the potential for study participants to figure out the purpose of the intervention and evaluate contact positively because they have learned the socially desirable answer. When pretest evaluations are collected some weeks before the intervention, and where outcome measures are proxies for behavioral (rather than attitudinal) change, they offer more compelling information, although they are more difficult studies to undertake. Also, it is important to note that some studies have demonstrated a lasting effect of contact-based interventions over several months (Henderson, 2020).

A plausible theory of change and the ability to point to "key ingredients" strengthens any inferences that can be made about the underlying mechanism of action for antistigma initiatives. For example, Knaak and colleagues (2014) used a mixed methods design to identify program characteristics that predicted positive change among healthcare providers in 22 interventions partnering with the Opening Minds initiative in Canada. All of the studies used a common rating scale to assess outcomes. An emphasis on and demonstration of recovery and multiple forms of social contact were two of the six elements that were most predictive of positive change. Other elements included personal recovery stories, an emphasis on behavioral change through skills training, an emphasis on myth-busting, and an enthusiastic presenter who modeled a person-centered approach. Programs with all six elements demonstrated superior outcomes to those with fewer elements.

Chen and colleagues (2016) evaluated 18 contact-based educational programs that targeted high school students in order to identify critical domains. Information was gathered from key program stakeholders as well as field observations. Three broad domains emerged as important: the characteristics of the speaker, the message, and the interaction. The most important criterion was having a speaker who was in recovery from a mental illness and who was psychologically ready to share their personal story, not as a therapeutic opportunity for the speaker, but as an educational opportunity for the students. Speakers had to be well equipped with presentation skills, which also required program support. Speakers needed to learn communication skills and public speaking skills and have a basic knowledge of mental health and mental illnesses (in case questions were asked), as well as other skills needed to deliver an effective presentation. During the presentation, speakers had to act as role models who embodied recovery. With respect to the message, speakers had to be adept at crafting a recovery message, correct misperceptions, and connect students with additional teaching resources. With respect to the interaction, speakers had to be ready to conduct a question-and-answer period following their presentation. They had to engage students and encourage open dialogue. Finally, speakers had to empower students to access resources and to help reduce stigma in their schools and wider communities. The extent to which speakers are supported in this role varies from program to program, accounting for variations in results.

Education

Educational approaches are based on a factual exchange. They try to challenge inaccurate depictions with accurate information. Educational approaches have included a broad array of interventions including fact sheets, public service announcements, flyers, web pages, podcasts, and books (Corrigan et al., 2012). Some educational approaches, such as Mental Health First Aid, aim to increase the mental health literacy of members of the public so that they better understand the signs and symptoms of mental illnesses, improve their attitudes, and help others take appropriate actions in the face of a mental health crisis (Jorm et al., 2004). Mental Health First Aid is delivered face to face in a classroom setting by a trained facilitator working from a standardized manual and so provides an intensive educational experience. Less intensive experiences, such as the provision of facts in a leaflet or through a public service advertisement, may be considerably less effective. A meta-analysis of 15 studies that examined the effects of Mental Health First Aid showed that the program is effective in improving knowledge and attitudes and increasing help-providing behaviors, though effects varied considerably from study to study (Hadlaczky et al., 2014).

An underlying assumption of many awareness and literacy initiatives is that they lead to behavioral change and subsequently reduce discrimination and social inequity in the broader community. This assumption may not be valid, particularly where there are entrenched structural inequities. Stuart and colleagues (2012) highlighted the important distinction between misconceptions and prejudices. Misconceptions are amenable to correction through factual knowledge, such as that delivered through a literacy program. Prejudices are emotionally based antipathies that are deeply entrenched and highly resistant to change. When prejudices are confronted with countervailing perspectives, people may become highly emotional and resistant. While it is yet unclear what proportion of stigmatizing behaviors are inadvertent and the result of genuine misconceptions and what degree reflect true prejudice, it is clear that people who have a high degree of knowledge can still express highly stigmatizing beliefs and act in discriminatory ways—healthcare workers being a good example. Therefore, it is important to carefully target literacy-based programs to areas and groups where additional knowledge can modify attitudes and behaviors.

Social marketing campaigns are an educational strategy targeted to entire populations. Typically, the information is factual and brief—something that could be conveyed in a 15- or 30-second infobyte or commercial. "Nuggets of knowledge" form the currency of social marketing campaigns. Often, such messaging assumes that the acquisition of an important fact (or factoid, e.g., One in five people will experience mental illness in their lifetime; Depression is treatable) will reduce public stigma and ultimately improve behaviors. However, there is no supporting evidence from social psychology that deep-seated prejudices or resulting discriminatory actions can be changed with improved information. Thus, although literacy can be improved with information, it is unlikely that a small fact is potent enough to unseat a fear-based prejudice. Further, while social marketing campaigns may pave the way for more targeted antistigma efforts, they have not been evaluated in this light. Also, these programs are typically expensive and beyond the budget of most grass-roots initiatives (Stuart et al., 2012). Finally, it is unclear how long the brief messages of social marketing campaigns last after their conclusion.

Stigma Self-Management

Self-stigma refers to the internalization of negative stereotypes about mental illnesses and is associated with low levels of hope, reduced quality of life, less adherence to treatment recommendations, decreased help seeking, and poor recovery. The idea of stigma self-management is consistent with the recovery paradigm that calls for services and supports to empower people who have a mental illness to overcome their illness identities and to find new personal meaning and valued social roles and relationships (Amering & Schmolke, 2009). Mittal and colleagues (2012) conducted a comprehensive literature review and identified 14 interventions designed to reduce self-stigma in people with mental illnesses and substance use disorders (though only

1 study focused on people with a substance use disorder). The most common type of intervention was psychoeducational, which ranged from printed material to training sessions (ranging from 1 to 23 sessions) delivered by a trainer. Three interventions combined psychoeducation with cognitive behavioral therapy and three studies used more complex multimodal interventions. Eight studies reported positive outcomes, although effect sizes were generally small. Substantive and methodological difficulties identified in this review serve as an important impetus for developing best practices in the field. For example, studies differed in their definition of self-stigma, so clarity in conceptualization is needed. The majority of studies evaluated outcomes using a scale that measured the extent to which someone was aware of public stereotypes, rather than a scale that directly measured the extent to which these stereotypes had been internalized. Finally, few studies developed an intervention that was based on a clear conceptual model. Despite these problems, cognitive behavioral interventions were deemed to have the best potential.

Yanos and colleagues (2015) reviewed six intervention approaches that targeted self-stigma. To be included in the review, interventions had to explicitly target negative views about the self that were related to receiving a diagnosis or as a result of being in treatment, as distinct from beliefs about others' negative stereotypes. Although the interventions were diverse, several common mechanisms provided suggestions about the most promising practices. For example, all programs used psychoeducation and factual information to counteract myths about mental illnesses. Knowledge acquisition was important to correct misconceptions and develop critical thinking skills that could be used to reject rather than internalize negative stereotypes. Cognitive techniques that offered opportunities to learn and practice skills to identify and combat self-stigmatizing thoughts were central to many of the programs. Interventions also tended to emphasize narration and its potential to help individuals make sense and create meaning out of past experiences. The aim was to empower program participants to be active agents. Finally, interventions tended to include some degree of behavioral decision-making as well as tools and experiences to promote hope, empowerment, and motivation to act toward one's goals and values.

The Coming Out Proud program (Rüsch et al., 2014) is an example of a peer-led program with many ideal characteristics. It is delivered over three sessions in a group format. The program supports people with mental illnesses in their decisions surrounding disclosure and secrecy in different settings. The efficacy of this program was examined in a pilot randomized trial of 100 participants with a mental illness, randomly assigned to the Coming Out Proud program or a treatment-as-usual control condition. The intervention did not modify the primary or secondary outcomes of interest, which were self-stigma and empowerment, respectively. However, it did have significant positive effects on the cognitive appraisal of stigma as a stressor, disclosure-related distress, perceived benefits of disclosure, and secrecy. It is possible that self-stigma and empowerment are broad and stable attributes and therefore less amenable to short-term change, whereas the remaining variables were process oriented and more sensitive to a brief intervention. These preliminary results support the use of the

Coming Out Proud program in clinical and mutual support settings to help reduce the stress related to disclosure and secrecy, though more evaluation is needed.

The BRIDGES program (Building Recovery of Individual Dreams and Goals) (Pickett et al., 2012) is an example of a longer, 8-week, peer-led program focusing on empowerment. The course teaches about the biological causes of mental illnesses, medications and common side-effects, and treatment services. A self-advocacy component focuses on how to talk with providers, discuss preferred treatment options, and develop collaborative skills. Results of a randomized controlled trial of 428 consumers indicated that participation in the program enhanced self-reported feelings of empowerment and self-advocacy and increased assertiveness in interactions with treatment providers. Results were maintained at 6 months.

Peer support programs are not explicitly antistigma interventions, but they do have important antistigma effects and deserve mention for their potential to reduce self-stigma and improve social inclusion. Peer support roles have been introduced in a variety of mental health organizations and peer workers have developed a broad range of functions. What is distinctive about peer support is its value base, which stands in juxtaposition to traditional mainstream medical models emphasizing impairments and disabilities (Gillard et al., 2017). Peer support interventions are provided by individuals who have lived experience of a mental illness or substance use disorder, who are in recovery, and who coach and support others who are experiencing similar challenges. By example, peer support workers highlight the potential for people with a mental or substance use disorder to adopt meaningful social roles. A key aspect of peer support and the recovery paradigm is stigma reduction. Peer support workers are often more successful in promoting hope, a belief in recovery, empowerment, a positive self-concept, and social inclusion than professionally trained mental health workers (Repper & Carter, 2011).

With respect to their specific role in the stigma process, peer support workers can help individuals gain important insights about stigma and the various manifestations of self-stigma. Peer support can help participants identify methods to address stigma-related problems. They can help the individual consider different and more effective ways to confront stigma and help them to rehearse various ways to handle stigma encounters (Verhaeghe et al., 2008). Further, there is evidence that peer support workers teach nonpeer staff about recovery-oriented care and can become key drivers of cultural change within health settings (Stein et al., 2013). Thus, by heralding recovery-oriented principles, peer support workers can promote a socially accepting and less stigmatizing healthcare environment.

Discussion

Evidence supporting the effectiveness of antistigma programs is still somewhat limited, with some strategies garnering more research interest than others. What evidence does exist may be overlooked by program developers in their enthusiasm to promote their own initiatives. Indeed, many interventions proceed without evidence on the assumption that programmers know what needs to be done and can deliver a successful intervention (Stuart et al., 2012). This chapter has reviewed six approaches that may be used to disrupt the process of stigmatization. Because stigma is multifactorial and pervasive, no single approach will be sufficient to eradicate stigma. Rather a concerted, multilevel plan is necessary, which can be maintained over time. Solitary interventions will not engender the cultural change needed to reduce stigma for people with mental and substance use disorders.

Broad legislative change is important to set the parameters to protect the rights and freedoms of people with mental and substance use disorders, guarantee their equitable access to care, and promote social equity in areas such as housing and employment. However, legislation alone is not sufficient to create behavioral change. Strong advocacy is needed to ensure that people can access the social entitlements promised in legislation and gain avenues for redress when barriers emerge. Protest is a useful strategy when the goal is to remove a specific negative representation or modify individual or organizational behavior. Contact-based education has been used widely to create an engaging educational experience that has the capacity to transform individual attitudes, prejudices, and feelings of social acceptance. It works best when it is targeted to specific groups, with active interactions and speakers who are well trained and able to model recovery. Didactic educational interventions are best suited to improve mental health literacy and raise awareness about the importance of help seeking or the efficacy of treatment. Stigma-self management programs help people with lived experiences overcome self-imposed barriers to social exclusion and increase empowerment and self-esteem. Finally, peer support programs are important for helping to change healthcare cultures to be less stigmatizing and for helping peers understand stigma and develop tools for addressing it in their lives.

Ultimately, decreasing mental health and substance use stigma will require a concerted effort that will involve many players over a long time. Large-scale coordinated efforts are relatively uncommon, although a number of countries have implemented national antistigma initiatives. Still, there is considerable fragmentation across national, regional, and local efforts and not every intervention is successful. Thus, there is great potential for disparate programs to be inconsistent with each other or to unnecessarily duplicate efforts. It is important to ensure that people with lived experience, as well as their family members, have a strong and meaningful voice in the development, implementation, and evaluation of antistigma activities. It is also important to develop strong community and university research alliances to critically reflect on and understand the inner workings of antistigma programs. These alliances are essential to build bridges among the consumer/survivor, academic, policy, and practitioner communities.

Key Considerations

- When determining what strategy may best disrupt the stigmatization process, it is important to tailor the intervention to the nature of the problem, the needs of the target audience, and the specific outcomes to be achieved.
- Antistigma approaches vary greatly, from structural to individual interventions. Stigma reduction is enhanced when multilayered approaches are created to simultaneously address individual, organizational, cultural, and structural change.
- The evidence base for stigma interventions is under development. It is therefore important for programmers to work with local researchers to implement methods that systematically evaluate program impacts, both anticipated and unanticipated.
- To maximize success, interventions must be based on a plausible theory of change so that it is possible to discern if the underlying mechanism coincides with available evidence or whether it is based on strongly held beliefs about what might or might not work.

References

Amering, M., & Schmolke, M. (2009). *Recovery in mental health.* Wiley–Blackwell.

Arboleda-Flórez, J., & Stuart, H. (2012). From sin to science: Fighting the stigmatization of mental illnesses. *Canadian Journal of Psychiatry, 57*(8), 457–463. https://doi.org/10.1177/070674371205700803

Callard, F., Sartorius, N., Arboleda-Flórez, J., Bartlett, P., Helmchen, H., Stuart, H., Taborda, J., & Thornicroft, G. (2012). *Mental illness, discrimination and the law: Fighting for social justice.* Wiley–Blackwell. https://doi.org/10.1002/9781119945352

Chen, S. P., Koller, M., Krupa, T., & Stuart, H. (2016). Contact in the classroom: Developing a program model for youth mental health contact-based anti-stigma education. *Community Mental Health Journal, 52*(3), 281–293. https://doi.org/10.1007/s10597-015-9944-7

Collier, R. (2012). Person-first language: Noble intent but to what effect? *CMAJ: Canadian Medical Association Journal. Journal de l'association medicale canadienne, 184*(18), 1977–1978. https://doi.org/10.1503/cmaj.109-4319

Corrigan, P. W., & Kosyluk, K. A. (2013). Erasing the stigma: Where science meets advocacy. *Basic and Applied Social Psychology, 35*(1), 131–140. https://doi.org/10.1080/01973533.2012.746598

Corrigan, P. W., Morris, S. B., Michaels, P. J., Rafacz, J. D., & Rusch, N. (2012). Challenging the public stigma of mental illness: A meta-analysis of outcome studies. *Psychiatric Services, 63*(10), 963–973. https://doi.org/10.1176/appi.ps.005292011

Funk, M., Minoletti, A., Drew, N., Taylor, J., & Saraceno, B. (2006). Advocacy for mental health: Roles for consumer and family organizations and governments. *Health Promotion International, 21*(1), 70–75. https://doi.org/10.1093/heapro/dai031

Gillard, S., Foster, R., Gibson, S., Goldsmith, L., Marks, J., & White, S. (2017). Describing a principles-based approach to developing and evaluating peer worker roles as peer support moves into mainstream mental health services. *Mental Health and Social Inclusion, 21*(3), 133–143. https://doi.org/10.1108/MHSI-03-2017-0016

Hadlaczky, G., Hökby, S., Mkrtchian, A., Carli, V., & Wasserman, D. (2014). Mental health first aid is an effective public health intervention for improving knowledge, attitudes, and behaviour: A meta-analysis. *International Review of Psychiatry, 26*(4), 467–475. https://doi.org/10.3109/09540261.2014.924910

Henderson, C. (2020). Commentary on "Effect of contact-based interventions on stigma and discrimination." *Psychiatric Services, 71*(7), 738–739. https://doi.org/10.1176/appi.ps.202000210

Johnson, M. E., & Dowling-Guyer, S. (1996). Effects of inclusive vs. exclusive language on evaluations of the counselor. *Sex Roles, 34*(5–6), 407–418. https://doi.org/10.1007/BF01547809

Jorm, A. F. (2020). Effect of contact-based interventions on stigma and discrimination: A critical examination of the evidence. *Psychiatric Services, 71*(7), 735–737. https://doi.org/10.1176/appi.ps.201900587

Jorm, A. F., Kitchener, B. A., O'Kearney, R., & Dear, K. B. G. (2004). Mental Health First Aid training of the public in a rural area: A cluster randomized trial [ISRCTN53887541]. *BMC Psychiatry, 4*, 1–9. https://doi.org/10.1186/1471-244X-4-33

Knaak, S., Modgill, G., & Patten, S. B. (2014). Key ingredients of anti-stigma programs for health care providers: A data synthesis of evaluative studies. *Canadian Journal of Psychiatry. Revue canadienne de psychiatrie, 59*(10), S19–S26. https://doi.org/10.1177/070674371405901s06

Mittal, D., Sullivan, G., Chekuri, L., Allee, E., & Corrigan, P. W. (2012). Empirical studies of self-stigma reduction strategies: A critical review of the literature. *Psychiatric Services, 63*(10), 974–981. https://doi.org/10.1176/appi.ps.201100459

Moncrieff, J., & Steingard, S. (2019). What is critical psychiatry? In L. Cosgrove & A. Vaswani (Eds.), *Critical psychiatry: Controversies and clinical implications* (pp. 1–16). Springer Nature Switzerland.

Pickett, S. A., Diehl, S. M., Steigman, P. J., Prater, J. D., Fox, A., Shipley, P., Grey, D. D., & Cook, J. A. (2012). Consumer empowerment and self-advocacy outcomes in a randomized study of peer-led education. *Community Mental Health Journal, 48*, 420–430. https://doi.org/10.1007/s10597-012-9507-0

Repper, J., & Carter, T. (2011). A review of the literature on peer support in mental health services. *Journal of Mental Health, 20*(4), 392–411. https://doi.org/10.3109/09638237.2011.583947

Rüsch, N., Abbruzzese, E., Hagedorn, E., Hartenhauer, D., Kaufmann, I., Curschellas, J., Ventling, S., Zuaboni, G., Bridler, R., Olschewski, M., Kawohl, W., Rössler, W., Kleim, B., & Corrigan, P. W. (2014). Efficacy of Coming Out Proud to reduce stigma's impact among people with mental illness: Pilot randomised controlled trial. *British Journal of Psychiatry, 204*(5), 391–397. https://doi.org/10.1192/bjp.bp.113.135772

Sayce, L. (2000). *From psychiatric patient to citizen.* Macmillan.

Sayce, L. (2003). Beyond good intentions. Making anti-discrimination strategies work. *Disability and Society, 18*(5), 625–642. https://doi.org/10.1080/0968759032000097852

Stein, C. H., Aguirre, R., & Hunt, M. G. (2013). Social networks and personal loss among young adults with mental illness and their parents: A family perspective. *Psychiatric Rehabilitation Journal, 36*(1), 15–21. https://doi.org/10.1037/h0094744

Stuart, H. (2007). Employment equity and mental disability. *Current Opinion in Psychiatry, 20*(5), 486–490. https://doi.org/10.1097/YCO.0b013e32826fb356

Stuart, H. (2016a). Global mental health reducing the stigma of mental illness. *Global Mental Health, 3*(e17), 1–14. https://doi.org/10.1017/gmh.2016.11

Stuart, H. (2016b). What has proven effective in anti-stigma programming. In W. Gaebel, W. Rossler, & N. Sartorius (Eds.), *The stigma of mental illness—End of the story?* (pp. 497–514). Springer International. https://doi.org/10.1007/978-3-319-27839-1_27

Stuart, H., Arboleda-Flórez, J., & Sartorius, N. (2012). *Paradigms lost: Fighting stigma and the lessons learned.* Oxford University Press.

Varghese, P. J. (2015). Advocacy in mental health: Offering a voice to the voiceless. *Indian Journal of Social Psychiatry, 31*(1), 4. https://doi.org/10.4103/0971-9962.161987

Verhaeghe, M., Bracke, P., & Bruynooghe, K. (2008). Stigmatization and self-esteem of persons in recovery from mental illness: The role of peer support. *International Journal of Social Psychiatry, 54*(3), 206–218. https://doi.org/10.1177/0020764008090422

World Health Organization. (2003). *Advocacy for mental health.*

Yanos, P. T., Lucksted, A., Drapalski, A. L., Roe, D., & Lysaker, P. (2015). Interventions targeting mental health self-stigma: A review and comparison. *Psychiatric Rehabilitation Journal, 38*(2), 171–178. https://doi.org/10.1037/prj0000100

4

Measuring Structural Stigma

Thomas Ungar and Stephanie Knaak

Stigma has been identified as a major barrier to access to healthcare services and recovery for people with mental health or substance use problems. It operates at multiple levels and in multiple domains, including the healthcare system. Stigmatizing processes influence all levels of the design and delivery of care for mental health and substance use disorders and impact all organizational areas (Henderson et al., 2014; Livingston, 2020). Increasingly, there is an interest in understanding how stigmatization processes work at the structural or institutional level, as being embedded in the policies, practices, and culture of healthcare organizations (Hatzenbuehler, 2016; Knaak et al., 2020; Livingston, 2020). More specifically, structural stigma refers to the accumulated activities of organizations that deliberately or inadvertently create and maintain social inequalities for people with mental health or substance use problems. It is located in the formal and informal rules and practices of social institutions and is "reinforced in laws, the internal policies and procedures of private or public institutions and systems, and the practices of professionals" (Livingston, 2020, p. 4).

Much of the current measurement of stigma in healthcare environments focuses on capturing attitudes, behaviors, knowledge, and skills of health providers and other healthcare staff and on understanding the experiences and perspectives of people with lived experience of a mental illness or substance use problem in their interactions with the health system (Henderson et al., 2014; Knaak et al., 2020; Livingston, 2020). Because these approaches are used to capture aspects of the cultural environment in which care is delivered, they can be useful as indicators of structural stigma. Also important for the measurement of structural stigma is capturing normative behaviors, as well as the formal and informal policies, processes, and practices of organizations and groups. Determining how to approach measurement of structural stigma and trying to decide what to measure are challenges. This chapter describes key considerations for measuring mental illness–related stigma within healthcare contexts.

Approaching the Measurement of Structural Stigma

One way to approach measuring structural stigma is to think of it as a way to "make visible" what is currently hidden in the culture and policies of healthcare that leads to poorer quality or less equitable care for people with mental health or substance use problems. We have argued elsewhere that structural stigma is an implicit systemic cognitive bias and an unperceived learning need within healthcare contexts (Ungar & Knaak, 2013). From this, we understand stigma as a cultural phenomenon with a hidden curriculum, requiring contextual understanding and transformative learning approaches when designing interventions (Sukhera et al., 2020; Ungar & Knaak, 2013; Ungar et al., 2016). In this understanding, measurement in and of itself becomes a potential antistigma intervention as it begins to make visible that which is often implicit, below the level of conscious awareness. It also means that a required first step may be one of transformative learning and awareness-raising for healthcare providers, policy makers, and decision-makers about how to see and think about structural stigma. As we conceptualize measurement in this way, we are conscious that our intentions are beyond the obvious analytic benefits of empirical measurement. As we are at the earliest stages of creating and deciding on measures, we are intentionally using measurement of structural stigma as a strategic transformative action and as a catalyst for change in the hopes of improved equity and rights and to stimulate attitude, behavior, and policy changes to quality of care.

There is also the question of how to measure. A recent environmental scan initiated by the Mental Health Commission of Canada contacted 13 agencies across a sampling of the health regulatory and performance measurement field, including Canada, as well as the United States and the United Kingdom more selectively (Ungar & Moothathamby, 2020). The results revealed that there is currently no measurement tool or process specific to structural stigma for mental health and substance use (MHSU) (Ungar & Moothathamby, 2020). This absence is an opportunity for the creation of new tools and processes.

We believe that the greatest impact may be realized by leveraging existing systems for tracking and performance. To this end, we suggest that existing quality standards and regulatory, oversight, and monitoring frameworks and processes may be used to think about our approach to the measurement of structural stigma. For example, many health delivery systems use the Institute of Medicine's six pillars of quality of care as an organizing framework (Institute of Medicine, 2006; Knaak et al., 2015). Quality frameworks are used by hospital boards, quality-of-care committees, incident reviews, coroners' inquests, and public quality reporting methods. Also, a quality-of-care framework encompasses key categories important for structural stigma, such as access, wait times/timeliness, equity, patient centeredness, safety, and effectiveness. The equity pillar may be especially useful to help reveal structural stigma in the context of resource allocation and the availability and delivery of services (Knaak & Ungar, 2017).

We also suggest using a human factor approach in thinking about how to capture structural stigma (Vicente, 2006). Unlike technoscientific models of performance and quality measurement, human factor models acknowledge human limitations and biases, including cognitive bias and implicit stigma, and account for them in the design of services, policies, and processes with a goal to minimize risk and improve quality. The old approach to clinical medical error was to blame the individual for the error. The new approach is to expect error, including human and structural factors as contributors, and to review all aspects of a clinical process to find opportunities for improvement well beyond the individual but also within the system. Human system engineers and quality-of-care professionals use multifactor capturing processes such as the "Swiss cheese" model of error, the Ishikawa or Fishbone diagram, and root cause analyses, which attempt to capture all inputs and factors to a clinical outcome including systemic structural factors beyond the individual (e.g., see Ishikawa, 1990; Reason, 2000).

Finally, in designing indicators and methods of measurement for structural stigma of mental health and substance use, it will be imperative to meaningfully include persons with lived experience and their family members and significant others in all measurement design and development processes so that the outcomes they find important are captured in the tools and approaches developed. In addition to involvement in the coproduction and guidance of measures and processes, the perspectives of people with lived experience will be central to helping determine measurement priorities. For example, a recent qualitative study revealed wait times, deaths by suicide, client satisfaction ratings, and levels of peer support as key structural stigma metrics to track (Knaak et al., 2020; see also Chapter 7). It will be particularly valuable if people with personal experiences of a MHSU problem (either directly or through a family member or loved one) also have insight into various aspects of the health system, such as with respect to service availability, access pathways, governance, policies, training, or decision-making.

Eight Possible Prototypes

There are many ways to measure structural stigma within the healthcare context. Because structural stigma is a "wicked" problem hidden from view (Buchanan, 1992; Henderson & Gronholm, 2018), this section uses a human-centered design approach to identify several rapid prototypes for structural stigma measurement products and processes. Rapid prototyping design methods are analogous to a proof-of-concept process. The process begins by quickly creating a future state of a product or process to imperfectly begin the design process and thereafter iteratively redesign by validating and testing with a group of users, stakeholders, developers, and other designers. Our prototypes are possibilities that could be used as indicators or manifestations of observed structural stigmatization outcomes. The value of a rapid prototype approach is to help transform awareness, stimulate discussion, and encourage novel ideas for what is an unconscious implicit phenomenon (Roberts et al., 2016). Sharing innovative prototype possibilities also can help widen the frame of possibility for improvement, disruption, and transformation. Next we will discuss potential structural stigma prototype measures and measurement interventions developed through participant observation, discussion and consultation, empathic ethnographic insight, scholarly expertise, clinical experience, and administrative leadership experience within healthcare.

Creation of a Novel Structural Stigma Implicit Cognitive Bias Training Module

Implicit bias, also known as unconscious bias, is "the bias in judgment and/or behavior that results from subtle cognitive processes (e.g., implicit attitudes and implicit stereotypes) that often operate at a level below conscious awareness and without intentional control" (Institute for Healthcare Improvement, 2017). Although it is not a direct measurement activity, we believe this is an important component to achieve the awareness-raising and transformative learning goal that will allow policy makers and decision-makers to see structural stigma where they did not see it before. We believe such training could increase the capacity of decision-makers to conceptualize stigma as a deficit in structural performance and outcomes and identify where it exists and how to look for it within their organization or department (Devine et al., 2012; Forscher et al., 2017). It is our hope that this precursor activity to measurement could lead to greater organizational buy-in by boards of directors and chief executive officers and improve uptake and willingness to tackle structural stigma in healthcare.

The educational module content could include ways to view structural stigma through a quality-of-care lens as a structural area of concern beyond an issue of individual attitudes or knowledge. Given the effectiveness of social contact as an approach to stigma reduction (Corrigan et al., 2012), curriculum design components could include testimonials and real-life examples of persons with lived experience and health providers who have been affected by structural stigma, as well as examples of potential exemplars or new designs to measure stigma to stimulate curious, inquisitive, creative measurement tool choices and designs. Describing critical incidents and/or scenarios where structural stigma has been a component or root cause but was not properly identified is recommended. Examples of diagnostic overshadowing—a process in which medical conditions are ignored or undertreated or diagnoses are delayed because a person has had a mental health or substance use problem—leading to critical incidents that garner the attention of boards of directors, malpractice and risk insurance, and shareholders/people with learned experience are high-fidelity, powerful stories with impact (Ungar et al., 2020).

A simple, all-too-common scenario could be a person with mental illness or substance use presenting to an emergency room. They are prematurely referred to the mental health service without adequate physical assessment or investigation. Shortly after, their concurrent physical health problem results in a tragic, unexpected, sudden death. This example of diagnostic overshadowing is familiar to most health leaders and practitioners, but perhaps generally thought of not as a problem of structural systemic bias within healthcare, but as a "one off" or a case of individual clinical error. Framing this example in the context of structural stigma and implicit cognitive bias would point out deficits in established processes that allow this overshadowing to occur, such as the need to change mandatory workflows, introduce standard pathway emergency room algorithms for medical stability clearance, or improve standardization of triage.

A structural stigma training program could also include concrete structural stigma-focused examples, including gaps in funding, resource allocation, service availability, and physical environment for persons with mental illnesses and substance use problems. The use of social contact through the telling of real-world stories and sharing of concrete structural examples could assist transformative learning and reflection for decision-makers (Corrigan et al., 2012).

To evaluate such a structural stigma training program, we believe the measurement outcome target could be focused on the extent to which leaders and decision-makers: (a) increase their awareness and understanding of structural stigma within a transformative learning framework (Mezirow, 2003; Sukhera et al., 2020; Ungar, 2012); (b) are able to see examples of structural stigma where they did not before; (c) are motivated to introduce structural stigma measures within their own department, organization, or institution, with the intention of implementing changes where inequities or quality-of-care deficits are identified; and (d) result in real-world behavior change to structures such as policy or practice change in their own healthcare context. Transformative learning is a theory of adult education that focuses not on content acquisition, but on transforming the learner's perspective, paradigms, or the way they conceptualize things. As such, it seeks to transform their perspective and worldview. Mezirow (2003, p. 58) describes transformative learning as "learning that transforms problematic frames of reference to make them more inclusive, discriminating, reflective, open, and emotionally able to change." The learning process involves critical thinking and reflection, grappling with disorienting dilemmas, examining one's assumptions, seeking out additional perspectives, and acquiring new knowledge.

We hope that implicit structural stigma systemic bias training for MHSU becomes a mandatory training requirement for healthcare leaders and decision-makers, similar to other mandatory implicit bias training undertaken by health providers and staff, because the downstream effects of such a training may include a greater desire to measure structural systemic bias of MHSU and improved policies, resource allocation, and care practices. Best practices in governance would also include a structural stigma/implicit/cognitive bias training module as a requirement for boards of directors or other governors in hopes of improved ethical and equitable decision-making and improved quality of care (e.g., see Devine et al., 2012; Forscher et al., 2017).

Audit Tools and Audit Process Enhancements

Most organizations and health systems use accreditation and audit processes. In Canada, these activities are primarily undertaken by Accreditation Canada/Health

Standards Organization (see https://accreditation.ca). Currently, there are relatively few items, measures, and required organizational practices developed for MHSU and none that we are aware of that could be defined as targeting or capturing structural stigma (Ungar & Moothathamby, 2020). This provides an opportunity to develop and embed new audit measurement items within existing accreditation processes that strategically enable capturing key inequities in care and quality for MHSU. The thoroughness of accreditation audits means there would be numerous areas for placement of structural stigma measures.

Also, current items likely do not work well as indicator measures for structural stigma. For example, the current Canadian accreditation item for mental health, "there is a process to ensure a response to requests for services in a timely way" (Accreditation Canada, 2015, p. 36), is too vague to protect against structural bias for MHSU. At most hospitals, a person with a fracture in the emergency room will usually be seen the next working day in a well-staffed fracture clinic. However, a person with a MHSU emergency presentation may have to wait weeks or months for a follow-up visit after an emergency room visit, with far fewer providers available to meet the need. Within the current framing, the accreditation audit question likely would not capture this structural inequity of access to care resources. An alternative prototype example for a measure that addresses this quality issue through a structural stigma–informed lens may include something like "mental health patients' wait time for post emergency room assessment is equivalent to that for physical health concerns of similar acuity," which would be more certain to capture and address structural inequities in post–emergency room staffing resources and low MHSU prioritization. Other examples for potential new accreditation items to capture structural stigma in healthcare include the following:

- Is the condition of the physical plant care environment for MHSU equivalent to physical health services?
- Are "code white" procedures (i.e., when a patient exhibits aggressive behavior) led by a clinician with support from security as opposed to led by a security person? This would address the implicit cognitive bias that patients with mental health or substance use problems are behaving badly and need coercive control or punishment, rather than the fact that they have symptoms of an illness, are in distress, and need healthcare.
- Is triage level assignment for MHSU by staff done according to the Canadian Triage and Acuity (CTAS) categories (Bullard et al., 2017), along with well-developed standard care pathways for mental health and substance use care, with clarity of "most responsible service" guidelines (e.g., see Ungar et al., 2017)? Early research evidence has shown that an electronic CTAS process is more accurate because it automatically helps individual triage staff assign a correct triage score based on the presenting problem, which may otherwise have been prioritized lower for MHSU presentations (McLeod et al., 2020).

Quality and Performance Dashboard Enhancements

It is common practice in hospitals and other healthcare organizations to have a reporting performance dashboard for quality (Dowding et al., 2015). A quality dashboard is an easy-to-evaluate summary that provides high-level assessment of a curated set of measures for system performance, similar to a summative report card. Typically, these have a select synthesized list of tracked items with adjacent metrics, trends, and targets with easy to review, at-a-glance visual scoring—such as a green, yellow, or red light—beside each item. Dashboards are reviewed regularly by quality-of-care committees and presented to hospital governance boards (Kroch et al., 2006). Healthcare system governance structures include public dashboards and/or mandatory reporting to their funding agencies (Kroch et al., 2006). These dashboards are increasingly organized under the six pillars of quality of care with minor modifications or customizations by local organizations. Common indicators include hospital standard mortality ratio, percentage of completion of the surgical safety checklist in the operating room, hand hygiene compliance rates as a percentage, emergency room time to physician initial assessment, and rates of harmful and critical falls (Dowding et al., 2015).

Upon review of several system and organization quality dashboards, it is apparent there are few, if any, indicators related to MHSU, which, in our opinion, may itself be an example of a taken-for-granted, unnoticed manifestation of structural stigma. While measuring outcomes for MHSU can be challenging, some measurement inclusion for MHSU quality is certainly achievable. Some possible considerations include the following:

- Under the quality pillar of timeliness, include an item that monitors emergency room follow-up care for persons with MHSU problems who have presented with a CTAS 1 or 2[1] (including persons with acute suicidal ideation, intent, or behaviors) (Bullard et al., 2017), with a target time to receive follow-up care within 14 days (or according to what best evidence guidelines recommend). This type of indicator is used for cancer care follow-up wait time targets (Health Quality Ontario, n.d.).
- Under the safety pillar of quality, add an indicator for percentage of documented physical examination assessments of admitted mental health patients, along with a target percentage. This indicator would help counteract the phenomenon of diagnostic overshadowing and the tendency to miss concurrent physical health disorders among patients with a history of mental health or substance use problems (e.g., see Atzema et al., 2011).
- Under the quality pillar of patient and family centeredness, add a new indicator for patient/family satisfaction scores for persons admitted or treated for MHSU problems, relative to comparator satisfaction rates for those receiving

medical and surgical services within the same institution or system, with a target. Standard satisfaction scales are available and already in use by many systems or organizations (e.g., see Hadibhai et al., 2018).

Embedding a small number of strategically curated and selected quality indicators will help inform boards and decision-makers of areas of concern and underperformance of outcomes of structural stigma, because they would appear as a red light or low score compared to other indicators. This could catalyze action and motivation to improve care, spark oversight and governance concern, and encourage decision-makers to allocate institutional energy, attention, and resources to help address MHSU structural quality gaps.

Policy and Legislation Interventions

Structural stigma not only manifests in clinical behaviors and services, but also is "baked into" the architecture of policies and legislation. Reviewing policies through a structural stigma lens will allow for revisions and improvements to reduce the negative impacts and outcomes of MHSU structural stigma. In some cases, this may mean improving existing policies as part of an organization's routine schedule and policy review process. In other cases, it will mean the creation of new policies or legislation targeting structural inequity and structural stigma for MHSU.

Some countries have started these legislative interventions. In 1996, the United States passed the Mental Health Parity Act, requiring annual benefit limits for mental health to be no lower than those for medical or surgical care (Canadian Mental Health Association, 2018). In 2012, the United Kingdom enacted similar "parity of esteem" legislation, requiring the National Health Service of England to provide parity of mental and physical health services through its mandate (Canadian Mental Health Association, 2018). Unfortunately, adherence to parity legislation remains weak (Canadian Mental Health Association, 2018).

While legislation to undermine structural stigma is not in itself a measurement tool, it provides a policy direction that requires additional measurement and monitoring (Funk & Drew, 2017; Hoffman et al., 2016; Morrissey, 2012; O'Reilly & Gray, 2014). For example, enforcing existing conventions and laws on social justice and autonomy—including the UN Convention on the Rights of Persons With Disabilities, disability rights such as Mental Disability and the European Convention on Human Rights, the Canadian Charter of Rights and Freedoms, and the World Health Organization's QualityRights movement—can be an important way of institutionalizing the need for more equitable monitoring and performance within the healthcare context (Funk & Drew, 2017; Hoffman et al., 2016; Morrissey, 2012; O'Reilly & Gray, 2014).

Client/Patient/People With Learned Experience Satisfaction and Engagement Surveys

Under the quality pillar of patient (and family) centeredness, most health organizations attempt or are required to measure patient satisfaction of care received. A number of standard satisfaction or engagement surveys exist (e.g., see Hadibhai et al., 2018). These satisfaction surveys contain some general elements that broadly apply to MHSU services, which may be used as indicators for structural stigma such as the following:

- "The physical care environment supports my treatment and recovery."
- "I was given clear information and recommendations about follow-up care."
- "Care providers were courteous, empathic, and understanding."
- "I would recommend this care organization to friends and family."

However, such surveys can be enhanced by adding purposely developed items that better target or identify structural stigma from the perspective of patients. This may include new prototype question examples, such as, "I was offered harm reduction services or opioid agonist therapy treatment in a timely manner" or "It was clear and easy for me to access care and navigate services."

Last, as described under "Quality and Performance Dashboard Enhancements," quality dashboards often report a global patient and family satisfaction score. Further stratifying patient satisfaction scores from MHSU patients versus patients receiving medical or surgical care services may be another useful way to measure structural differences in care. Of special note in this context is the importance of capturing the voices of caregivers. Some serious mental illnesses, such as schizophrenia, commonly have an onset in late adolescence and early adulthood. For schizophrenia as well as many other MHSU conditions, the impact and involvement of family is thus a central, yet rarely measured or spoken of, quality concern. Developing and tracking satisfaction scores for family centeredness of MHSU care is another measurement opportunity and an important gap to address.

Economic, Financial, and Resource Equity Scorecard

Social and cultural values are often enacted through economic and financial decisions, including budgets, remuneration, and allocation of resources. Mental health and substance use disorders are well reported to be inequitably underfunded compared to other health conditions and compared to their burden of disease (Canadian Mental Health Association, 2018; Livingston, 2020; Mental Health Commission of Canada, 2017). Measurement of financial budgets and other resource allocations could be reported via a visual scorecard to highlight structural economic gaps and inequities. This measurement approach would be similar to those that highlight gender inequities in pay, for example.

One could also measure courtesy stigma or stigma by association as a structural problem, particularly as it exists within healthcare environments among those who provide care to people with mental health or substance use problems. For example, psychiatrists are often the lowest paid medical specialty relative to other medical specialties despite similar years of training and equal work. In some cases, specialist psychiatrist providers are paid less than a family physician, a discipline that requires fewer years of professional training (Canadian Institute for Health Information, 2017). Measuring and monitoring relative financial remuneration of mental health providers (medical, nursing, etc.) compared to physical health providers could help identify gaps and assess structural inequities. Interestingly, within medicine there is a growing movement for gender-based pay equity because female physicians are paid less than males, even when controlling for multiple variables (Cohen & Kiran, 2020). Measuring and further exploring the potential intersections of structural stigmas of MHSU could be illuminating because psychiatry has a relatively high percentage of female practitioners. Making transparent to society these values-based unconscious economic and financial MHSU inequities may also lead to human rights or civil litigation challenges. Measurement indicator items to develop for a resource equity scorecard for MHSU could include items such as:

- the percentage of the overall health budget for MHSU,
- the relative ranking of pay for MHSU providers compared to physical health providers,
- the percentage of the research budget allocated to MHSU research by funding agencies,
- the percentage of charitable donations within a healthcare organization or system donated to MHSU relative to physical health disorders,
- the percentage of continuing health education training budgets directed to MHSU, and
- spending parity targets or benchmarks for MHSU versus other physical health conditions.

Creation of an economic and financial resource scorecard for MHSU could be most effective and powerful if it originated from health insurance providers, justice organizations, or financial decision-makers and regulators. Depending on each nation's local governance and financial decision-making processes, this could be an auditor general's office, a government finance committee, or perhaps human rights and justice regulators. It could be public or private health insurance regulatory bodies or a ministry of health. It could be an ideal activity for national public health regulatory agencies and for international organizations such as the World Health Organization, independent international policy groups and think tanks, and economic and financial policy and development groups such as the Organisation for Economic Co-operation and Development or the World Bank Group.

Health Equity Impact Assessment Add-Ons

Healthcare organizations are increasingly focusing on health equity diversity and inclusion and attempts to minimize disparities based on sexual orientation, gender, and ethnoracial background. Health impact equity assessment templates capture a number of possible marginalized statuses, such as being a member of a racial minority, an indigenous population, a particular religious background, a low-income population, or a language minority (Heller et al., 2014). Adding new categories for MHSU would acknowledge these statuses as also being key concerns for health equity, which would be in keeping with recent arguments that MHSU should be considered a health disparity in its own right (Bartels & DiMilia, 2017).

Structural Stigma MHSU Global Measure

Creating a de novo original global measurement standard specifically targeting structural stigma toward mental illnesses and substance use is our final consideration. Such a measurement tool would likely contain elements selected from a curated compilation of previously mentioned items. This is perhaps a more ambitious approach, because it would require a greater commitment within healthcare organizations to adopt and implement an entirely new measurement tool and process. The previous measurement strategies, by contrast, generally present ways to embed new elements within existing structures for ease of adoption and likelihood of successful implementation and impact.

As a future goal, a de novo, stand-alone MHSU structural stigma measure could be worth pursuing. It could be designed to give an overall score or grade or quality seal for organizations, with a high score or rating being a desirable achievement for healthcare organizations to be able to show that they have addressed structural inequities in quality and services for MHSU. Establishing a global MHSU structural stigma measurement and scoring system also could be useful as an incentive program, offering a seal of approval or recognition for organizations who score well, similar to those by Consumer Reports, J. D. Power rankings, or Best Managed Companies awards.

Conclusions and Key Considerations

Because the measurement of mental illness and substance use–related structural stigma is still in its infancy, this chapter has provided a number of discussion points for thinking about how to proceed. We have proposed the following main ideas:

- Ensuring meaningful involvement of people with lived experience of MHSU problems and their family members is necessary to ensure that the outcomes most important to them are captured in the tools and approaches developed.
- Measures and approaches that can be easily embedded into existing processes and structures will be the most efficient and effective way to achieve change. This approach is consistent with design methods, marketing, and elements of social engineering (strategic collusion). Hacking structural stigma within healthcare culture will not be easy. It is necessary to measure gaps and inequities, because many aspects of structural stigma exist beyond the immediate conscious awareness of the organization's agents, stakeholders, and decision-makers.
- Given that structural stigma is often considered a problem that is "hidden in plain sight," we believe there is tremendous value in developing awareness-raising and training modules to illuminate the problem of structural stigma, particularly among those who have the power to make changes within their organizations and within systems. We encourage an approach that frames structural stigma as an unconscious cognitive bias or implicit systemic inequity to minimize resistance and increase the likelihood for transformative learning to occur.
- Given its hidden nature within healthcare, we believe a human-centered design approach to selecting measures is well suited. There will be no single bullet measure to singularly address the complex phenomenon of MHSU structural stigma. Instead, measurement that combines the best of evidence-based analytic inquiry and methods of participant observation, cultural, and social inquiry are optimal for deep insights and a more thorough understanding. This productive balance could be ideal in guiding where to look and what to select as measures and indicators of stigma outcomes. This approach was used to develop the eight prototype measurement ideas expressed in this chapter.

Note

1. Canadian Triage Acuity Scale is a Canada-wide process to standardize the acuity and urgency of persons presenting to an emergency room. The triage level assigned determines prioritization of care. This includes how quickly the physician and nurse will attend to a patient and the physical areas and resources allocated to the patient's care. The highest urgency (CTAS 1) would be for an imminent, life-threatening condition such as a person not breathing or vital signs absent. Minor concerns such as a sore throat would be a CTAS 5. Suicidal thoughts or plans are categorized as a CTAS 2.

References

Accreditation Canada. (2015). *Standards: Mental Health Services, v. 10.*

Atzema, C. L., Schull, M. J., & Tu, J. V. (2011). The effects of a charted history of depression on emergency department triage and outcomes in patients with acute myocardial infarction. *Canadian Medical Association Journal, 183*(6), 663–669.

Bartels, S., & DiMilia, S. (2017). Why serious mental illness should be designated a health disparity and the paradox of ethnicity. *The Lancet Psychiatry, 4*(5), 351–352. https://doi.org/10.1016/S2215-0366(17)30111-6

Buchanan, R. (1992). Wicked problems in design thinking. *Design Issues, 8*(2), 5–21.

Bullard, M. J., Musgrave, E., Warren, D., Unger, B., Skeldon, T., Grierson, R., van der Linde, E., & Swain, J. (2017). Revisions to the Canadian Emergency Department Triage and Acuity Scale (CTAS) Guidelines 2016. *Canadian Journal of Emergency Medicine, 19*(S2), S18–S27. https://doi.org/10.1017/cem.2017.365

Canadian Institute for Health Information. (2017). *Physicians in Canada, 2016: Summary report.* https://secure.cihi.ca/free_products/Physicians_in_Canada_2016.pdf

Canadian Mental Health Association. (2018). *Mental health in the balance: Ending the health care disparity gap in Canada.*

Cohen, M., & Kiran, T. (2020) Closing the gender pay gap in Canadian medicine. *Canadian Medical Association Journal, 192*(35), E1011–E1017. https://doi.org/10.1503/cmaj.200375

Corrigan, P. W., Morris, S. B., Michaels, P. J., Rafacz, J. D., & Rüsch, N. (2012). Challenging the public stigma of mental illness: A meta-analysis of outcome studies. *Psychiatric Services, 63*(10), 963–973. https://doi.org/10.1176/appi.ps.201100529

Devine, P. G., Forscher, P. S., Austin, A. J., & Cox, W. T. (2012). Long-term reduction in implicit race bias: A prejudice habit-breaking intervention. *Journal of Experimental Social Psychology, 48*(6), 1267–1278. https://doi.org/10.1016/j.jesp.2012.06.003

Dowding, D., Randell, R., Gardner, P., Fitzpatrick, G., Dykes, P., Favela, J., Hamer, S., Whitewood-Moores, Z., Hardiker, N., Borycki, E., & Currie, L. (2015). Dashboards for improving patient care: Review of the literature. *International Journal of Medical Informatics, 84*(2), 87–100. https://doi.org/10.1016/j.ijmedinf.2014.10.001

Forscher, P. S., Mitamura, C., Dix, E. L., Cox, W., & Devine, P. G. (2017). Breaking the prejudice habit: Mechanisms, timecourse, and longevity. *Journal of Experimental Social Psychology, 72,* 133–146. https://doi.org/10.1016/j.jesp.2017.04.009

Funk, M., & Drew, N. (2017). WHO QualityRights: Transforming mental health services. *The Lancet Psychiatry, 4*(11), 826–827. https://doi.org/10.1016/S2215-0366(17)30271-7

Hadibhai, S., Lacroix, J., & Leeb, K. (2018). Developing the first pan-Canadian acute care patient experiences survey. *Patient Experience Journal, 5*(3), Article 5. https://doi.org/10–35680/2372-0247.1227

Hatzenbuehler, M. L. (2016). Structural stigma: Research evidence and implications for psychological science. *The American Psychologist, 71*(8), 742–751. https://doi.org/10.1037/amp0000068

Health Quality Ontario. (n.d.). *Indicator library.* Retrieved August 31, 2020, from https://www.hqontario.ca/System-Performance/Measuring-System-Performance/Indicator-Library

Heller, J., Givens, M. L., Yuen, T. K., Gould, S., Jandu, M. B., Bourcier, E., & Choi, T. (2014). Advancing efforts to achieve health equity: Equity metrics for health impact assessment practice. *International Journal of Environmental Research and Public Health, 11*(11), 11054–11064. https://doi.org/10.3390/ijerph111111054

Henderson, C., & Gronholm, P. C. (2018). Mental health related stigma as a "wicked problem": The need to address stigma and consider the consequences. *International*

Journal of Environmental Research and Public Health, 15(6), 1158. https://doi.org/10.3390/ijerph15061158

Henderson, C., Noblett, J., Parke, H., Clement, S., Caffrey, A., Gale-Grant, O., Schulze, B., Druss, B., & Thornicroft, G. (2014). Mental health-related stigma in health care and mental health-care settings. *Lancet Psychiatry, 1*, 467–482. https://doi/10.1016/S2215-0366(14)00023-6

Hoffman, S. J., Sritharan, L., & Tejpar, A. (2016). Is the UN Convention on the Rights of Persons With Disabilities impacting mental health laws and policies in high-income countries? A case study of implementation in Canada. *BMC International Health and Human Rights, 16*(1), 28. https://doi.org/10.1186/s12914-016-0103-1

Institute for Healthcare Improvement (2017, September 28). *How to reduce implicit bias.* http://www.ihi.org/communities/blogs/how-to-reduce-implicit-bias

Institute of Medicine. (2006). *Improving the quality of health care for mental and substance-use conditions.* National Academies Press.

Ishikawa, K. (1990). *Introduction to quality control* (J. H. Loftus, Trans.). 3A Corporation.

Knaak, S., Livingston, J., Stuart, H., & Ungar, T. (2020). *Combating mental illness- and substance use-related structural stigma in health care.* Mental Health Commission of Canada.

Knaak, S., Patten, S., & Ungar, T. (2015). Mental illness stigma as a quality-of-care problem. *The Lancet Psychiatry, 2*(10), 863–864. https://doi.org/10.1016/S2215-0366(15)00382-X

Knaak, S., & Ungar, T. (2017). Towards a mental health inequity audit. *The Lancet Psychiatry, 4*(8), 583. https://doi.org/10.1016/S2215-0366(17)30281-X

Kroch, E., Vaughn, T., Koepke, M., Roman, S., Foster, D., Sinha, S., & Levey, S. (2006). Hospital boards and quality dashboards. *Journal of Patient Safety, 2*(1), 10–19.

Livingston, J. D. (2020). *Structural stigma in health-care contexts for people with mental health and substance use issues: A literature review.* Mental Health Commission of Canada.

McLeod, S. L., McCarron, J., Ahmed, T., Grewal, K., Mittmann, N., Scott, S., Ovens, H., Garay, J., Bullard, M., Rowe, B. H., Dreyer, J., & Borgundvaag, B. (2020). Interrater reliability, accuracy, and triage time pre- and post-implementation of a real-time electronic triage decision-support tool. *Annals of Emergency Medicine, 75*(4), 524–531. https://doi.org/10.1016/j.annemergmed.2019.07.048

Mental Health Commission of Canada. (2017). *Strengthening the case for investing in Canada's mental health system: Economic considerations.*

Mezirow, J. (2003). Transformative learning as discourse. *Journal of Transformative Education, 1*(1): 58–63. https://doi.org/10.1177/1541344603252172

Morrissey, F. (2012). The United Nations Convention on the Rights of Persons with Disabilities: A new approach to decision-making in mental health law. *European Journal of Health Law, 19*(5), 423–440. https://doi.org/10.1163/15718093-12341237

O'Reilly, R. L., & Gray, J. E. (2014). Canada's mental health legislation. *International Psychiatry, 11*(3), 65–67.

Reason, J. (2000). Human error: Models and management. *British Medical Journal (Clinical Research Edition), 320*(7237), 768–770. https://doi.org/10.1136/bmj.320.7237.768

Roberts, J. P., Fisher, T. R., Trowbridge, M. J., & Bent, C. (2016). A design thinking framework for healthcare management and innovation. *Healthcare, 4*(1), 11–14. https://doi.org/10.1016/j.hjdsi.2015.12.002

Sukhera, J., Watling, C. J., & Gonzalez, C. M. (2020). Implicit bias in health professions: From recognition to transformation. *Academic Medicine, 95*(5), 717–723. https://doi.org/10.1097/ACM.0000000000003173

Ungar, T. (2012, April 24). Reducing stigma in mental illness with transformative learning [Letter to the Editor]. *CMAJ.* https://www.cmaj.ca/content/178/10/1320/tab-e-letters#reducing-stigma-in-mental-illness-with-transformative-learning

Ungar, T., & Knaak, S. (2013). The hidden medical logic of mental health stigma. *Australian & New Zealand Journal of Psychiatry, 47*(7), 611–612. https://doi.org/10.1177/0004867413476758

Ungar, T., Knaak, S., & Mantler, E. (2020, September). Making the implicit explicit: A visual model for lowering the risk of implicit bias of mental/behavioural disorders on safety and quality of care. *Healthcare Management Forum*, *34*(2), 72–76. https://doi.org/10.1177/0840470420953181

Ungar, T., Knaak, S., & Szeto, A. C. (2016). Theoretical and practical considerations for combating mental illness stigma in health care. *Community Mental Health Journal*, *52*(3), 262–271. https://doi.org/10.1007/s10597-015-9910-4

Ungar, T., & Moothathamby, N. (2020). *Structural stigma in health care for mental health and substance use: Networking for the design, development, and implementation of an audit tool.* Mental Health Commission of Canada.

Vicente, K. (2006). *The human factor: Revolutionizing the way people live with technology.* Routledge.

5

The Assessment of Mental Health Stigma in the Workplace

Keith S. Dobson and Andrew C. H. Szeto

It has been increasingly recognized that mental health problems can manifest themselves in the workplace and potentially cause significant distress for the affected employee, as well as impacts for others in the work setting. As humans, it is not typically possible to simply distinguish mental health concerns between home and the workplace. Mental health issues are therefore important to recognize and address in whatever context they arise. In this chapter we emphasize the measurement of mental health stigma in the workplace, but recognize that many of the same principles and even some of the same measures may apply across settings.

Mental illnesses in the workplace have a number of potential consequences for the employee, the people with whom they work, and the organization more generally. At the personal level, mental health concerns may lead an employee to feel less connected to the organization, limit their involvement, and even reduce participation in development opportunities such as training programs, advancements, or promotions (Harder et al., 2014). Some of these consequences are a result of appraisals from others, but some may also be caused by self-stigma and self-limitation. At the group level, individuals who have mental health concerns and illnesses may be perceived more negatively by coworkers and may face either negative attitudes and opinions or even social exclusion and discriminatory behavior (Baldwin & Marcus, 2006). Finally, organizations that fail to appropriately respond to the mental health concerns of their workers risk potential consequences, including increased sick leave, increased healthcare benefits and disability insurance costs, the need to recruit and train new workers, lower business morale and productivity, and reduced or lost business opportunities (Dyck, 2013; Harder et al., 2014).

Employer responses to these concerns can take various forms. In some workplace settings employees with mental health problems may be considered to present an unacceptable workplace risk, and efforts may be made to either not hire such individuals or place them in less risky roles. Examples of such situations include airplane pilots, individuals in certain heavy equipment or construction roles, and first-responder positions. Employers for these types of employment roles often have well-developed recruitment and screening programs, which are legally defensible. The major challenge in such circumstances are employees who did meet the criteria for employment or advancement at one time, but who then develop mental health problems while in these roles, such as individuals who experience operational stress injuries. Such employees may limit disclosure of their mental health problems because of real or perceived consequences for their career and/or social relations in an organization (Dewa et al., 2020; Irvine, 2011; Jones, 2011).

Although, in some instances, there may be bona fide reasons not to hire or retain employees with mental health problems, such circumstances are rare. In recognition of this fact, Canadian human rights law (Government of Canada, 1985) generally upholds the need to provide reasonable accommodations to individuals with physical and mental disorders, to allow for meaningful engagement in society, to maximize their productivity, and to achieve life goals. It is further recognized that some employment positions are inherently stressful and that the nature of work itself may increase stress and personal challenges. For example, police and other first responders, members of the military, and medical and front-line healthcare workers, to name a few occupations, have a relatively high risk of stress, exposure to trauma, and burnout (Benedek et al., 2007; Garbern et al., 2016; Stanley et al., 2016). In such cases, it can be reasonably argued that employers have a duty to provide their employees access to programs to maintain mental and physical health, appropriate services for employees who require care, and extended health, disability, and retirement benefits to compensate for the nature of the risks that are inherent in such positions. A recent voluntary occupational health standard published by the Canadian Standards Association Group, in concert with the Mental Health Commission of Canada (Canadian Standards Association, 2013) in Canada invites employers to provide psychologically safe work environments and provides guidance about areas to evaluate and address, if necessary. Several Canadian provinces have also recently revised their occupational health and safety legislation to ensure that psychological safety is considered by employers (for example, see https://www.alberta.ca/workplace-harassment-violence.aspx and https://www.princeedwardisland.ca/sites/default/files/legislation/o01-01-3-occupational_health_and_safety_act_workplace_harassment_regulations_0.pdf).

As this brief discussion makes clear, it is critical for employers to address mental health and mental illnesses in the workplace (Harder et al., 2014). One of the primary concerns in this regard is the risk of potential stigma directed to workers who have either suspected or substantiated mental health problems. Workplaces can be the site for structural stigma, public stigma, and self-stigma (see Chapter 1 for discussion of these concepts; see also Knaak et al., 2017), any or all of which can have unfortunate consequences for the affected worker or the workplace in general. It therefore becomes important to address stigma related to mental health in the workplace because its reduction can help affected employees to function better in the workplace and allow them to develop to their maximal potential. The reduction of stigma also undermines such insidious potential effects as socially isolating individuals with mental health problems and the office gossip mill. Addressing mental health stigma also helps to fulfill the social obligation of employers to provide a psychologically (and physically) safe workspace and to assume responsibility for either essential aspects of the workplace that increase the risk for mental challenges (e.g., exposure to trauma) or unfortunate workplace incidents that can cause mental disturbance (e.g., harassment and bullying, accidents, and injury).

As described elsewhere in this volume, a number of existing workplace programs have the goals of exposing workplace mental health risks, discussing stigma and how to best discuss mental health problems in the workplace, the management of critical incidents, and duties of accommodation and disability in the contemporary workplace. When the coauthors of this chapter began to examine stigma in the workplace with the Mental Health Commission of Canada, we began with a literature review of existing programs and their outcomes (Szeto & Dobson, 2010; see also Szeto, Dobson, Luong, et al., 2019). That review made it clear that, although several programs existed, their evaluations were generally weak and consisted mostly of attendance figures at events or satisfaction ratings. It also became clear that although mental health was being increasingly addressed in the workplace, stigma was rarely considered as a target of these programs and we could find no program that assessed potential reductions in stigma as an outcome of workplace programs.

As discussed elsewhere in this book (see also Yang & Link, 2016), a large number of mental health stigma measures have been developed for a broad number of situations and settings. Most of these measures assess the negative attitudes that are broadly held toward individuals with mental illnesses. These include measures for the general community, mental health consumers and family measures of perceived stigma and discrimination, and measures of self-stigma (Modgill, et al., 2014; Yang & Link, 2016). Several scales related to mental health stigma exist for health professionals. These tools include self-report measures of beliefs, stereotypes, and attitudes; emotional responses to others with mental illness; the desire for social distance (an indirect measure of social rejection); sematic differential tools; and perceived devaluation/discrimination toward people with mental illness (Yang & Link, 2016). As described next, however, there are several measures related to mental illness stigma in the workplace.

Measuring Workplace Constructs

As we have suggested, it is important to measure mental illness stigma in the workplace for several reasons. Workplaces are where most adults spend the majority of their time outside the home, and employment and careers are primary sources of personal identity and social valuation. Thus, in addition to the legal issues inherent in personal rights, national guidelines, and occupational and health standards, there is a moral imperative to maximize mental health and well-being in the workplace. The recognition that stigma plays an important role in the exclusion of workers with mental health problems implies a coincident need to measure workplace stigma, examine its effects, and monitor changes associated with antistigma programs. As noted in Chapter 1, and in the brief description given previously, it is possible to conceive of a variety of measures related to mental illness stigma in the workplace. These measures could include attitudinal, emotion-related, and behavioral indices as related to public stigma, self-stigma, and structural stigma. As we will show, however, there are relatively few measures in this area. We discuss a recent attitude measure related to workplace stigma and opportunities in the domains of structural stigma and self-stigma. Further, because absenteeism (being away from the workplace) and presenteeism (being in the workplace but not fully engaged or productive) can be taken as behavioral indicators of health concerns, we also discuss how such measurement could be applied within these domains.

Workplace Stigma

Although a large number of social stigma measures exist (Cohen & Struening, 1962; Karidi et al., 2014; King et al., 2007; Todor, 2013; Yang & Link, 2016), the majority of these scales focus on attitudes and behavioral intentions (e.g., social distance) toward people with mental illness in general. Some scales do include work-related items (e.g., "Do you believe that people suffering from chronic illnesses have no chance of finding a job?" from the Stigma Inventory for Mental Illnesses; Karidi et al., 2014). These items, however, are often embedded in a scale that reflects generally negative beliefs about the efficacy of individuals with mental illness. As an example, the 28-item Stigma Scale (King et al., 2007) has three factors (discrimination, disclosure, and positive aspects). There is 1 item related to employment issues within the 13 items on the discrimination factor ("I have been discriminated against by employers because of my mental health problems") and only 2 items on the entire scale that focus on workplace stigma (the other is a reverse-coded disclosure item: "I would say I have had mental health problems if I was applying for a job").

To our knowledge, only a single measure exists that directly evaluates stigma in the workplace. This scale is the Opening Minds Scale for Workplace Attitudes (OMS-WA; see Appendix 5.1; Dobson et al., 2019; Szeto, Dobson, & Knaak, 2019; Szeto, Luong, & Dobson, 2013). The impetus to develop this measure was the lack of evaluations of workplace stigma reduction programs for efficacy and effectiveness (as opposed to satisfaction) and the lack of a measure to assess stigma in the workplace setting (see Szeto, Dobson, Luong, et al., 2019). As well, the development of this measure was consistent with Opening Mind's approach to stigma reduction in other target groups (Stuart et al., 2014a, 2014b) and reflected a general interest in the development of evidence-based programs.

The development of the OMS-WA began with the adaptation of Koller and Stuart's (2016) 22-item measure of stigmatizing attitudes toward people with mental illnesses in general. Koller and Stuart's measure can be divided into two subscales that assess behavioral intentions, including a desire for social distance and social responsibility attitudes toward others with mental illnesses and general attitudes toward people with mental illnesses in three domains (i.e., controllability, recovery potential, violence/responsibility). These items were contextualized to the workplace setting, such as referring to coworkers, supervisors, or the workplace. As well, the Opening Minds workplace researchers generated additional workplace-related items based on their experience in the sector and previous research (e.g., Krupa et al., 2009). These additional items focused on perceptions of competency in the workplace setting.

Once the initial pool of items had been created, it was administered in a pilot study to a large sample of undergraduate students. Exploratory factor analysis showed that 23 of the 27 items fit within five distinct factors: avoidance/social distance (6 items), danger/unpredictability (5 items), work-related beliefs/competency (5 items), helping behaviors (4 items), and perceptions of responsibility (3 items). The internal consistency for the 23 items was high (Cronbach's α = .90), and four of the five subscales had at least acceptable internal consistencies (i.e., Cronbach's α ≥ .73). The exception was the perceptions of responsibility subscale with a marginal internal consistency (Cronbach's α = .66), which was also the smallest subscale, with only 3 items. Subsequent testing with the OMS-WA in workplace samples indicated that one item from the avoidance/social distance subscale was not acceptable in workplace settings. Some participants indicated that the item "If I knew a co-worker who had a mental illness, I would not date them" was not applicable, because they either were in a relationship or would never date someone from work. This item was subsequently dropped from use in workplace settings.

The OMS-WA has been used in all Opening Minds workplace antistigma program evaluations and has been adapted for use in other samples. For example, Dobson et al. (2019) and Szeto, Dobson, Luong, et al. (2019) used the OMS-WA as one of their primary outcome measures to assess stigma reduction in the Working Mind and the Road to Mental Readiness (now called the Working Mind for First Responders) programs, respectively. These two studies demonstrated that the OMS-WA was able to detect changes across three timepoints (i.e., pre, post, and 3-month follow-up) and changes that ranged between small and large effect sizes. Similarly, Szeto et al. (2020) used a version of the OMS-WA adapted for the postsecondary context to examine the efficacy of the Inquiring Mind Post-Secondary program to reduce mental illness–related stigma. This study found comparable results to the workplace programs. Beyond program evaluations, the OMS-WA also has been used in other contexts. For example, Szeto et al. (2015) examined personality (e.g., Big Five) and other individual measures (e.g., intergroup anxiety, empathy) as correlates of mental illness stigma as measured by the OMS-WA and a traditional social distance measure. Although the OMS-WA has not been formally validated, it did demonstrate good internal consistency. It also has been used in various samples and has been sensitive to change over time in meta-analyses (Dobson et al., 2019; Szeto, Dobson, Luong, et al., 2019). The OMS-WA developers are in the process of validating the measure's factor structure and assessing various validities (e.g., convergent) and reliabilities (e.g., test–retest).

Experiences of Discrimination or Stigma

In addition to using attitudinal stigma scales as a convenient way to assess the levels of stigma within particular samples, as well as a way to measure efficacy or effectiveness of stigma reduction programs using statistical analyses, other types of measures also have been used to assess various aspects of stigma in workplaces. Some of these measures are more quantitative, while others are more qualitative. For example, Baldwin and Marcus (2006) examined data from the 1994–1995 National Health Interview Survey–Disability in the United States for experiences of employment-related discrimination. For this survey, participants were asked if they were experiencing a specific illness, whether it limited their participation in employment or other work, and what that illness was. If the participant was experiencing limitations, they were also asked a set of work history questions on whether "they had been refused employment, a promotion, a transfer, or access to training programs. Additionally, persons were asked whether the condition made it difficult to change jobs, made it difficult to advance in their current job, or ever caused them to lose a job" (Baldwin & Marcus, 2006, p. 398). Baldwin and Marcus found that 20% of their sample had experienced one of the listed experiences, with 29% of those with psychotic disorders having had one of the listed experiences. Additionally, 14% of those with a psychotic disorder compared to only 7% of those with mood or anxiety disorders had a job loss as a result of their condition.

In another study, Yoshimura et al. (2018) used the Discrimination and Stigma Scale 12 (DISC-12; Brohan et al., 2013) to examine experiences of workplace discrimination and anticipated workplace discrimination. The DISC-12 contains two direct questions assessing workplace discrimination: "Have you been treated unfairly in finding a job?" and "Have you been treated unfairly in keeping a job?" that are rated on a 4-point scale from *not at all* to *a lot*. Additionally, the DISC-12 assesses anticipated workplace discrimination (i.e., Have you stopped yourself from applying for work?). Yoshimura and colleges found that 16% of their sample had experienced discrimination while trying to find a job because of their mental health problem, while 15% had experienced discrimination while trying to keep their job. Forty-five percent also reported that anticipated discrimination had prevented them from applying for a job.

More qualitative approaches to workplace discrimination or stigmatizing experiences may include interviews or open-ended survey questions. For example, Wahl (1999) interviewed 100 participants and asked about their experiences of discrimination. Thirty-six of the interviewees described stigmatizing experiences with colleagues at work, while 22 interviewees described stigmatizing experiences with supervisors and employers. In another study, Waugh et al. (2017) interviewed healthcare providers about disclosing a mental illness at work. These researchers found various perceptions, including the risk of being fired from the job and the potential negative social consequences (e.g., stigma from coworkers). Joyce et al. (2009), similarly, interviewed nurses and their experiences navigating the workplace with a mental illness and found that their workplace was not supportive of nurses who had a mental illness.

Experiences or behavioral outcomes, as opposed to quantitative scales, also have been used to examine the impact of stigma reduction programming. For example, Moll et al. (2015) conducted a randomized trial to compare a contact-based education program with a mental health literacy program on various outcomes. In addition to quantitative stigma scale measures, these researchers also evaluated behavioral outcomes such as help-seeking behavior from a list of 10 services from the 2012/2013 Canadian Community Health Survey (Statistics Canada, 2012), with the addition of several others (e.g., employee and family assistance program) and "outreach behaviors," such as listening to a coworker discuss their mental health problem or recommending employee and family assistance. Similarly, Dobson et al. (2019) and Szeto, Dobson, Luong, et al. (2019) asked their participants 3 months after completing the Working Mind and Road to Mental Readiness programs, respectively, if they had used any of the skills or knowledge taught in the program and, if so, to elaborate on what was used in an open-ended question. Fully 69% of the Working Mind participants and 59% the Road to Mental Readiness participants reported the use of what they had learned 3 months after completing the program. In the open-ended questions, participants reported using various components of the programs, as well as seeking help themselves or supporting a colleague to seek help.

Structural Stigma

Hatzenbuehler and Link (2014) defined the concept of structural stigma as "societal-level conditions, cultural norms, and institutional practices that constrain the opportunities, resources, and wellbeing for stigmatized populations" (p. 2; see also Chapter 4 in this volume). The concept of structural stigma is evolving within the field of stigma, but up to the present, most of the research has examined issues such as interpersonal isolation and restriction, media reporting (Corrigan et al., 2005; Klin & Lemish, 2008), and biases within the healthcare system that delimit timely or appropriate access to care (Corrigan et al., 2004; Wahl, 1999), biases within the legal and penal systems that disadvantage people with mental illness (Blitz et al., 2008; Sarteschi, 2013; Wolff et al., 2007), and housing inadequacies (Callard et al., 2012).

A discussion about structural stigma within employment settings has emerged in different ways. There has been some discussion about employment as a civic right and that discrimination in the workplace based on either physical or mental disability may constitute a legally indefensible action as a form of discrimination (Ellemers & Barreto, 2015; Ellemers & Rink, 2016; Stuart, 2006). In the United States, the Americans with Disabilities Act prohibits unjust discrimination in employment and other sectors, and a number of court challenges have forced increased services and employment protections for people with mental disabilities (Scheid, 2005). Within

Canada, the Charter of Rights and Freedoms prohibits indefensible acts of discrimination based on several factors, including "disability." Based on these pieces of legislation, efforts are under way both to establish limits on defensible discrimination and to recognize the need for employers to provide work settings that are psychologically safe and protective of employees with mental health challenges (Sipe et al., 2015).

In Canada, a voluntary employment standard entitled Psychological Health and Safety in the Workplace (or the Standard) (Canada Standards Association, 2013; Shain et al., 2012) has been created to encourage employers to recognize excessive work demands, facilitate maximal employee engagement, encourage effort, and recognize and reward appropriately, among other roles. The Standard recognizes that some workplaces have inherent stress and risk, but that employers have responsibilities to prevent, mitigate, or provide postvention to these risks. It is also recognized (Shain & Suurvali, 2006; Shain et al., 2012) that the costs associated with a psychologically risky workplace environment can be measured using a number of parameters (e.g., workplace injury, absenteeism and presenteeism, short- and long-term disability, mental health injury, employee loyalty, retention, and worker replacement).

The Standard uses a framework of 13 psychosocial factors that have been found in the research literature to relate to employee well-being. These factors include psychological support; organizational culture; clear leadership and expectations; civility and respect; psychological job demands; growth and development; recognition and reward; involvement and influence; workload management; engagement; work/life balance; psychological protection from violence, bullying, and harassment; and protection of physical safety (see Canada Standards Association, 2013, p. 8). Guarding Minds@Work (see https://www.guardingmindsatwork.ca) is an online tool that organizations can use to assess and address the 13 psychosocial factors. At the heart of the tool is a 73-item measure that assesses where an organization stands on each of the 13 psychosocial factors. After a sufficient number of employees complete the survey, a detailed report outlines how employees perceived each psychosocial factor, as well as how the organization compares to a national sample. Resources are offered on how to improve each psychosocial factor within the organization. The survey itself is viewed by the developers as a quality improvement tool and does not seem to appear in the research literature.

The development of a measure of structural stigma in the workplace remains a direction for future development. Some current methods may help inform this development or offer promising avenues to measure structural stigma. In addition to interviewing key workplace informants about full participation of individuals with mental illnesses in the workforce, Krupa et al. (2009) analyzed over 400 documents from various sources and scopes (e.g., academic, government, legal) with regard to work-related stigma. Through this process, they developed a schematic related to the process of mental illness stigma within the work setting. Presumably, this type of document analysis could be used within an organization to examine the existence of structural stigma.

A related but more pragmatic approach to structural stigma in the workplace may be policy review through a mental health lens (see Olding & Yip, 2014; see also Chapter 11 in this volume). Although this process may not be geared toward research or act as an outcome measure, it could be adapted to identify policies or practices (e.g., hiring process, accommodations, return to work) that unfairly impact, discriminate against, or otherwise stigmatize employees with mental health problems and may yield policies that promote or support mental health. Finally, using administrative data may hold promise for examining structural stigma. For example, anonymized organizational data such as salary, promotions, benefits usage, and short- and long-term disability claims might be analyzed to uncover systematic inequalities in employees with or who have sought help for mental health problems.

Absenteeism/Presenteeism

Both physical and mental health problems significantly affect the ability of an employee both to attend the workplace and to be fully engaged while there (Johns, 2009; Kessler et al., 2004; Lohaus & Habermann, 2019). The constructs of absenteeism and presenteeism have been recognized for some time (Kessler et al., 2003; Ospina et al., 2015), and scales have been developed to assess the extent of these constructs. Thus, while this construct is not a literal index of stigma related to mental illness in the workplace, such measures could be deployed as a proxy for the engagement of employees with mental health problems and could thus be taken as a peripheral indicator of stigma.

The most studied presenteeism instruments are the Stanford Presenteeism Scale, the Endicott Work Productivity Scale, and the Health and Work Performance Questionnaire (HQP). Of these, the most often employed of these scales is the HQP, developed by the World Health Organization (see Appendix 5.2). It is described here as an exemplar of this type of measurement tool. The HQP is a brief questionnaire that asks employees about absence from the workplace as a result of illness, reduced workplace effectiveness, and the presence of critical incidents. The measurement of absenteeism is relatively objective, because it is related to the percentage or number of days in the recent past that an employee could not attend their workplace. In contrast, presenteeism is often measured as a subjective experience on the part of the employee and their own evaluation of how effective or productive they have been in the recent past. Studies of the reliability and validity of the HQP suggest that it has good reliability and validity (Kawakami et al., 2020; Ospina et al., 2015) and that it has correspondence with employee attendance records (Kessler et al., 2004).

The HQP can be used to examine absenteeism and presenteeism in relationship to all forms of illness, but several studies have documented that there are implications in both areas for mental health problems (Al-Hamzawi et al., 2014; Cardoso et al., 2017; Suzuki et al., 2015). For example, employees with depression are more likely to be absent from the workplace, and they report less engagement while at work (Al-Hamzawi et al., 2014; Suzuki et al., 2015).

Self-Stigma

Although it is widely recognized that self- or internalized stigma is a common outcome of experiencing mental illness (see Chapter 1; Evans-Lacko et al., 2012), to our knowledge there is no scale that exists to measure self-stigma within the workplace. Further, scales that do measure self-stigma do not typically include items related to the workplace, even though self-limitations such as self-censoring, self-isolation, failure to seek training or promotion opportunities, or even early departure and/ or retirement from the workplace could all be envisioned as aspects of self-stigma. Indeed, the most common measure of self-stigma, the Internalized Stigma of Mental Illness Inventory (ISMI; see Boyd et al., 2014, for a review) has no items that directly assess the occurrence of self-stigma in the work context. Appendix 5.3 includes the original 29 items of the ISMI (available at https://mirecc.va.gov/visn/training/docs/Handout_ISMI.pdf). The scale has been factor analyzed into more focused and efficient forms and has been translated into multiple languages and revalidated in diverse cultures (Boyd et al., 2014). As such, its use in the workplace could help to discern its value in that context or if a more specialized version of the ISMI or even a novel measure perhaps is warranted.

The development of a self-stigma scale for the workplace would be an important development in the field. Such a scale could be compared with general measures of self-stigma to see if there is a specificity to workplace self-stigma. This hypothetical measure could also be examined in the context of structural stigma in the workplace and the general attitudes of employees toward people with mental illnesses in the workplace. It can be easily imagined that workplaces that have higher levels of structural or general stigma toward people with mental health challenges would also find that employees tend to self-limit and internalize such stigmatizing beliefs and/or discriminating behaviors. Future research could also examine internalized stigma in various types of workplaces. Some workplaces, such as military and first-responder organizations, often foster an attitude of resilience and strength (Bartone, 2000; Dolan & Adler, 2006), and it may be that people with mental illnesses in such organizations adopt a stronger sense of self-stigma, and possibly even shame, than do people in other organizations that are more tolerant or respectful of mental health challenges and illnesses.

Summary

This chapter has presented a series of constructs related to mental illness stigma that can be measured in the workplace. As the chapter demonstrates, there are relatively few well-defined and validated measures in this area. In particular, measures related to structural stigma and self-stigma are needed. This chapter therefore presents a series of opportunities for future theory and measurement development.

Conclusions and Key Considerations

This chapter has examined the issues related to the measurement of mental health stigma in the workplace. As the chapter details, although stigma measures have been deployed in workplace studies, few measures have been developed specifically for that context. The following key recommendations derive from the current review:

- The only specific measure of negative workplace attitudes and stigma toward mental illness is the OMS-WA. This scale has not been formally validated, and while this validation work is strongly encouraged, the scale is recommended as an interim benchmark for programs that have the expressed goal of stigma reduction in the workplace, because it has been used extensively and in meta-analyses.
- It is important to examine the relationship between stigma and a variety of workplace issues, such as workplace safety, harassment, and policies related to mental illness–related stigma. This examination may yield other constructs that can be integrated into future measurement.
- Although measures of absenteeism and presenteeism are not direct measures of stigma, these and other organization measures (e.g., short- and long-term disability rates, employee turnover, complaints) are important to analyze in association with measures of workplace stigma.
- Measures of both structural stigma and self-stigma in the workplace context are needed. Such measures could be compared with public stigma such as the OMS-WA and, once validated, can be used as outcome measures for programs that have the goal of stigma reduction in the workplace.

References

Al-Hamzawi, A. O., Rosellini, A. J., Lindberg, M., Petukhova, M., Kessler, R. C., & Bruffaerts, R. (2014). The role of common mental and physical disorders in days out of role in the Iraqi general population: Results from the WHO World Mental Health Surveys. *Journal of Psychiatric Research, 53*, 23–29. https://doi.org/10.1016/j.jpsychires.2014.02.006

Baldwin, M. L., & Marcus, S. C. (2006). Perceived and measured stigma among workers with serious mental illness. *Psychiatric Services (Washington, D.C.), 57*(3), 388–392. https://doi.org/10.1176/appi.ps.57.3.388

Bartone, P. T. (2000). Hardiness as a resiliency factor for United States forces in the Gulf War. In J. M. Violanti, D. Paton, & C. Dunning (Eds.), *Posttraumatic stress intervention: Challenges, issues, and perspectives* (pp. 115–133). Thomas.

Benedek, D. M., Fullerton, C., & Ursano, R. J. (2007). First responders: Mental health consequences of natural and human-made disasters for public health and public safety workers. *Annual Review of Public Health, 28,* 55–68. https://doi.org/10.1146/annurev.publhealth.28.021406.144037

Blitz, C. L., Wolff, N., & Shi, J. (2008). Physical victimization in prison: The role of mental illness. *International Journal of Law and Psychiatry, 31*(5), 385–393. https://doi.org/10.1016/j.ijlp.2008.08.005

Boyd, J. E., Adler, E. P., Otilingam, P. G., & Peters, T. (2014). Internalized Stigma of Mental Illness (ISMI) Scale: A multinational review. *Comprehensive Psychiatry, 55,* 221–231. http://dx.doi.org/10.1016/j.comppsych.2013.06.005

Brohan, E., Rose, D., Clement, S., Coker, E., van Bortel, T., Sartorius, N., Farrelly, S., & Thornicroft, G. (2013). *Discrimination and Stigma Scale (DISC) version 12: Manual version 3.* King's College London. https://www.kcl.ac.uk/ioppn/depts/hspr/archive/cmh/CMH-Stigma-Measures/2DISC12manualversion3MAY2013.pdf

Callard, F., Sartorius, N., Arboleda-Flórez, J., Bartlett, P., Helmchen, H., Stuart, H., Taborda, J., & Thornicroft, G. (2012). Housing. In *Mental illness, discrimination and the law: Fighting for social justice* (pp. 99–108). John Wiley & Sons.

Canadian Standards Association. (2013). *National Standard of Canada on Psychological Health and Safety in the Workplace.* CAN/CSA-Z1003-13/BNQ 9700-803/2013. http://www.csagroup.org/documents/codes-and-standards/publications/CAN_CSA-Z1003-13_BNQ_9700-803_2013_EN.pdf

Cardoso, G., Xavier, M., Vilagut, G., Petukhova, M., Alonso, J., Kessler, R. C., & Caldas-de-Almeida, J. M. (2017). Days out of role due to common physical and mental conditions in Portugal: Results from the WHO World Mental Health Survey. *British Journal of Psychology Open, 3*(1), 15–21. https://doi.org/10.1192/bjpo.bp.115.002402

Cohen, J., & Struening, E. L. (1962). Opinions about mental illness in the personnel of two large mental hospitals. *Journal of Abnormal and Social Psychology, 64*(5), 349–360.

Corrigan, P. W., Markowitz, F. E., & Watson, A. C. (2004). Structural levels of mental illness stigma and discrimination. *Schizophrenia Bulletin, 30*(3), 481–491. https://doi.org/10.1093/oxfordjournals.schbul.a007096

Corrigan, P. W., Watson, A. C., Gracia, G., Slopen, N., Rasinski, K., & Hall, L. L. (2005). Newspaper stories as measures of structural stigma. *Psychiatric Services (Washington, D.C.), 56*(5), 551–556. https://doi.org/10.1176/appi.ps.56.5.551

Dewa, C. S., van Weeghel, J., Joosen, M., & Brouwers, E. P. M. (2020). What could influence workers' decisions to disclose a mental illness at work? *International Journal of Occupational and Environmental Medicine, 11*(3), 119–127. https://doi.org/10.34172/ijoem.2020.1870

Dobson, K. S., Szeto, A. C. H., & Knaak, S. (2019). The Working Mind: A meta-analysis of a workplace mental health and stigma reduction program. *Canadian Journal of Psychiatry, 64* (Suppl.), 39S–47S.

Dolan, C., & Adler, A. (2006). Military hardiness as a buffer of psychological health on return from deployment. *Military Medicine, 171*(2), 93–98. https://doi.org/10.7205/MILMED.171.2.93

Dyck, D. (2013). *Disability management: Theory, strategy & industry practice* (5th ed.). LexisNexis Canada.

Ellemers, N., & Barreto, M. (2015). Modern discrimination: How perpetrators and targets interactively perpetuate social disadvantage. *Current Opinions in Behavioral Science, 3,* 142–146. https://doi.org/10.1016/j.cobeha.2015.04.001

Ellemers, N., & Rink, F. (2016). Diversity in work groups. *Current Opinions in Psychology, 11,* 49–53. https://doi.org/10.1016/j.copsyc.2016.06.001

Evans-Lacko, S., Brohan, E., Mojtabai, R., & Thornicroft, G. (2012). Association between public views of mental illness and self-stigma among individuals with mental illness in 14 European countries. *Psychological Medicine, 42*(8), 1741–1752.

Garbern, S. C., Ebbeling, L. G., & Bartels, S. A. (2016). A systematic review of health outcomes among disaster and humanitarian responders. *Prehospital and Disaster Medicine, 31*(6), 635–642. https://doi.org/10.1017/s1049023x16000832

Government of Canada. (1985). *Canadian Human Rights Act* (R.S.C., 1985, c. H-6). https://laws-lois.justice.gc.ca/eng/acts/h-6/

Harder, H. G., Wagner, S. L., & Rash, J. A. (2014). *Mental illness in the workplace: Psychological disability management.* Gower.

Hatzenbuehler, M. L., & Link, B. G. (2014). Introduction to the special issue on structural stigma and health. *Social Science & Medicine, 103*, 1–6. https://doi.org./10.1017/S0033291711002558

Irvine, A. (2011). Something to declare? The disclosure of common mental health problems at work. *Disability & Society, 26*(2), 179–192. https://doi.org/10.1080/09687599.2011.544058

Johns, G. (2009). Presenteeism in the workplace: A review and research agenda. *Journal of Organizational Behavior, 31*(4),519–542. https://doi.org/10.1002/job.630

Jones, A. M. (2011). Disclosure of mental illness in the workplace: A literature review. *American Journal of Psychiatric Rehabilitation, 14*(3), 212–219. https://doi.org./10.1080/15487768.2011.598101

Joyce, T., McMillan, M., & Hazelton, M. (2009). The workplace and nurses with a mental illness. *International Journal of Mental Health Nursing, 18*(6), 391–397.

Karidi, M. V., Vasilopouloua, D., Savvidou, E., Vitoratou, S., Rabavilas, A. D., & Stefanis, C. N. (2014). Aspects of perceived stigma: The Stigma Inventory for Mental Illness, its development, latent structure and psychometric properties. *Comprehensive Psychiatry, 55*(7), 1620–1625. https://doi.org/10.1016/j.comppsych.2014.04.002

Kawakami, N., Inoue, A., Tsuchiya, M., Watanabe, K., Imamura, K., Iida, M., & Nishi, D. (2020). Construct validity and test–retest reliability of the World Mental Health Japan version of the World Health Organization Health and Work Performance Questionnaire Short Version: A preliminary study. *Individual Health, 58*(4), 375–387. https://doi.org./10.2486/indhealth.2019-0090.

Kessler, R. C., Ames, M., Hymel, P. A., Loeppke, R., McKenas, D. K., Richling, D., Stang, P. E., & Üstün, T. B. (2004). Using the WHO Health and Work Performance Questionnaire (HPQ) to evaluate the indirect workplace costs of illness. *Journal of Occupational and Environmental Medicine, 46*(Suppl. 6), S23–S37.

Kessler, R. C., Barber, C., Beck, A., Berglund, P., Cleary, P. D., McKenas, D., Pronk, N., Simon, G., Stang, P., Ustun, T. B., & Wang. P. J. (2003). The World Health Organization Health and Work Performance Questionnaire (HPQ). *Occupational and Environmental Medicine, 45*(2), 156–74. https://doi.org./10.1097/01.jom.0000052967.43131.51

King, M., Dinos, S., Shaw, J., Watson, R., Stevens, S., Passetti, F., Weich, S., & Serfaty, M. (2007). The Stigma Scale: Development of a standardised measure of the stigma of mental illness. *The British Journal of Psychiatry, 190*(3), 248–254.

Klin, A., & Lemish, D. (2008). Mental disorders stigma in the media: Review of studies on production, content, and influences. *Journal of Health Communication, 13*(5), 434–49. https://doi.org/10.1080/10810730802198813

Knaak, S., Mantler, E., & Szeto, A. C. H. (2017). Mental illness–related stigma in healthcare: Barriers to access and care and evidence-based solutions. *Healthcare Management Forum, 30*, 111–116.

Koller, M., & Stuart, H. (2016). Reducing stigma in high school youth. *Acta Psychiatrica Scandinavica, 135* (Suppl. 446), 63–70. https://doi.org/10.1111/acps.12613

Krupa, T., Kirsh, B., Cockburn, L., & Gewurtz, R. (2009). A model of stigma of mental illness in employment. *Work, 33*, 413–425.

Lohaus, D., & Habermann, W. (2019). Presenteeism: A review and research directions. *Human Resource Management Review, 29*(1), 43–58. https://doi.org/10.1016/j.hrmr.2018.02.010

Modgill, G., Patten, S.B., Knaak, S., Kassam, A., & Szeto, A. C. H. (2014). Opening Minds Stigma Scale for Health Care Providers (OMS-HC): Examination of psychometric properties and responsiveness. *BMC Psychiatry,* 14, 120. https://doi.org/10.1186/1471-244X-14-120

Moll, S., Patten, S. B., Stuart, H., Kirsh, B., & MacDermid, J. C. (2015). Beyond silence: Protocol for a randomized parallel-group trial comparing two approaches to workplace mental health education for healthcare employees. *BMC Medical Education, 15*(1), 1–9.

Olding, M., & Yip, A. (2014). *Policy approaches to post-secondary student mental health.* OCAD University & Ryerson University Campus Mental Health Partnership Project. https://campusmentalhealth.ca/wp-content/uploads/2018/04/Policy-Approaches-to-PS-student-MH.FINAL_April15-2014.pdf

Ospina, M. B., Dennett, L., Waye, A., Jacobs, P., & Thompson, A. H. (2015). A systematic review of measurement properties of instruments assessing presenteeism. *American Journal of Management Care, 21*(2), e171–e185.

Sarteschi, C. M. (2013). Mentally ill offenders involved with the U.S. criminal justice system: A synthesis. *SAGE Open, 3*(3). https://doi.org/10.1177/2158244013497029

Scheid, T. L. (2005). Stigma as a barrier to employment: Mental disability and the Americans with Disabilities Act. *International Journal of Law and Psychiatry, 28*(6), 670–690. https://doi.org/10.1016/j.ijlp.2005.04.003

Shain, M., Arnold, I., & GermAnn, K. (2012) The road to psychological safety: Legal, scientific, and social foundations for a Canadian National Standard on Psychological Safety in the Workplace. *Bulletin of Science, Technology & Society, 32*(2), 142–162. https://doi.org/10.1177/0270467612455737

Shain, M., & Suurvali, H. (2006). Work-induced risks to mental health: Conceptualization, measurement and abatement. *International Journal of Mental Health Promotion, 8*(2), 12–22.

Sipe, T. A., Finnie, R. K. C., Knopf, J. A., Qu, S., Reynolds, J. A., Thota, A. B., Hahn, R. A., Goetzel, R. Z., Hennessy, K. D., McKnight-Eily, L. R., Chapman, D. P., Anderson, C. W., Azrin, S., Abraido-Lanza, A. F., Gelenberg, A. J., Vernon-Smiley, M. E., Nease, D. E., & Community Preventive Services Task Force. (2015). Effects of mental health benefits legislation. *American Journal of Preventive Medicine, 48*(6), 755–766. https://doi.org/10.1016/j.amepre.2015.01.022

Stanley, I. H., Hom, M. A., & Joiner, T. E. (2016). A systematic review of suicidal thoughts and behaviors among police officers, firefighters, EMTs, and paramedics. *Clinical Psychology Review, 44*, 25–44. https://doi.org/10.1016/j.cpr.2015.12.002

Statistics Canada. (2012). *The 2011/2012 Canadian Community Health Survey.* http://www.statcan.gc.ca/daily-quotidien/131113/dq131113c-eng.htm

Stuart, H. (2006). Mental illness and employment discrimination. *Current Opinion in Psychiatry, 19*(5), 522–526. https://doi.org/10.1097/01.yco.0000238482.27270.5d

Stuart, H., Chen, S-P., Christie, R., Dobson, K. S., Kirsh, B., Knaak, S., Koller, M., Krupa, T., Lauria-Horner, B., Luong, D., Modgill, G., Patten, S., Pietrus, M., Szeto, A. C. H., & Whitley, R. (2014a). Opening Minds in Canada: Background and rationale. *Canadian Journal of Psychiatry, 59* (Suppl.), S8–S12.

Stuart, H., Chen, S-P., Christie, R., Dobson, K. S., Kirsh, B., Knaak, S., Koller, M., Krupa, T., Lauria-Horner, B., Luong, D., Modgill, G., Patten, S., Pietrus, M., Szeto, A. C. H., & Whitley, R. (2014b). Opening Minds in Canada: Targeting change. *Canadian Journal of Psychiatry, 59* (Suppl.), S13–S18.

Suzuki, T., Miyaki, K., Song, Y., Tsutsumi, A., Kawakami, N., Shimazu, A., Takahashi, M., Inoue, A. & Kurioka, S. J. (2015). Relationship between sickness presenteeism (WHO-HPQ) with depression and sickness absence due to mental disease in a cohort of Japanese workers. *Journal of Affective Disorders, 180*, 14–20. https://doi.org/10.1016/j.jad.2015.03.034

Szeto, A. C. H., & Dobson, K. S. (2010) Reducing the stigma of mental disorders at work: A review of current workplace anti-stigma intervention programs. *Applied and Preventive Psychology, 14*, 41–56. https://doi.org/10.1016/j.appsy.2011.11.002

Szeto, A. C. H., Dobson, K. S., Luong, D., Krupa, T., & Kirsh, B. (2019). Workplace anti-stigma programs at the Mental Health Commission of Canada: Part—processes and projects. *Canadian Journal of Psychiatry, 64*(Suppl.), 5S–12S.

Szeto, A. C. H., Dobson, K. S., & Knaak, S. (2019). The Road to Mental Readiness for First Responders: A meta-analysis of program outcomes. *Canadian Journal of Psychiatry, 64*(Suppl.), 18S–29S.

Szeto, A. C. H., Henderson, L., Lindsay, B., Knaak, S. & Dobson, K. S. (2020). *Increasing resiliency and reducing mental illness stigma in post-secondary students: A meta-analytic evaluation of the Inquiring Mind Program.* [Manuscript submitted for publication].

Szeto, A. C. H., Luong, D., & Dobson, K. S. (2013). Does labeling matter? An examination of attitudes and perceptions of labels for mental disorders. *Social Psychiatry and Psychiatric Epidemiology, 48*, 659–671. https://doi.org/10.1007/s00127-012-0532-7

Szeto, A. C. H., O'Neill, T., & Dobson, K. S. (2015). The association between personality and stigmatizing attitudes towards people with mental disorders. *American Journal of Psychiatric Rehabilitation, 18*, 303–332.

Todor, I. (2013). Opinions about mental illness. *Procedia—Social and Behavioral Sciences, 82*, 209–214. https://doi.org/10.1016/j.sbspro.2013.06.247

Wahl, O. F. (1999). Mental health consumers' experience of stigma. *Schizophrenia Bulletin, 25*(3), 467–478. https://10.1093/oxfordjournals.schbul.a033394

Waugh W., Lethem, C., Sherring, S., & Henderson C. (2017). Exploring experiences of and attitudes towards mental illness and disclosure amongst health care professionals: A qualitative study. *Journal of Mental Health, 26*(5), 457–463. doi:10.1080/09638237.2017.1322184

Wolff, N., Blitz, C. L., & Shi, J. (2007). Rates of sexual victimization in prison for inmates with and without mental disorders. *Psychiatric Services (Washington, D.C.), 58*(8), 1087–1094. https://doi.org/10.1176/appi.ps.58.8.1087

Yang, L., & Link, B. G. (2016). *Measurement of attitudes, beliefs, and behaviors of mental health and mental illness.* National Academy of Sciences. https://nyuscholars.nyu.edu/en/publications/measurement-of-attitudes-beliefs-and-behaviors-of-mental-health-and-mental-illness/dbasse_170048.pdf

Yoshimura, Y., Bakolis, I., & Henderson, C. (2018). Psychiatric diagnosis and other predictors of experienced and anticipated workplace discrimination and concealment of mental illness among mental health service users in England. *Social Psychiatry and Psychiatric Epidemiology, 53*(10), 1099–1109.

6
Measuring Opioid-Related Stigma

Stephanie Knaak and Heather Stuart

Many countries are experiencing an opioid crisis characterized by high rates of opioid use problems, overdose, poisoning, and death (Vojtila et al., 2019). In Canada, the crisis has claimed over 15,393 lives between 2016 and 2019 and has led to a decrease in life expectancy in Canada's hardest-hit province, British Columbia (Government of Canada, 2020; Orpana et al., 2019). Stigmatization toward people with opioid use problems has been identified as a major concern in this context, with negative impacts that include lower rates of help seeking because of shame, hiding and system mistrust among people who use drugs, lower quality of care and response, poor availability of services across the continuum of care, and higher morbidity and mortality (Knaak et al., 2019a; Livingston, 2020; Lloyd, 2013; Luoma, 2010; McGinty & Barry, 2020; Stuart, 2019; van Boekel et al., 2020).

Research shows that people with substance use problems tend to be viewed as untrustworthy and as less deserving of care (Knaak et al., 2019a; Livingston, 2020; Lloyd, 2013; Luoma, 2010; McGinty & Barry, 2020; Stuart, 2019; van Boekel et al., 2013; Volkow, 2020). Also, whether the substance in question is legal or illegal, people with drug problems are frequently blamed for their addictions and viewed as untreatable and unable to recover (Knaak et al., 2019a; Livingston, 2020; Lloyd, 2013; Luoma, 2010; McGinty & Barry, 2020; Stuart, 2019; van Boekel et al., 2013; Volkow, 2020). A recent American study found that 90% of the general public would not want a person with a drug use problem to marry into their family (compared to 59% sharing this view if that person were to have a mental illness), and 79% would not want a person with a drug use problem to work closely with them on a job (compared to 38% sharing this view if that person were to have a mental illness) (McGinty & Barry, 2020). In that study, people were also much more likely to endorse discrimination toward people with drug use problems. For example, 64% endorsed denial of employment to a person with a drug use problem and 54% thought that landlords would be right to deny renting to such a person. Further, 43% opposed insurance parity for people with drug use problems, and 49% opposed increased government spending on drug addiction treatment. The study also found low belief in recovery and a general view that treatment for substance use problems was largely ineffective, because only 28% believed that a person with a drug use problem could get well with treatment and return to living a productive life.

Health and public policy decisions, including how health crises are framed, prioritized, and addressed, are inherently shaped by public opinion. As such, these findings illuminate a core challenge with respect to the stigma toward people with substance use problems. Negative public perceptions are of concern because they can seep into professional and organizational practices, where they have the potential to undermine effective healthcare responses (Lloyd, 2013; Volkow, 2020). In the case of substance use problems, the dominant cultural norm in countries such as the United States and Canada has been a mix of criminal and disease perspectives. Despite longstanding attempts to embed substance use disorders into a public health model, they continue to carry a heavy load of negative symbolism and are highly stigmatized (Corrigan & Nieweglowski, 2018; Volkow, 2020).

Negative views about people with substance use problems abound in the healthcare sector and among health professionals (Kennedy-Hendricks et al., 2016; Knaak et al., 2019b; Livingston, 2020; Stuart, 2019; van Boekel et al., 2013). For example, a 2013 systematic review (van Boekel et al., 2013) found generally negative attitudes among health professionals toward patients with substance use problems across nearly all 28 studies reviewed, and providers' preference for working with patients with substance use problems was considerably lower than their preference for other patient groups. Patients who used illegal drugs were viewed particularly negatively. Encouragingly, the review did find studies that reported more positive attitudes among some health professionals toward people with substance use problems, with the general finding being that professionals who had more personal or professional social contact and involvement with people with substance use problems reported more positive attitudes.

There is much less research with respect to stigma toward opioid use than toward drug use in general. However, studies that have attempted to differentiate across substances have found that intravenous drug use is particularly stigmatized (Kulesza et al., 2013). A recent review completed by Stuart (2019) found considerable stigmatization toward people with opioid use problems, both for prescription and for illicit opioid users. Opioid use stigma had unique qualities not necessarily shared by other substances. These issues were observed especially in the realm of help seeking and treatment (e.g., harm reduction services, methadone maintenance therapy [MMT], other opioid agonist therapies), where "even among health professionals, the understanding of opioid use disorder as a medical problem remains overshadowed by its portrayal as a moral weakness or willful choice" (Stuart, 2019, p. 2).

Qualitative research with people with lived experience of opioid use problems supports this view (Brener et al., 2010; Earnshaw et al., 2013; Knaak et al., 2019a; Woo et al., 2017). For example, one recent Canadian study (Woo et al., 2017) found that most people on MMT experienced stigma from friends, family, and health providers on a regular basis. The most commonly endorsed stereotypes included the view that methadone was a way to get high (as opposed to a treatment), that people on MMT were incompetent and untrustworthy, that they lacked willpower, and that they were choosing to be addicted. Participants reported that the stigma they experienced resulted in lower self-esteem; relationship conflicts; reluctance to initiate, access, or continue MMT; and distrust toward the healthcare system. Other research has identified stigma as a major barrier to help seeking, recovery, retention in treatment, and access and use of harm reduction services and practices (Knaak et al., 2019a; Livingston, 2020; Lloyd, 2013; Luoma, 2010; McGinty & Barry, 2020; Stuart, 2019; van Boekel et al., 2013; Volkow, 2020).

Taken together, research paints a grim picture for people with opioid use problems in terms of the stigma they experience, including in their interactions with family, social contacts, health and social care professionals, and first responders. It was in this context that the Mental Health Commission of Canada, under direction from Health Canada, undertook a research project to better understand how to combat stigma among health and social care providers, and first responders toward people with opioid use problems and people at risk of opioid-related poisoning or overdose (Knaak et al., 2019a).

A key component of this project was to develop a scale that could be used to measure stigma in this population, because no such scale existed. The rationale for the design of such a scale was that it could be used to gauge attitudes and behaviors of direct service providers specific to opioid-related stigma. Such a validated scale would be indispensable for the purposes of evaluation to assess the impact of programs designed to address stigmatizing attitudes or behaviors toward people with opioid use problems and people at risk of opioid-related poisoning/overdose.

The remainder of this chapter describes the process undertaken to develop the scale called the Opening Minds Provider Attitudes Towards Opioid Use Scale (OM-PATOS) and provides some considerations for its use in the field. The process undertaken to build the OM-PATOS followed established procedures for scale development (Boateng et al., 2018). First, findings from a qualitative key informant study were used to identify key attitudinal and behavioral domains. Then, a review of existing scales was undertaken to help generate an item pool. Once the first iteration of the new scale was complete, expert consultation meetings were undertaken to examine and refine the items and response anchors. Upon completion of this phase, cognitive interviews ensured that interpretation of the proposed items was as designed. A pilot test and subsequent psychometric testing of the proposed scale items with a larger sample followed. The main steps are described in more detail next.

Development of the OM-PATOS

Phase 1: Identification of Key Domains and Item Pool Generation

The development of the OM-PATOS was part of a larger project completed by the Mental Health Commission of Canada (Knaak et al., 2019a). The project, entitled Stigma & the Opioid Crisis, was an 18-month research study that investigated the problem of stigmatization on the front lines of Canada's opioid crisis, with specific attention to opioid-related overdoses and poisoning. The study was a qualitative key informant study, which included focus groups and interviews with first responders (e.g., paramedics, fire services, police services), health providers, social service and outreach workers, policy and program staff, and people with lived and living experience of substance use problems across Canada. The research addressed four main questions:

1. What does opioid-related stigma look and feel like?
2. How does it get in the way of providing quality service, response, and care?
3. Where does stigma come from/what are the sources or contributing factors?
4. What are the most promising ideas or strategies for addressing opioid-related stigma in the context of direct service provision?

The themes identified through the qualitative research provided the foundation for the development of the OM-PATOS because they articulated the main attitudinal and behavioral domains that the new measure would need to capture. *Attitudes* were defined as cognitive and conceptual dispositions and beliefs used to think about someone or a group of people in a certain way. These concepts primarily included opinions, judgments, and perceptions based on misconception and stereotypical thinking. The behavioral domain was viewed as a caring orientation characterized by a low motivation to help or that expressed a preference for emotional and behavioral distance from people with opioid use problems in the context of helping.

Based on the results from the qualitative research (Knaak et al., 2019a, 2019b), four key attitudinal themes and two main behavioral themes were identified for inclusion in the scale. These themes are listed here, with extracted respondent comments from the qualitative research to help illustrate each theme.

Attitudinal Domain

1. Negative attitudes toward treatment, recovery, and belief in recovery—including seeing addiction as a "master status":
   - "The . . . hospital has an acronym for people with overdose and addictions issues, ANDY. Anybody heard that? ANDY? Addict Not Dead Yet. So, he's an ANDY." (focus group participant)
   - "I've been [in recovery] for a few years now and I still am flagged at a hospital. So, when I go in, I'm treated really well upon presentation. As soon as my name goes into that system, it's a completely different story. It's shitty. It really sucks." (focus group participant)
   - "Huge stigma regarding methadone and other medication treatment . . . they see it that you are using a crutch—substituting one drug for another. So, there is a lot of stigma around it even in the recovery community, like you are not 'doing the work.'" (key informant interview)

- "[When relapse happens] the belief is that you've failed, you know? Our language has to change. The way we view recovery has to change." (key informant interview)

2. Negative beliefs about a person's responsibility for their illness, including the notion of addiction as a choice:
   - "I mean, as soon as somebody is labelled as an addict or a user they're just written off. Not probably everybody but for the most part they're written off and the reason why is they say because that person had a choice.... So, I think that's what we find, kind of, front-line, is these people are just simply written off because they made a crappy choice. Not appreciating the gambit of reasons why they went down that drug road, right?" (focus group participant)
   - "We still see addiction as being a choice or just this bad thing and . . . why should I be paying for your lifestyle choices that you're making? . . . But the reality is that every day people are in hospitals getting treated for lifestyle related—right, people are—you know we don't shame people who have diabetes because you ate too much ice cream or too much sugar. We don't shame people who have cancer because of smoking. We just treat them." (key informant interview)
   - "We're not treating addiction the same way we would treat cancer or that you have an illness. We're treating it as you have a failing." (focus group participant)

3. Judgments about the deservingness/worthiness of people with opioid use problems:
   - "'. . . those people don't deserve treatment as much as others'—that was actually articulated [in a hospital I visited]. Like think of all the things that weren't said when things like that are actually said, right?" (key informant interview)
   - "I think that one of the big stereotypes, one of the biggest problems we have it's that . . . in the eyes of society, [people with drug use problems], they're not worth much. Some might even say, 'one less drug addict is one less financial drain on society.'" (focus group participant)
   - "This population is seen as more difficult, hard to treat, maybe even less deserving of care." (key informant interview)

4. Negative perceptions as to the integrity or trustworthiness of people with opioid use problems:
   - "They treat us like criminals . . . it shouldn't be a law issue, it's a health issue." (focus group participant)
   - "I think the first assumption that people make . . . is, you're misusing . . . and so, anybody with an addiction issue is suspect." (focus group participant)
   - "[My husband] missed a lot of appointments, I get it. But they need to understand the symptoms that come with the condition and work with them. Being able to recognize when a client or patient is lying to you is not impressive. Creating an environment where someone feels safe enough to not lie—that's impressive." (key informant interview)

Behavioral Domain

1. Negative behaviors—for example, use of demeaning language, delivering lower quality care or response:
   - "There are a lot of staff in our department that don't care, they couldn't give two craps about it and they treat people probably worse than people treat their animals." (focus group participant)
   - "[When someone arrives at a place to get help], you know that [staff] are throwing dirty looks. They're not welcomed or accepted ... they're judged and sent away." (focus group participant)
   - "There's this perception and language floating around these days in paramedic and other circles is that the opioid crisis is part of the process of natural selection." (key informant interview)
2. A caring orientation characterized by low motivation to help or to justify the delivery of inequitable care:
   - "I think there's a sense of—I don't know what you say, apathy at times in regard to treating opiate overdoses in general like, 'Oh, here's another one. Here's another one.'" (focus group participant)
   - "If I only have X number of minutes or time to give to people, well, why should I give it to that person who's choosing to do that thing that hurts them, whereas you know, that kid fell and broke his arm and he didn't mean to do that, right?" (focus group participant)
   - "In emerg ... [if] an IV drug user is there with their cellulitis, or some older gentleman is there with cellulitis maybe because he's a diabetic, and you got one space, I can tell you who's going to get it, right, even if that IV drug user's cellulitis is much worse, because that is a druggie [sic]. He did it to himself." (focus group participant)

These main domains—along with a review of existing measures on substance use stigma (Chappel et al., 1985; Christison et al., 2002; Kennedy et al., 2017; Luoma et al., 2010; Smith et al., 2016) and measures for helping professionals toward people with substance use problems or mental illnesses (Charles & Bentley, 2018; Modgill et al., 2014; Netemeyer et al., 2003; Watson et al., 2007)—were used to generate an item pool for the new scale. Through this process, 47 items were generated for potential inclusion.

Phase 2: Scale Refinement

Following the initial generation of the 47 scale items, expert consultation meetings were undertaken for examination and review of proposed items and response anchors. These meetings involved input from first responders, health and social care providers, people with lived experience of opioid use, and research experts. Three expert consultation meetings were held, each comprising between five and eight participants. Based on the results of these consultations, the number of items was reduced to 32 to reduce redundancy of concepts, and there were refinements and changes in question wording. This process also determined the preference for a 5-point agree/disagree Likert scale response set.

Four one-on-one cognitive interviews were completed with the 32-item version to ensure that interpretation of the items was as designed. One interview was completed with a person with lived experience of opioid use, while the others were with direct service providers—a police officer, a health provider, and an addictions counselor. A few wording adjustments were made based on the feedback obtained through the interviews, but no item was removed or added. Expert consultation meetings and cognitive testing took place between September 2018 and January 2019.

Phase 3: Scale Testing

The next phase was to undertake a pilot test of the 32-item scale. The pilot test was administered in February and March 2019 as an anonymous online survey to a convenience sample of 56 providers and responders in different jurisdictions across the country. The sample included police officers, healthcare providers, paramedics, and firefighters.

Analysis of the pilot-test data used low item-total correlations (under .30), very low mean scores (which may be indicative of a social desirability response), and respondent feedback as the main criteria for determining the suitability of tested items. The results of the pilot test led to further refinements to the scale, with 8 items being removed and 2 items being reworded. Cronbach's α for the revised 24-item version of the scale was .87, indicating an acceptable level of reliability.

In March 2020, an exploratory factor analysis was completed on the 24-item scale with a sample of over 460 health providers and first responders who had participated in an online antistigma training program. Participant baseline data were used to complete the factor analysis. The results indicated the adoption of a single-factor scale with 19 items as the preferred solution, which explained 56.9% of the variance. Replication of the analysis with another participant sample from this same program ($n = 457$) revealed highly similar results. Cronbach's α for the 19-item version of the scale was .96 for both the initial exploratory factor analysis sample and the replication sample.

A test–retest analysis was completed on the 19 items with a convenience sample of $n = 37$ respondents who completed the scale approximately 4 weeks apart. The intraclass correlation coefficient from the test–retest was .81, indicating satisfactory test–retest stability. A more complete description of the psychometric testing of the OM-PATOS is the subject of another publication, currently in progress.

Key Considerations and Recommendations for Implementation

The OM-PATOS is a 19-item self-report scale that assesses attitudes and behaviors of health and social care providers and first responders toward people with opioid use problems (see Appendix 6.1). Respondents indicate the extent to which they agree or disagree with each item. Items are rated on a 5-point scale: *strongly agree, agree, neither agree nor disagree, disagree,* or *strongly disagree.* Item scores can range from 1 to 5, with lower scores indicating more positive attitudes (i.e., less stigma). No items are reverse coded. A total scale score is the simple sum of all item scores and can range from 19 to 95, with lower scores indicating lower levels of stigma. Mean scores can also be used. Some considerations for use of the OM-PATOS and further research include the following:

- The scale is designed for use with people who work in helping professions who may respond to or care for people with opioid use problems or who may be at risk of experiencing an overdose or poisoning (e.g., paramedics, fire services, police services, health providers, social workers, pharmacists, counselors).
- Opioid use encompasses both legal and illegal substances; it is therefore recommended that a preamble be included when the OM-PATOS is administered to specify what aspects of opioid use respondents should consider when completing the scale (see Appendix 6.1 for an example).
- The OM-PATOS has been used in multiple Canadian studies to help assess the impact of substance and opioid use–related antistigma interventions targeting direct service providers. The scale has shown good reliability and responsiveness to change (Community Addictions Peer Support Association, 2020; Knaak et al., 2021; Knaak et al., 2020), and it is recommended as an evaluation tool to assess change.
- Further psychometric testing with more varied samples would be beneficial because the samples on which the initial factor analysis and replication analysis are based included a disproportionate representation of health professionals. Confirmatory factor analysis also could be used to examine the feasibility of shortening the scale somewhat, because the very high Cronbach α scores observed in the exploratory factor analysis samples suggest the possibility of some item redundancy (Streiner, 2003).
- Adaptations of the existing scale may be of use. For example, it might be adapted to capture attitudes and behaviors toward people with substance use problems more generally or in capturing attitudes and behaviors toward other specific substances. The scale might also be adapted for other target audiences, such as for the general public. For any of these possible adaptions, additional qualitative research and psychometric testing are required to assess validity and reliability.

References

Boateng, G. O., Neilands, T. B., Frongillo, E. A., Melgar-Quiñonez, H. R., & Young, S. L. (2018). Best practices for developing and validating scales for health, social, and behavioral research: A primer. *Frontiers in Public Health, 6*, 149. https://doi.org/10.3389/fpubh.2018.00149

Brener, L., von Hippel, W., von Hippel, C., Resnick, I., & Treloar, C. (2010). Perceptions of discriminatory treatment by staff as predictors of drug treatment completion: Utility of a mixed methods approach. *Drug and Alcohol Review, 29*(5), 491–497. https://doi.org/10.1111/j.1465-3362.2010.00173.x

Chappel, J. N., Veach, T. L., & Krug, R. S. (1985). The substance abuse attitude survey: An instrument for measuring attitudes. *Journal of Studies on Alcohol, 46*(1), 48–52. https://doi.org/10.15288/jsa.1985.46.48

Charles, J., & Bentley, K. J. (2018). Measuring mental health provider-based stigma: Development and initial psychometric testing of a self-assessment instrument. *Community Mental Health Journal, 54*(1), 33–48. https://doi.org/10.1007/s10597-017-0137-4

Christison, G. W., Haviland, M. G., & Riggs, M. L. (2002). The Medical Condition Regard Scale: Measuring reactions to diagnoses. *Academic Medicine: Journal of the Association of American Medical Colleges, 77*(3), 257–262. https://doi.org/10.1097/00001888-200203000-00017

Community Addictions Peer Support Association, Canadian Centre on Substance Use and Addiction & Mental Health Commission of Canada. (2020). *Stigma ends with me: Results from the evaluation of a contact-based substance use stigma reduction intervention.* Mental Health Commission of Canada.

Corrigan, P. W., & Nieweglowski, K. (2018). Stigma and the public health agenda for the opioid crisis in America. *International Journal of Drug Policy, 59*, 44–49.

Earnshaw, V., Smith, L., & Copenhaver, M. (2013). Drug addiction stigma in the context of methadone maintenance therapy: An investigation into understudied sources of stigma. *International Journal of Mental Health and Addiction, 11*(1), 110–122. https://doi.org/10.1007/s11469-012-9402-5

Government of Canada. (2020). *Opioid-related harms in Canada.* https://health-infobase.canada.ca/substance-related-harms/opioids/

Kennedy, S. C., Abell, N., & Mennicke, A. (2017). Initial validation of the Mental Health Provider Stigma Inventory. *Research on Social Work Practice, 27*(3), 335–347. https://doi.org/10.1177/1049731514563577

Kennedy-Hendricks, A., Busch, S. H., McGinty, E. E., Bachhuber, M. A., Niederdeppe, J., Gollust, S. E., Webster, D. W., Fiellin, D. A., & Barry, C. L. (2016). Primary care physicians' perspectives on the prescription opioid epidemic. *Drug and Alcohol Dependence, 165*, 61–70. https://doi.org/10.1016/j.drugalcdep.2016.05.010

Knaak, S., Billet, M., Besharah, J., Karphal, K., & Patten, S. (2021). *Nursing education and the value of personal story: Measuring the impact of curricular content versus social contact on substance use stigma* [Manuscript submitted for publication].

Knaak, S., Christie, R., Mercer, S., & Stuart, H. (2019a). Stigma and the opioid crisis—final report. Mental Health Commission of Canada. https://www.mentalhealthcommission.ca/English/media/4271 24

Knaak, S. Christie, R., Mercer, S., & Stuart, H. (2019b). Harm reduction, stigma and recovery: Tensions on the front-lines of Canada's opioid crisis. *Journal of Mental health and Addiction Nursing, 3*(1). https://doi.org/10.22374/jmhan.v3i1.37

Knaak, S., Sandrelli, M., & Patten, S. (2020). How a shared humanity model can improve provider wellbeing and client care: An evaluation of Fraser Health's Trauma and Resiliency Informed Practice (TRIP) training program. *Healthcare Management Forum, 34*(2), 87–92 https://doi.org/10.1177/0840470420970594

Kulesza, M., Larimer, M. E., & Rao, D. (2013). Substance use related stigma: What we know and the way forward. *Journal of Addictive Behaviors, Therapy & Rehabilitation, 2*(2), 782. https://doi.org/10.4172/2324-9005.1000106

Livingston, J. D. (2020). *Structural stigma in health-care contexts for people with mental health and substance use issues: A literature review.* Mental Health Commission of Canada.

Lloyd, C. (2013). The stigmatization of problem drug users: A narrative literature review. *Drugs: Education, Prevention and Policy, 20*(2), 85–95.

Luoma, J. B. (2010). Substance use stigma as a barrier to treatment and recovery. In B. Johnson (Ed.), *Addiction medicine* (pp. 1195–215). Springer. https://doi.org/10.1007/978-1-4419-0338-9_59

Luoma, J. B., O'Hair, A. K., Kohlenberg, B. S., Hayes, S. C., & Fletcher, L. (2010). The development and psychometric properties of a new measure of perceived stigma toward substance users. *Substance Use & Misuse, 45*(1–2), 47–57. https://doi.org/10.3109/10826080902864712

McGinty, E. E., & Barry, C. L. (2020). Stigma reduction to combat the addiction crisis— developing an evidence base. *New England Journal of Medicine, 382*(14), 1291–1292. https://doi.org/10.1056/nejmp2000227.

Modgill, G., Patten, S. B., Knaak, S., Kassam, A., & Szeto, A. C. (2014). Opening Minds Stigma Scale for Health Care Providers (OMS-HC): Examination of psychometric properties and responsiveness. *BMC Psychiatry, 14*, 120. https://doi.org/10.1186/1471-244X-14-120

Netemeyer, R. G., Bearden, W., & Sharma, S. C. (2003). *Scaling procedures: Issues and applications.* Sage.

Orpana, H. M., Lang, J. J., George, D., & Halverson, J. (2019). At-a-glance—the impact of poisoning-related mortality on life expectancy at birth in Canada, 2000 to 2016. *Health Promotion and Chronic Disease Prevention in Canada: Research, Policy and Practice, 39*(2), 56–60.

Smith, L. R., Earnshaw, V. A., Copenhaver, M. M., & Cunningham, C. O. (2016). Substance use stigma: Reliability and validity of a theory-based scale for substance-using populations. *Drug and Alcohol Dependence, 162*, 34–43. https://doi.org/10.1016/j.drugalcdep.2016.02.019

Streiner, D. L. (2003). Starting at the beginning: An introduction to coefficient alpha and internal consistency. *Journal of Personality Assessment, 80*, 99–103.

Stuart, H. (2019). Managing the stigma of opioid use. *Healthcare Management Forum, 32*(2), 78–83.

van Boekel, L. C., Brouwers, E. P., van Weeghel, J., & Garretsen, H. F. (2013). Stigma among health professionals towards patients with substance use disorders and its consequences for healthcare delivery: Systematic review. *Drug and Alcohol Dependence, 131*(1–2), 23–35. https://doi.org/10.1016/j.drugalcdep.2013.02.018

Vojtila, L., Pang, M., Goldman, B., Kurdyak, P., & Fischer, B. (2019). Non-medical opioid use, harms and interventions in Canada—a 10-year update on an unprecedented and unabating substance use-related public health crisis. *Drugs: Education, Prevention & Policy, 27*(2), 118–122.

Volkow, N. D. (2020). Stigma and the toll of addiction. *New England Journal of Medicine, 382*(14), 1289–1290.

Watson, H., Maclaren, W., & Kerr, S. (2007). Staff attitudes towards working with drug users: Development of the Drug Problems Perceptions Questionnaire. *Addiction (Abingdon, England), 102*(2), 206–215. https://doi.org/10.1111/j.1360-0443.2006.01686.x

Woo, J., Bhalerao, A., Bawor, M., Bhatt, M., Dennis, B., Mouravska, N., Zielinski, L., & Samaan, Z. (2017). "Don't judge a book by its cover": A qualitative study of methadone patients' experiences of stigma. *Substance Abuse: Research and Treatment, 11*, 1178221816685087. https://doi.org/10.1177/1178221816685087

7

Stereotype and Social Distance Scales for Youth

Michelle Koller and Heather Stuart

Background

Antistigma programs vary widely in content, and because of the lack of psychometrically tested instruments for youth populations, program staff often find it necessary to adapt existing instruments or develop new ones to assess the outcomes of specific program content. Unfortunately, poorly developed and untested instruments are often biased toward a finding of no effect for a given program. This chapter describes the creation and validation of two scales to evaluate contact-based youth antistigma programs offered in middle and secondary schools. As well as providing useful psychometric information for individuals wishing to use these scales, we profile the steps that are required to develop and test novel instruments.

Adolescents have become an important target for antistigma programs. Yet, there are few validated outcome measures for this group. In their review, Link et al. (2004) found research focused on adolescents accounted for only 4% of all research on mental illness stigma, and no stigma measure was designed and psychometrically validated for use with adolescent populations. While some measures have been developed for and used in adolescent studies (Rahman et al., 1998; Rickwood et al., 2004), they often have poor or untested reliability.

Because our work was intervention oriented, we focused on elements of stigma that were targeted by the contact-based programs in our research network. These elements were stereotypical attitudes and social distance. Stereotypes were defined as negative expectations about a person with a mental illness, for example, dangerousness, unpredictability, or incompetence (Corrigan, River, et al., 2001; Martin et al., 2000). Social distance measures capture an individual's self-report of their willingness to participate in different types of relationships of varying degrees of intimacy with a person who has a stigmatized identity (Corrigan, Edwards, et al., 2001; Link et al., 2004). Social distance measures have been widely used and are considered a fair (but imperfect) proxy for behavioral intent. The desire for social distance toward people with mental illnesses is considered one of the key indicators for individual discrimination (Dietrich et al., 2004) and an important target for change.

The Opening Minds initiative of the Mental Health Commission of Canada partnered with a network of 22 youth antistigma programs (offering 25 interventions) from across Canada that used some form of contact-based education. Programs varied in the intensity and duration of their interventions, from 1-hour classroom sessions, to large assembly presentations, to 5-day intensive programs. Many programs used direct, face-to-face contact, but some used indirect contact through storytelling or artistic performances. Our goal was to evaluate their results and then replicate the most promising approaches as part of a national scale-up.

Most of these programs collected pre- and posttest data. Unfortunately, the measures were typically homegrown, not psychometrically tested, and not comparable across programs, making it impossible to determine which programs were the most effective. Therefore, before we could evaluate program effectiveness, we had to develop and field test standardized outcome instruments to be used by all programs in the network. Fundamental requirements for such instruments included the ability to capture the important dimensions of stigma addressed by the program partners, brevity and flexibility to use in school settings in the context of brief programs (e.g., 1 hour) and at an age-appropriate language (defined as a Grade 6 reading level).

Item Development

All of the outcome measures used by program partners were collected and the main constructs associated with each question were identified. Promising items from the literature were added. Two outcomes emerged as important across all program partners: negative stereotypic attitudes and feelings of social acceptance. Candidate items for each dimension were created from the many variants appearing on the program surveys. The most promising items were chosen based on their relevance to underlying constructs of interest and their relative simplicity (DeVellis, 2003).

The goal of content validation is to determine whether the scale items covered the constructs adequately, were easy to follow, and flowed (Nunnally & Bernstein, 1994). Experts assessed the appropriateness of the overall content of the scales, and items were further reviewed by program staff, an advisory committee composed of those with lived experience of a mental illness, family members, and researchers. Once there was agreement on the initial pool of items, the Flesch–Kincaid grade level for each question was calculated and, using an iterative process, items were reworded until they were accessible to a Grade 6 reading level. Some items were reverse phrased to avoid response sets. We chose a 5-point agreement scale as recommended in the literature (Lissitz & Green, 1975), with response options ranging from *strongly disagree*, *disagree*, *unsure*, and *agree* to *strongly agree*. All items were numerically coded from 1 to 5 so that higher values indicated higher levels of stigma. This required reverse-phrased items to be reverse coded. The result yielded 15 items that measured negative stereotypic attitudes and 17 items measuring social acceptance.

The Validation Process

In the second step, data were collected to illuminate different aspects of validity. In this context, validity was defined as the degree of confidence that could be placed on inferences about change using the test scores (Landy, 1986) under different circumstances (Streiner & Norman, 2008), such as different programs and target groups. Validation data were then collected on three separate samples. Table 7.1 summarizes the nature of the sample and identifies the component of the research for which that sample was used.

Table 7.1 *Characteristics for the Exploratory, Confirmatory, and Test–Retest Samples*

Characteristic	Exploratory Factor Analysis % (N = 1,352)	Confirmatory Factor Analysis % (N = 576)	Test–retest Reliability % (N = 190)
Gender			
• Male	38.9 (521)	28.7 (68)	42.2 (78)
• Female	61.1 (817)	71.3 (169)	57.8 (107)
• Missing (no.)	14	339[b]	5
Grade			
• 8	4.8 (64)	20.4 (103)	—
• 9	9.5 (127)	33.9 (171)	—
• 10	3.7 (49)	25.2 (127)	99.5 (189)
• 11	52.7 (713)	11.1 (56)	0.5 (1)
• 12	28.4 (378)	9.3 (47)	0
• Missing (no.)	21	72	
Age			
• 12	0·1 (1)	0.4 (1)	—
• 13	2.0 (27)	30.8 (72)	—
• 14	7.5 (100)	16.2 (38)	—
• 15	7.0 (93)	12.0. (28)	60.5 (115)
• 16	30.1 (402)	19.7 (46)	38.6 (73)
• 17	38.2 (510)	15.8 (37)	0.5 (1)
• 18+	15.1 (201)	5.1 (11)	—
• Missing (no.)	18	342[c]	1
Does someone you know have a mental illness?[a]			
• I do	23.7 (313)	26.2 (149)	23.1 (43)
• Family member	24.5 (323)	17.6 (100)	13.4 (25)
• Close friend	17.0 (225)	10.7 (61)	18.3 (34)
• Somebody else	21.8 (288)	21.4 (122)	22.6 (42)
• Uncertain	20.3 (268)	21.3 (121)	23.7 (44)
• No	11.4 (151)	13.0 (74)	10.8 (20)
• Missing (no.)	32	7	4

[a] Multiple responses accepted, so items will not sum to 100%.

[b] One program did not ask about gender.

[c] One program did not ask about age.

The first sample included 1,352 students in Grades 8–12 who received antistigma interventions from six programs in four provinces (Alberta, Saskatchewan, Ontario, and Nova Scotia). Pre- and posttest data using the new instrument were collected by program staff and provided to researchers at Queen's University. This sample was used to assess the distribution of scores across each item. The underlying structure of the data was investigated using exploratory factor analysis. The second sample was 576 students in Grades 8–12 who had received antistigma interventions from four programs in Ontario. This sample was used to confirm the two-factor structure that we had identified in the exploratory phase of the analysis and to identify any further weaker items that could be eliminated from the scales (Brown, 2015). Finally, we collected data on a smaller sample of students in Grades 10 and 11 from one program Ontario to assess test–retest reliability, or the stability of scores over a short period. The survey was administered 2 weeks apart without an intervention (Bland & Altman, 1986). Females outnumbered males in all samples, although the precise proportions varied from sample to sample. Approximately one-quarter of respondents indicated that they had a mental illness, and approximately two-thirds thought that they knew someone with a mental illness (see Table 7.1 for detailed characteristics of the three samples).

Descriptive Analysis and Exploratory Factor Analysis

First, the distributions of item scores were explored using descriptive statistics. There were few missing values (less than 1.5% for any item). Item means ranged from 1.85 to 3.31 for the stereotype scale and from 1.97 to 3.52 for the social acceptance scale. All item scores were well distributed, with no apparent floor or ceiling effects (scores that were clustered at either extreme of the scale).

An exploratory factor analysis was conducted for each scale separately following standard procedures outlined in the literature (Bartlett, 1950; Horn, 1965; Kiaser, 1960; Thompson & Daniel, 1996), allowing for potential correlation between the scales. More detailed information on the statistical analysis can be found elsewhere (Koller, 2018). Items that loaded weakly on their putative factor (with factor loadings of less than 0.40) were eliminated. Eleven items were retained for each scale such that total scores could range from 11 (least stigmatizing) to 55 (most stigmatizing). The resulting stereotypic attribution scale contained 4 items pertaining to controllability of the illness, 2 pertaining to recovery, and 5 pertaining to violence and unpredictability. The social acceptance scale contained 7 items pertaining to the desire for social distance and 4 items related to feelings of social responsibility for mental health issues. As expected, the two scales had a moderate correlation with each other (Spearman rank order correlation of 0.48, $p < .001$), indicating that they measured largely unique constructs.

Confirmatory Factor Analysis

Two confirmatory factor analyses were carried out following procedures outlined in the literature (Bentler & Chou, 1987; Brown, 2015; Browne & Cudeck, 1993; Hu & Bentler, 1999; Joreskog, 1969) (see Tables 7.2 and 7.3). The first model assumed no correlation between scales but did not fit the data well. The second model allowed for correlation. Model fit statistics showed acceptable results for this model. All factor loadings were above 0.40. Reverse-scored items had lower factor loadings, potentially indicating that students had some difficulty interpreting them. Internal consistency was high for both scales, with coefficient α's for stereotypic attribution and social acceptance scales of .80 and .85, respectively.

Table 7.2 Stereotypic Attribution Factor Loadings: Confirmatory Factor Analysis (CFA1) and Respecified Confirmatory Factor Analysis (CFA2) (N = 576)

	Nonstigmatizing[a] % (N)	CFA1[b]	CFA2[c]
Most people with a mental illness are too disabled to work.	61.0 (350)	0.558	0.585
People with a mental illness tend to bring it on themselves.	63.2 (361)	0.586	0.617
People with mental illnesses often don't try hard enough to get better.	66.9 (384)	0.664	0.702
People with a mental illness could snap out of it if they wanted to.	76.7 (438)	0.570	0.602
People with a mental illness are often more dangerous than the average person.	43.1 (248)	0.633	0.496
People with a mental illness often become violent if not treated.	28.5 (164)	0.660	0.495
Most violent crimes are committed by people with a mental illness.	59.4 (340)	0.564	0.499
You can't rely on someone with a mental illness.	57.6 (330)	0.654	0.634
You can never know what someone with a mental illness is going to do.	23.3 (133)	0.539	0.436
Most people with a mental illness get what they deserve.	69.4 (396)	0.648	0.680
People with serious mental illnesses need to be locked away.	72.3 (415)	0.665	0.693

[a]Percent giving a nonstigmatizing response: *disagree* or *strongly disagree*. Missing values ranged from 0 to 5.
[b]CFA1: χ^2 model = 314, df = 44, $p < .001$; root mean square error of approximation = .106; comparative fit index =.91; Tucker–Lewis index = 0.89; standardized root mean squared residual = .065.
[c]CFA2: χ^2 model= 129, df = 34, $p < .001$; root mean square error of approximation = .072; comparative fit index = .97; Tucker–Lewis index = 0.95; standardized root mean squared residual = .043.

Table 7.3 Social Acceptance Factor Loading From Confirmatory Factor Analysis (CFA1) and Respecified Confirmatory Factor Analysis (CFA2) (N = 576)

	Nonstigmatizing[a] % (N)	CFA1[b] (N = 576)	CFA2[c] (N = 576)
I would be upset if someone with a mental illness always sat next to me in class.	66.5 (383)	0.768	0.808
I would not be close friends with someone I knew had a mental illness.	71.5 (412)	0.805	0.845
I would visit a classmate in hospital if they had a mental illness.	67.3 (380)	0.652	0.532
I would try to avoid someone with a mental illness.[c]	74.7 (426)	0.793	0.838
I would not mind it if someone with a mental illness lived next door to me.	74.7 (429)	0.585	0.559
If I knew someone had a mental illness I would not date them.[c]	29.4 (169)	0.651	0.690
I would not want to be taught by a teacher who had been treated for a mental illness.[c]	57.0 (326)	0.598	0.635
I would tell a teacher if a student was being bullied because of their mental illness.	79.8 (458)	0.603	0.400
I would stick up for someone who had a mental illness if they were being teased.	80.9 (466)	0.709	0.530
I would tutor a classmate who got behind in their studies because of their mental illness.	57.8 (333)	0.755	0.603
I would volunteer my time to work in a program for people with a mental illness.	46.1 (265)	0.768	0.659

[a]Percent giving a nonstigmatizing response: *disagree* or *strongly disagree* or *agree* or *strongly agree* for reverse-phrased items. Missing values ranged from 0 to 11.

[b]CFA1: χ^2 model 642, df = 44, p < .001; root mean square error of approximation = .15; comparative fit index = .90; Tucker–Lewis index = 0.95; standardized root mean squared residual = .078.

[c]CFA2: χ^2 model 86, df = 29, p < .001; root mean square error of approximation = .06; comparative fit index = .99; Tucker–Lewis index = 0.95; standardized root mean squared residual = .024.

Test–Retest Reliability

Test–retest reliability was examined following standard procedures outlined in the literature (Bland & Altman, 1986; Koo & Li, 2016; McGraw & Wong , 1996; Shrout & Fleiss, 1979). Items were aggregated to provide a scale score and mean scale scores were compared across the two administrations. Mean scores on both scales did not significantly differ for either scale for the two administrations. Correlations were strong (.73 and .82) and coefficient α's were high (.79 and .86). Paired *t* tests for a difference of means were nonsignificant for both scales (p = .093 and p = .065), indicating no statistically significant differences between the two measurement periods. More detailed results can be found in Koller (2018).

Discussion

This chapter has described the procedures taken to develop and test two new scales to measure outcomes in antistigma interventions targeting youth from middle and secondary schools across Canada. Prior to this work, there were no standardized and psychometrically tested scales that could be used to evaluate these outcomes. Rigorous procedures were employed in three different samples to develop an 11-item stereotype attribution scale measuring student attitudes toward people with a mental illness and an 11-item social acceptance scale. Multiple sources of evidence assessing validity were collected and the scales performed well in all circumstances.

A particular strength of our approach was that extensive stakeholder consultations were held about the items to be included. As a result, the scales contained items that were of interest to program staff and represented the two broad measurement domains that were major targets of program activities. The 11-item stereotypic attributions scale included items pertaining to controllability of the illness, potential for recovery, and potential for violence or unpredictability. The 11-item social acceptance scale included items pertaining to desire for social distance from someone with a mental illness and general feelings of social responsibility. Because the confirmatory factor analysis for the social acceptance scale highlighted some potential difficulties for the reverse-worded items, we suggest not reverse phrasing any items. These modifications are contained in the Youth Opinion Survey found in Appendix 7.1.

Because there is no gold standard to assess the attitudes of Canadian youth toward people with mental illnesses, the scales described in this chapter provide an important means to collect consistent data across antistigma programs. They offer the potential to identify the most potent interventions and set the stage for a more detailed examination of key ingredients. They also provide the opportunity for further validation work among researchers and program evaluators across a broad array of programs in different geographic, demographic, and cultural groups.

In conclusion, the scales described in this chapter were systematically developed, were extensively tested, and provide a sound basis for further validation work. They are recommended as tools for use in the evaluation of programs aimed at reducing mental illness–related stigma in adolescents. Given the growing recognition of the need to reduce the stigma toward those with a mental illness, these tools can be used by programs to evaluate their effectiveness in increasing positive attitudes and social acceptance of the mentally ill. The use of these tools will enable programs to further validate, develop, and tailor their interventions to optimally suit students' needs.

Key Considerations

There are a number of key considerations to keep in mind for anyone who wishes to make significant alterations to an existing scale or develop one from the beginning, as follows:

- There must be clearly conceptualized and defined domains of interest. The current work focused on an attitudinal dimension (negative stereotypes) and a behavioral proxy (social acceptance).
- Items must cover areas that are relevant to the program's content and come from multiple sources, including other programs, people with lived experience, researchers, and other content experts.
- An expert review of the items will provide a scale that has face and content validity and help to ensure that items are relevant, feasible to administer, and age appropriate.
- Newly developed surveys cannot be assumed to be reliable and valid. Considerable testing is required before evaluators can be sure that the scales capture relevant outcomes precisely and are sensitive to change. For this reason, it is useful to use previously tested scales if available, rather than something homegrown without psychometric testing.
- Program staff should consider partnerships between local researchers and program evaluators because of the considerable statistical analysis that is required for validation work. This partnership model was employed in the current project.

References

Bartlett, M. S. (1950). Tests of significance in factor analysis. *British Journal of Statistical Psychology, 3*(2), 77–85.

Bentler, P. M., & Chou, C. P. (1987). Practical issues in structural modeling. *Sociological Methods & Research, 16*(1), 78–117.

Bland, J., & Altman, D. (1986). Statistical methods for assessing agreement between two methods of clinical measurement. *Lancet, 327*(8476), 307–310.

Brown, T. A. (2015). *Confirmatory factor analysis for applied research* (2nd ed.). Guilford Press.

Browne, M. W., & Cudeck, R. (1993). Alternative ways of assessing model fit. In K. A. Bollen & J. S. Long (Eds.), *Testing structural equation models* (pp. 136–162). Sage.

Corrigan, P., Edwards, A., Green, A., Diwan, S., & Penn, D. (2001). Prejudice, social distance, and familiarity with mental illness. *Schizophrenia Bulletin, 27*, 219–225.

Corrigan, P., River, L. P., Lundin, R. K., Penn, D. L., Uphoff-Wasowski, K., Campion, J., Mathisen, J., Gagnon, C., Bergman, M., Goldstein, H., & Kubiak, M. A. (2001). Three strategies for changing attributions about severe mental illness. *Schizophrenia Bulletin, 27*(2), 187–195.

DeVellis, R. (2003). *Scale development—Theory and applications* (Vol. 26). Sage.

Dietrich, S., Beck, M., Bujantugs, B., Kenzine, D., Matschinger, H., & Angermeyer, M. (2004). The relationship between public causal beliefs and social distance toward mentally ill people. *Australia and New Zealand Journal of Psychiatry*, 183–200.

Horn, J. L. (1965). A rationale and test for the number of factors in factor analysis. *Psychometrika*, *30*, 179–185.

Hu, L., & Bentler, P. (1999). Cutoff criteria for fit indexes in covariance structure analysis: Conventional criteria versus new alternatives. *Structural Equation Modeling: A Multidisciplinary Journal*, *6*(1), 1–55.

Joreskog, K. G. (1969). A general approach to confirmatory factor analysis. *Psychometrika*, *34*, 183–202.

Kiaser, H. F. (1960). The application of electronic computers to factor analysis. *Educational and Psychological Measurement*, *20*, 141–151.

Koller, M. (2018). *A multi-site evaluation of contact-based anti-stigma programs for high school youth* [Doctoral dissertation]. Queen's University.

Koo, T. K., & Li, M. Y. (2016). A guideline of selecting and reporting intraclass correlation coefficients for reliability research. *Journal of Chiropractic Medicine*, *15*(2), 155–163.

Landy, F. J. (1986). Stamp collecting versus science: Validation as hypothesis testing. *American Psychologist*, *41*(11), 1183–1192.

Link, B., Yang, L., Phelan, J., & Collins, P. (2004). Measuring mental illness stigma. *Schizophrenia Bulletin*, *30*, 511–541.

Lissitz, R. W., & Green, S. B. (1975). Effect of number of scale points on reliability: A Monte Carlo approach. *Journal of Applied Psychology*, *60*, 10–13.

Martin, J., Pescosolido, B., & Tuch, S. (2000). Of fear and loathing: A role of "disturbing behavior," labels and causal attributions in shaping public attitudes toward people with mental illness. *Journal of Health and Social Behavior*, *41*, 208–223.

McGraw, K. O., & Wong, S. P. (1996). Forming inferences about some intraclass correlation coefficients. *Psychological Methods*, *1*, 30–46.

Nunnally, J. C., & Bernstein, I. H. (1994). *Psychometric theory* (3rd ed.). Applied Psychological Measurement.

Rahman, A., Mubbashar, M., Gater, R., & Goldberg, D. (1998). Randomised trial of impact of school mental-health programme in rural Rawalpindi, Pakistan. *Lancet*, *352*, 1022–1025.

Rickwood, D., Cavanagh, S., Curtis, L., & Sakrouge, R. (2004). Educating young people about mental health and mental illness: Evaluating a school-based programme. *International Journal of Mental Health Promotion*, *6*(4), 23–32. https://doi.org/10.1080/14623730.2004.9721941

Shrout, P. E., & Fleiss, J. L. (1979). Intraclass correlations: Uses in assessing reliability. *Psychological Bulletin*, *86*, 420–428.

Streiner, D., & Norman, G. (2008). *Health measurement scales: A practical guide to their development and use*. Oxford University Press.

Thompson, B., & Daniel, L. G. (1996). Factor analytic evidence for the construct validity of scores: A historical overview and some guidelines. *Educational and Psychological Measurement*, *56*(2), 197–208.

8

The Opening Minds Stigma Scale for Health Providers

Stephanie Knaak and Scott Patten

Mental illness–related stigmatization has been well identified as a key concern in healthcare environments (Henderson et al., 2014; Knaak, Mantler, et al., 2017). The problem of stigmatization within healthcare is increasingly being described as a system problem, embedded in the policies, practices, and culture of healthcare organizations (Knaak et al., 2020; Livingston, 2020, Public Health Agency of Canada, 2019). In this vein, much of the current measurement of stigma in healthcare environments—which most commonly relies on assessing the attitudes, behaviors, knowledge, and skills of health providers and other healthcare staff through qualitative research with people with lived experience of a mental illness—can be understood as a quality of the cultural environment in which care is delivered, as opposed to a problem of individual practitioners (Knaak, Mantler, et al., 2017; Livingston, 2020). Considerable research recognizes negative attitudes as a main driver of stigma within healthcare contexts and as a key barrier to care, and the measurement of attitudes is an important aspect of evaluating system changes when these are implemented (Henderson et al., 2014; Knaak, Mantler, et al., 2017; Livingston, 2020). Indeed, practitioners' attitudes and behaviors are central to the quality of healthcare interactions for people seeking help for mental health problems as they fundamentally shape therapeutic processes, care quality, and health outcomes.

Previous research has identified several key learning needs for health providers related to stigmatization, including a low belief in recovery, a lack of skills and confidence in working with patients with a mental illness, lack of awareness of one's own prejudices, and a tendency to see the label ahead of the person (Knaak & Patten, 2016). Addressing these issues is an important focus for stigma reduction within healthcare environments. In the context of training interventions for healthcare staff, strategies for effective content and delivery of anti-stigma initiatives also have been identified (Knaak et al., 2014; Knaak & Patten, 2016). For example, identified "key ingredients" for effective stigma reduction programming include the use of multiple forms of social contact, including first voice personal experience testimonies from people with lived experience of a mental illness, an emphasis on and demonstration of recovery, teaching skills (especially communication skills), educational myth-busting, and setting the tone through first-person language and messaging (Knaak et al., 2014).

Contact-based approaches are those that meaningfully involve people with lived experience of a mental illness who are living in recovery in the process of program development and delivery. Often, this approach includes the delivery of a personal testimony or sharing of personal experiences and stories as a key part of a training or intervention. Social contact approaches work best when some or all of Allport's (1954) four optimal contact conditions (i.e., equal status, cooperation, work toward a common goal, and support from authorities) are observed (Pettigrew & Tropp, 2008; Ungar et al., 2015).

The measurement of stigma is complex, given its multidimensionality. That said, attitude measures are a common approach to assessing stigma among healthcare providers and staff. Attitude scales are also commonly used tools in evaluation research, particularly where the goal is to determine the effectiveness of an anti-stigma program on the attitudes of healthcare staff and practitioners. The Opening Minds Stigma Scale for Health Care Providers (OMS-HC) is one such measure (Kassam et al., 2012; Modgill et al., 2014).

The OMS-HC was developed by a group of Canadian researchers in 2012, under the auspices of the Opening Minds initiative of the Mental Health Commission of Canada. The Opening Minds' philosophy was to scientifically evaluate the effectiveness of existing programs from across the country and build on their strengths by replicating effective programs nationally and developing new interventions as needed to address gaps in existing programs (Gabbidon et al., 2013; Stuart et al., 2014a). To achieve this goal within the context of healthcare, the Opening Minds initiative required a current, reliable, and valid tool that could be used to evaluate best practices and assess program outcomes in a variety of settings and with a variety of intervention approaches.

A common scale of measurement across many evaluative studies provides a means of improving the comparability of outcomes. The OMS-HC was developed in response to this need (Gabbidon et al., 2013; Kassam et al., 2012; Modgill et al., 2014; Stuart et al., 2014a, 2014b). When the OMS-HC was developed, there were no scales judged to be appropriate for mixed samples including multiple professional groups and/or students. Since that time, the MICA has been validated in diverse groups of health providers, and another scale called the Beliefs and Attitudes Towards Mental Health Service Users' Rights Scale has emerged (Eiroa-Orosa & Limiñana-Bravo, 2019). Yet, the OMS-HC remains widely used in evaluation of interventions for mental illness–related stigma.

The OMS-HC's development and initial psychometric evaluation results are described in a paper by Kassam and colleagues (2012). While this initial analysis suggested a 20-item scale, with the possible preference of a 12-item two-factor solution, a replication of this analysis with a larger and more diverse sample of healthcare practitioners in 2014 suggested that a 15-item scale with three factors (negative attitudes, providers' willingness to disclose or seek help for a mental illness, and preference for social distance) was superior (Modgill et al., 2014).

Since its development, the OMS-HC has been used and researched extensively. It has been widely used in evaluation studies to assess the effectiveness of anti-stigma interventions for health providers (e.g., Chang et al., 2017; Fernandez et al., 2016; Foster et al., 2019; Khenti et al., 2017, 2019; Knaak et al., 2014; Martin et al., 2020; Moll et al., 2018; Ng et al., 2017; Petkari, 2017). It has also been used in cross-sectional studies seeking to understand stigma within or across various provider groups, as well as in studies that investigate the relationship between stigmatizing attitudes and various clinical or professional decisions, behaviors, or preferences (Al Saif et al., 2019; Booke et al., 2020; Sandhu et al., 2019).

The scale has been translated for use into numerous languages, including French, German, Dutch, Italian, Portuguese, Hungarian, and Spanish (Destrebecq et al., 2018; Őri et al., 2020; Sapag et al., 2019). Separate validation studies have been undertaken on the scale for its use with nursing students and within community health settings (Happell et al., 2019; van der Mass et al., 2018). Also, adapted versions of the OMS-HC have been used to capture substance use–related stigma and stigma toward people with a borderline personality disorder (Knaak et al., 2015; Ronzani, 2020).

In 2019, a systematic psychometric review evaluated the measurement properties of instruments to assess mental health–related stigma among health professionals (Sastre-Rus et al., 2019). Among the 15 scales reviewed, the authors reported the OMS-HC was favorable in that it assessed "dimensions of stigma which have not been examined carefully to the present, such as emotional reactions, lack of social responsibility, empathy, or compassion towards people with mental illness" (Sastre-Rus et al., 2019, p. 1847), along with showing a positive strong level of evidence for content validity and structural validity, adequate evidence of reliability, and evidence of responsiveness to change. It also highlighted the OMS-HC as the best measure for associative stigma, which the authors of the review describe as stigma related to the practice of the mental health profession (Sastre-Rus et al., 2019).

The authors of the review study also recommended that future research focus on improvements of current instruments and continued validation studies to generate more evidence on their applicability and transferability (Sastre-Rus et al., 2019). To this end, we decided to undertake a confirmatory factor analysis of the OMS-HC on a sample of health providers in Canada, because we had not previously completed one. The remainder of this chapter reports the results of this analysis.

A Brief Description of the OMS-HC

A copy of the OMS-HC scale is provided in Appendix 8.1. The scale is designed to be used with people working in healthcare professions, including allied health professions and students within the health professions. This includes workers such as paramedics, social care providers, pharmacists, and counselors. It may also be used in student populations. To complete the scale, participants are asked the extent to which they agree or disagree with each item. Items are rated on a 5-point scale: *strongly agree, agree, neither agree nor disagree, disagree,* or *strongly disagree.* Scores can range from 1 to 5, with lower scores indicating more positive attitudes and beliefs (i.e., less stigma). As shown in Box 8.1, 5 items are reverse coded (Questions 2, 6, 7, 8, and 14).

To create a total scale score for the OMS-HC, the items are summed for each participant. Total scores can range from 15 to 75, with lower scores indicating less stigma. Mean average scores can be used to compute scale scores. Totals can also be computed for the three factors contained in the scale using the same approach. Based

---

Box 8.1 Opening Minds Stigma Scale for Health Care Providers Scale Items

1. I am more comfortable helping a person who has a physical illness than I am helping a person who has a mental illness.
2. If a colleague with whom I work told me they had a mental illness, I would be just as willing to work with him/her.
3. If I were under treatment for a mental illness I would not disclose this to any of my colleagues.
4. I would see myself as weak if I had a mental illness and could not fix it myself.
5. I would be reluctant to seek help if I had a mental illness.
6. Employers should hire a person with a managed mental illness if he/she is the best person for the job.
7. I would still go to a physician if I knew that the physician had been treated for a mental illness.
8. If I had a mental illness, I would tell my friends.
9. Despite my professional beliefs, I have negative reactions towards people who have mental illness.
10. There is little I can do to help people with mental illness.
11. More than half of people with mental illness don't try hard enough to get better.
12. I would not want a person with a mental illness, even if it were appropriately managed, to work with children.
13. Healthcare providers do not need to be advocates for people with mental illness.
14. I would not mind if a person with a mental illness lived next door to me.
15. I struggle to feel compassion for a person with mental illness.

on the 2014 analysis completed by Modgill and colleagues (2014), the three factors break down as follows:

- Items for the factor of "negative attitudes" include Questions 1, 9, 10, 11, 13, and 15.
- Items for the factor of preference for social distance include Questions 2, 6, 7, 12, and 14.
- Items for the providers' willingness to disclose or seek help for a mental illness include Questions 3, 4, 5 and 8.

Confirming the Factor Structure of the OMS-HC

To confirm the previously reported factor structure of the OMS-HC, we analyzed baseline data from a cohort of participants registered for an online anti-stigma training. The training program, called Understanding Stigma, is a nonaccredited, self-directed web-based stigma reduction intervention designed for health providers and others who work in healthcare environments. The course was adapted by the Mental Health Commission of Canada from a workshop created by the Central Local Health Integration Network in Ontario (see Knaak, Szeto, et al., 2017) and is hosted at https://www.understandingstigma.ca, on the Centre for Addiction and Mental Health's education website. The course is free, and registration is open to anyone interested in participating. As such, course registrants come from all across Canada; there are also international registrants. The course is available in both French and English.

The date range for the participant cohort spanned an approximate 22-month period, from February 14, 2018, to January 3, 2020, in which 7,662 participants enrolled in the program. This provided a set of $n = 3,856$ completed OMS-HC scales (scale completion is not a requirement for course completion). As highlighted in Table 8.1, the majority of respondents were female (3,188, 86.1%) and worked as nurses (1,121, 29.3%) or in allied health professionals (1,170, 30.6%).

A confirmatory factor analysis was initially conducted using a structural equation model with each of the 15 item responses as observed variables and 3 latent variables (and associated covariance), representing the three subscales reported by Modgill and colleagues (2014). The model was fit using maximum likelihood, and the results largely confirmed the previous factor structure. The root mean squared error of approximation was .067, lower than the .080 value generally regarded as evidence of a good fit. The comparative fit index was .90, with values of >.90 providing evidence of good fit. This index was preferred in this analysis over the Tucker–Lewis fit index because of the large sample size. The standardized root mean squared residual, which should be <.08, was .052. However, a likelihood ratio test for this model compared to a saturated model was highly significant (χ^2, $df = 87$, $p < .0001$), indicating that the fit of the model was not fully adequate.

Table 8.1 *Participant Characteristics*

Characteristic	*n*	Valid (%)
Gender		
Female	3,188	13.3
Male	492	86.1
Nonbinary	23	0.6
Missing	153	
Age		
20 and under	161	4.3
21–30	1.314	34.8
31–40	883	23.4
41–50	766	20.3
51–60	525	13.9
Over 60	129	3.4
Missing	78	
Occupation		
Nurse	1,121	29.3
Physician	52	1.4
Allied health	1,170	30.6
Healthcare administration/nonclinical	545	14.3
Student (in health discipline)	495	13.0
Support worker/peer support	202	5.3
Medical/lab technician	33	0.9
Other	203	5.3
Missing	35	

To explore the scale's performance further, a factor analysis of principal components (using a varimax rotation) was conducted. As in the previous analysis by Modgill et al. (2014), there were three factors with eigenvalues >1. These were similar to those previously reported, but with two differences. The first item, "I am more comfortable helping a person who has a physical illness than I am helping a person who has a mental illness," which in the previous analysis loaded heavily onto the "negative attitudes" factor, had similar weighting in the negative attitudes factor as in the social distance factor. Second, Item 12, "I would not want a person with a mental illness, even if it were appropriately managed, to work with children," loaded more strongly onto the negative attitudes factor than to the social distance factor. These differences were seen in both sexes, in younger and older respondents, and when nurses and nonnurses were examined separately.

Cronbach's α for the full scale was .84. Using the original subscales proposed by Modgill et al. (2014), Cronbach's α for negative attitudes (6 items) was .76, for willingness to disclose (4 items) it was .67, and for social distance (5 items) it was .74.

Based on the findings of the principal component analysis, the structural equation model was modified by attributing Item 12 to the latent characteristic of negative attitudes. This model had excellent fit, although the likelihood ratio test for fit remained significant ($\chi^2 = 1,274$, $df = 87$, $p < .0001$). The root mean squared error was .059, the comparative fit index was .922, and the standardized root mean squared residual was .048. The 7-item subscale for negative attitudes suggested by the structural equation model (which includes the previous 6 items plus Item 12) had a Cronbach α value of .80. The 4-item willingness to disclose subscale was unchanged at .67 and that for the social distance subscale, now 4 items, was .70.

Recommendations for Implementation

Based on the updated analysis, we make the following recommendations:

- In general, the results support the previously reported three-factor structure of the OMS-HC. It seems most appropriate that studies evaluating antistigma interventions continue to emphasize the overall score using the subscale scores, or their constituent items, as a basis for additional description.
- These new results suggest an alternative approach to scoring the scale in which the emphasis is placed on the overall scale score and a 7-item negative attitudes subscale that includes the above-noted items, as well as Item 12. The social distance subscale would now be calculated with the inclusion of only 4 items— Statements 2, 6, 7, and 14. The scoring of the willingness to disclose subscale would remain unchanged in scoring.
- Taking this new approach to scoring the subscales, we suggest cautious interpretation for both the (now shorter) social distance and the (already short) willingness to disclose subscales. Cronbach's α from the current study was at or near the generally considered acceptable threshold of .70. However, given that Cronbach's α is highly sensitive to the number of scale items, reliability could be impacted (Streiner, 2003). Researchers using the scale may wish to consider also using interitem correlations along with Cronbach's α to assess scale reliability (Streiner, 2003).
- The OMS-HC is a brief scale that is not intended to provide a detailed assessment of each of the psychological constructs that have been related to stigma. Rather, it is intended as a brief measure of stigmatizing attitudes, one that is practical to use in real-world evaluative studies and that is sensitive to change. Accumulating data indicate that the scale performs well in this context, especially the overall score, which provides a suitable index for assessing the efficacy and effectiveness of anti-stigma interventions.

References

Allport, G. W. (1954). *The nature of prejudice*. Addison–Wesley.

Al Saif, F., Al Shakhoori, H., Nooh, S., & Jahrami, H. (2019). Association between attitudes of stigma toward mental illness and attitudes toward adoption of evidence-based practice within health care providers in Bahrain. *PloS One, 14*(12), e0225738. https://doi.org/10.1371/journal.pone.0225738

Booke, S., Austin, J., Calderwood, L., & Campion, M. (2020). Genetic counselors' attitudes toward and practice related to psychiatric genetic counseling. *Journal of Genetic Counseling, 29*(1), 25–34. https://doi.org/10.1002/jgc4.1176

Chang, S., Ong, H. L., Seow, E., Chua, B. Y., Abdin, E., Samari, E., Teh, W. L., Chong, S. A., & Subramaniam, M. (2017). Stigma towards mental illness among medical and nursing students in Singapore: A cross-sectional study. *BMJ Open, 7*(12), e018099. https://doi.org/10.1136/bmjopen-2017-018099

Destrebecq, A., Ferrara, P., Frattini, L., Pittella, F., Rossano, G., Striano, G., Terzoni, S., & Gambini, O. (2018). The Italian version of the Opening Minds Stigma Scale for Healthcare Providers: Validation and study on a sample of bachelor students. *Community Mental Health Journal, 54*(1), 66–72. https://doi.org/10.1007/s10597-017-0149-0

Eiroa-Orosa, F. J., & Limiñana-Bravo, L. (2019). An instrument to measure mental health professionals' beliefs and attitudes towards service users' rights. *International Journal of Environmental Research and Public Health, 16*(2), 244. https://doi.org/10.3390/ijerph16020244

Fernandez, A., Tan, K. A., Knaak, S., Chew, B. H., & Ghazali, S. S. (2016). Effects of brief psychoeducational program on stigma in Malaysian pre-clinical medical students: A randomized controlled trial. *Academic Psychiatry, 40*(6), 905–911. https://doi.org/10.1007/s40596-016-0592-1

Foster, K., Withers, E., Blanco, T., Lupson, C., Steele, M., Giandinoto, J. A., & Furness, T. (2019). Undergraduate nursing students' stigma and recovery attitudes during mental health clinical placement: A pre/post-test survey study. *International Journal of Mental Health Nursing, 28*(5), 1065–1077. https://doi.org/10.1111/inm.12634

Gabbidon, J., Clement, S., van Nieuwenhuizen, A., Kassam, A., Brohan, E., Norman, I., & Thornicroft, G. (2013). Mental illness: Clinicians' Attitudes (MICA) scale-psychometric properties of a version for healthcare students and professionals. *Psychiatry Research, 206*(1), 81–87. https://doi.org/10.1016/j.psychres.2012.09.028

Happell, B., Platania-Phung, C., Scholz, B., Bocking, J., Horgan, A., Manning, F., Doody, R., Hals, E., Granerud, A., Jan van der Vaart, K., Allon, J., Lahti, M., Pulli, J., Vatula, A., Ellilä, H., Griffin, M., Russell, S., MacGabhann, L., Bjornsson, E., & Biering, P. (2019). Assessment of the Opening Minds Scale for use with nursing students. *Perspectives in Psychiatric Care, 55*(4), 661–666. https://doi.org/10.1111/ppc.12393

Henderson, C., Noblett, J., Parke, H., Clement, S., Caffrey, A., Gale-Grant, O., Schulze, B., Druss, B., & Thornicroft, G. (2014). Mental health-related stigma in health care and mental health-care settings. *Lancet Psychiatry, 1*, 467–482. https://doi/10.1016/S2215-0366(14)00023-6

Kassam, A., Papish, A., Modgill, G., & Patten, S. (2012). The development and psychometric properties of a new scale to measure mental illness related stigma by health care providers: The Opening Minds Scale for Health Care Providers (OMS-HC). *BMC Psychiatry, 12*, 62. https://doi.org/10.1186/1471-244X-12-62

Khenti, A., Bobbili, S. J., & Sapag, J. C. (2019). Evaluation of a pilot intervention to reduce mental health and addiction stigma in primary care settings. *Journal of Community Health, 44*(6), 1204–1213. https://doi.org/10.1007/s10900-019-00706-w

Khenti, A., Mann, R., Sapag, J. C., Bobbili, S. J., Lentinello, E. K., Maas, M. V., Agic, B., Hamilton, H., Stuart, H., Patten, S., Sanches, M., & Corrigan, P. (2017). Protocol: A cluster randomised control trial study exploring stigmatisation and recovery-based perspectives regarding mental illness and substance use problems among primary healthcare providers across Toronto, Ontario. *BMJ Open, 7*(11), e017044. https://doi.org/10.1136/bmjopen-2017-017044

Knaak, S., Livingston, J., Stuart, H., & Ungar, T. (2020). *Combating mental illness- and substance use-related structural stigma in health care*. Mental Health Commission of Canada.

Knaak, S. Mantler, E., & Szeto, A. (2017). Mental illness-related stigma in healthcare: Barriers to access and care and evidence-based solutions. *Healthcare Management Forum, 30*, 111–116. https://doi.org/10.1177/0840470416679413

Knaak, S., Modgill, G., & Patten, S. B. (2014). Key ingredients of anti-stigma programs for health care providers: A data synthesis of evaluative studies. *Canadian Journal of Psychiatry, 59*(Suppl. 1), s19–s26. https://doi/10.1177/070674371405901s06

Knaak, S., & Patten, S. (2016). A grounded theory for reducing stigma in health professionals in Canada. *Acta Psychiatrica Scandinavica, 134*(Suppl. 446), 53–62. https://doi.org/10.1111/acps.12612

Knaak, S., Szeto, A., Fitch, K., Modgill, G., & Patten, S. (2015). Stigma towards borderline personality disorder: Effectiveness and generalizability of an anti-stigma program for healthcare providers using a pre-post randomized design. *Borderline Personality Disorder and Emotion Dysregulation, 2*, 9. https://doi.org/10.1186/s40479-015-0030-0

Knaak, S., Szeto, A. S., Kassam, A., Hamer, A., Modgill, G., & Patten, S. (2017). Understanding stigma: A pooled analysis of a national program aimed at healthcare providers to reduce stigma towards patients with a mental illness. *Journal of Mental Health and Addictions Nursing, 1*(1), e19–e29.

Livingston, J. D. (2020). *Structural stigma in health-care contexts for people with mental health and substance use issues: A literature review*. Mental Health Commission of Canada.

Martin, A., Chilton, J., Gothelf, D., & Amsalem, D. (2020). Physician self-disclosure of lived experience improves mental health attitudes among medical students: A randomized study. *Journal of Medical Education and Curricular Development, 7*, 2382120519889352. https://doi.org/10.1177/2382120519889352

Modgill, G., Patten, S. B., Knaak, S., Kassam. A., & Szeto, A. C. (2014). Opening Minds Stigma Scale for Healthcare Providers (OMS-HC): Examination of psychometric properties and responsiveness. *BMC Psychiatry, 14*(1), 120. https://doi.org/10.1186/1471-244X-14-120

Moll, S. E., Patten, S., Stuart, H., MacDermid, J. C., & Kirsh, B. (2018). Beyond silence: A randomized, parallel-group trial exploring the impact of workplace mental health literacy training with healthcare employees. *Canadian journal of Psychiatry, 63*(12), 826–833. https://doi.org/10.1177/0706743718766051

Ng, Y. P., Rashid, A., & O'Brien, F. (2017). Determining the effectiveness of a video-based contact intervention in improving attitudes of Penang primary care nurses towards people with mental illness. *PloS One, 12*(11), e0187861. https://doi.org/10.1371/journal.pone.0187861

Őri, D., Rózsa, S., Szocsics, P., Simon, L., Purebl, G., & Győrffy, Z. (2020). Factor structure of the Opening Minds Stigma Scale for Health Care Providers and psychometric properties of its Hungarian version. *BMC Psychiatry, 20*(1), 504. https://doi.org/10.1186/s12888-020-02902-8

Petkari, E. (2017). Building Beautiful Minds: Teaching through movies to tackle stigma in psychology students in the UAE. *Academic Psychiatry, 41*(6), 724–732. https://doi.org/10.1007/s40596-017-0723-3

Pettigrew, T. F., & Tropp, L. R. (2008). How does intergroup contact reduce prejudice? Meta-analytic tests of three mediators. *European Journal of Social Psychology, 38*, 922–934.

Public Health Agency of Canada. (2019). *Addressing stigma: Towards a more inclusive health system. The Chief Public Health Officer's report on the state of public health in Canada* (Cat. No. HP2-10E-PDF). https://www.canada.ca/content/dam/phac-aspc/documents/corporate/publications/chief-public-health-officer-reports-state-public-health-canada/addressing-stigma-what-we-heard/stigma-eng.pdf

Ronzani, T. (2020, January 14–16). *Identifying evidence-based interventions that address the issue of stigma* [Paper presentation]. UNODC Technical Consultation on Stigma: Stigma Around Substance Use, Vienna, Austria.

Sandhu, H. S., Arora, A., Brasch, J., & Streiner, D. L. (2019). Mental health stigma: Explicit and implicit attitudes of Canadian undergraduate students, medical school students, and psychiatrists. *Canadian Journal of Psychiatry, 64*(3), 209–217. https://doi.org/10.1177/0706743718792193

Sapag, J. C., Klabunde, R., Villarroel, L., Velasco, P. R., Álvarez, C., Parra, C., Bobbili, S. J., Mascayano, F., Bustamante, I., Alvarado, R., & Corrigan, P. (2019). Validation of the Opening Minds Scale and patterns of stigma in Chilean primary health care. *PloS One, 14*(9), e0221825. https://doi.org/10.1371/journal.pone.0221825

Sastre-Rus, M., García-Lorenzo, A., Lluch-Canut, M. T., Tomás-Sábado, J., & Zabaleta-Del-Olmo, E. (2019). Instruments to assess mental health-related stigma among health professionals and students in health sciences: A systematic psychometric review. *Journal of Advanced Nursing, 75*(9), 1838–1853. https://doi.org/10.1111/jan.13960

Streiner, D. L. (2003). Starting at the beginning: An introduction to coefficient alpha and internal consistency. *Journal of Personality Assessment, 80*(1), 99–103. https://doi.org/10.1207/S15327752JPA8001_18

Stuart, H., Chen, S. P., Christie, R., Dobson, K., Kirsh, B., Knaak, S., Koller, M., Krupa, T., Lauria-Horner, B., Luong, D., Modgill, G., Patten, S. B., Pietrus, M., Szeto, A., & Whitley, R. (2014a). Opening Minds in Canada: Background and rationale. *Canadian Journal of Psychiatry, 59*(10, Suppl. 1), S8–S12. https://doi.org/10.1177/070674371405901s04

Stuart, H., Chen, S. P., Christie, R., Dobson, K., Kirsh, B., Knaak, S., Koller, M., Krupa, T., Lauria-Horner, B., Luong, D., Modgill, G., Patten, S. B., Pietrus, M., Szeto, A., & Whitley, R. (2014b). Opening Minds in Canada: Targeting change. *Canadian Journal of Psychiatry, 59*(10, Suppl. 1), S13–S18. https://doi.org/10.1177/070674371405901s05

Ungar, T., Knaak, S., & Szeto, A. C. (2015). Theoretical and practical considerations for combating mental illness stigma in healthcare. *Community Mental Health Journal, 52*(3), 262–271. https://doi.org/10-1007/s10597-015-9910-4

van der Maas, M., Stuart, H., Patten, S. B., Lentinello, E. K., Bobbili, S. J., Mann, R. E., Hamilton, H. A., Sapag, J. C., Corrigan, P., & Khenti, A. (2018). Examining the application of the Opening Minds Survey in the community health centre setting. *Canadian Journal of Psychiatry, 63*(1), 30–36. https://doi.org/10.1177/0706743717719079

9

Best Practices in Antistigma Programming Targeting Youth

Michelle Koller and Heather Stuart

Background

Mental illnesses are considered the most prevalent source of disability in adolescents. Fifty percent of people with a mental illness will experience its onset by age 11 and 75% before the age of 25 (Kessler et al., 2005). Further, it has been estimated that 14% to 25% of youth have some form of mental illness (Comeau et al., 2019; Gore et al., 2011; Health Canada, 2002; Waddell et al., 2002, 2013). More than 1 million Canadian youth live with a mental illness. By 2041, it is expected that there will be almost 1.2 million children and adolescents between the ages of 9 and 19 living with a mental illness in Canada (Smetanin et al., 2011).

There is evidence that Canadian youth experience higher levels of emotional distress than youth in other countries. In a multicountry study conducted by the World Health Organization, Canadian students were among the most likely to report feeling depressed for a week or more, with estimates ranging from one-quarter to over one-third of survey respondents, depending on age and gender (World Health Organization, 1996). Thirty-seven percent of high school students in one southeastern Ontario school district reported multiple symptoms of emotional distress (such as depression or anxiety) and 62% reported multiple stressors from school, work, parents, or friends (Stuart, 2006).

The Centre for Addiction and Mental Health's Ontario Student Drug Use and Health Survey (Boak et al., 2014) found that about one-fifth (21.9%) of students in Grades 7 through 12 reported visiting a professional about a mental health issue at least once in the past year (about 227,500 students), which was a significant increase from 1999 (12.4%) and 2011 (15.1%). The same study found that 15.3% of Ontario students (about 157,900) rated their mental health as fair or poor. The percentage of students who rated their mental health as fair or poor in 2013 (15.3%) did not significantly differ from 2011 (13.7%). However, the 2013 percentage was significantly worse than that found in 2007 (11.4%), the first year of monitoring (Boak et al., 2014).

Despite the high prevalence of mental disorders among adolescents, they are the least likely age group to seek help (Polanczyk et al., 2015). One of the most significant barriers to help seeking and continuing with treatment is the stigma associated with mental illnesses (Angermeyer & Dietrich, 2006; Boyd et al., 2010; Corrigan et al., 2014; Rüsch et al., 2005). Fear of stigmatization is one of the reasons reported by youth that reduces their willingness to seek help for a mental illness (Bowers et al., 2013; Chandra & Minkovitz, 2007; Corrigan, 2004; Gulliver et al., 2010; Rickwood et al., 2004). Many adolescents worry about negative perceptions from others and fear being judged as weak (Chandra & Minkovitz, 2007). In addition, youth who do receive treatment are most likely to report being stigmatized (Stuart et al., 2014).

Although much research has been devoted to the development and origins of stigma and its consequences, less is known about what makes a particular antistigma program successful. Growing evidence supports contact-based education as a promising strategy for improving knowledge, attitudes, and behavioral intent toward people with a mental illness (Kolodziej & Johnson, 1996; Pinfold et al., 2005; Rickwood et al., 2004; Sakellari et al., 2011; Stuart, 2006; Wei et al., 2013).

Inconsistencies among the various approaches used to investigate the outcomes of contact-based interventions have been an important barrier to understanding what works best, for whom, and under what circumstances (Schachter et al., 2008). For example, Corrigan and colleagues (2012) conducted a meta-analysis of 19 antistigma intervention studies targeting adolescents. Both traditional education and contact-based interventions led to significant changes in adolescent's attitudes and behavioral intentions. In-person contact showed greater effects than video contact. Unfortunately, a lack of standard measures and the variety of outcomes used across studies limited comparability of results. Also, the nature and quality of the interventions were unknown. Finally, the meta-analytic framework did not allow for an examination of student or intervention characteristics that were associated with outcome.

Figure 9.1 shows a logic model that has been used to describe the key ingredients for contact-based interventions (Chen et al., 2016). It includes four input

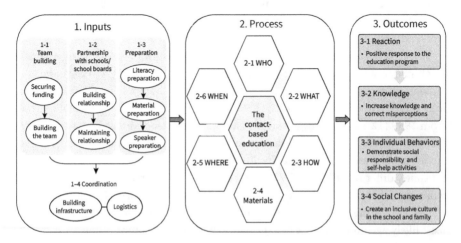

Figure 9.1 Program Logic Model
From Chen et al. (2016).

components, six process components, and four outcomes. The input components refer to the resources invested in a program that are necessary to form a supporting infrastructure for program activities, including team building, partnerships with schools, preparation, and coordination. Process components are the activities of the program in relation to the intervention delivered: who delivers it, what they say and do, how information is provided, whether materials are also provided, where the intervention is provided (e.g., a classroom setting, assembly, or summit), and when. Finally, the outcomes define the expected program effects. In this logic model the outcomes are based on a series of levels ranging from the simplest (student reaction to the program), to the most difficult to achieve (social changes).

This model was developed to help guide program activities along some logical course in order to maximize their chances of success. For example, the critical ingredients to engage students include speakers who are in recovery, who are well equipped and trained, and who are able to act as a role model. The message must be one of recovery that corrects misperceptions and connects students with important resources. The interaction is enhanced if students are prepared prior to the contact education, for example, if a teacher initiates in-class activities, if there is time allocated for connection and engagement (such as small-group discussions), and if the speaker promotes empowerment and advocacy.

Setting and Methods for the Study

Youth were identified by the Mental Health Commission of Canada as an important target for antistigma activities because of the high prevalence of mental illness and mental health–related disability and low access to treatment. Based on a request for interest and a subsequent international review of submissions, the team selected 20 youth stigma reduction programs to evaluate. All of the programs had an element of contact-based education involving people with lived experience of a mental illness.

Most of the selected programs were collecting data prior to and following their intervention. Unfortunately, instruments were not standardized across programs, and most were not psychometrically tested. In some cases, programs collected data but did not have the time or expertise to conduct statistical analyses. In consequence, programs were required to commit to standardized evaluation as part of the partnership agreement. Standardized assessment has the benefits of known outcomes, the ability to inform decisions about future programming, and support to seek funding. Network partners used a common data collection tool to capture the key dimensions of stigma addressed by the programs in conducting contact-based education (see Chapter 7). Change in behavioral intentions was the primary outcome of interest and was measured using an 11-item social acceptance scale. Changes in attitudes were measured using an 11-item stereotype scale. Other information included age, grade, gender, and prior contact with someone with a mental illness. At posttest, students were asked on a 5-point agreement scale whether they enjoyed learning about mental illnesses, whether they thought that more class time should be spent learning about mental illnesses, whether they thought about mental illnesses differently, and whether they would like to attend more presentations.

Using the metaphor of an "A grade" (highly approachable to program and school staff), a score of 80% or higher in nonstigmatizing responses on the social acceptance and attitude scales were employed to indicate program success. Changes in the proportion of students with an A grade from pretest (administered before the intervention) to posttest (administered immediately after the intervention) were evaluated. A unique anonymous identifier was employed to match the pretest to posttest surveys.

Results

Table 9.1 shows the characteristics of the evaluation samples. Females outnumbered males by approximately 10%. Fewer males provided matched posttest surveys.

Table 9.1 Sample Characteristics (N = 5,047)

Characteristic	% (*n*)[a]
Gender	
• Male	44.4 (2,146)
• Female	55.6 (2,691)
Grade	
• 9	26.3 (1,278)
• 10	17.1 (830)
• 11	37.9 (1,840)
• 12	18.6 (904)
Age	
• 13	0.7 (32)
• 14	17.7 (863)
• 15	21.7 (1,055)
• 16	32.5 (1,582)
• 17	21.7 (1,058)
• 18+	5.7 (278)
Does someone you know have a mental illness? (pretest)[b]	19.8 (951)
• I do	19.2 (923)
• Family member	10.6 (509)
• Close friend	20.6 (990)
• Somebody else	20.7 (993)
• Uncertain	19.3 (927)
• No	
Any contact with family or friends	43.8 (2,108)

From Koller and Stuart (2016).
[a]Missing data are not shown.
[b]Multiple responses were accepted, so items do not sum to 100%.

Grades ranged from 9 to 12. Ages ranged from 13 to over 18. Almost 20% of respondents indicated they had a mental illness. Almost half (43.8%) knew someone with a mental illness.

Forest plots graphically display the effects of multiple comparable interventions. Each line in Figure 9.2 represents the results of a single study. Boxes on the right side of the vertical line (at 1) show a positive outcome. Boxes on the left of the vertical line indicate an intervention that was not successful or had negative results. Boxes that cross the vertical line indicate that they had no statistically important effect. The bars indicate the precision of the estimate, and overlapping bars show that interventions are comparable. The red line with the diamond at the bottom of the plot shows the average or pooled estimate of effect. More detailed results of the statistical analysis are described elsewhere (Koller & Stuart, 2016). Programs varied in their effectiveness but all were on the right of the vertical line indicating that they all had a positive effect. The pooled estimate of effect across all of the interventions (shown as the

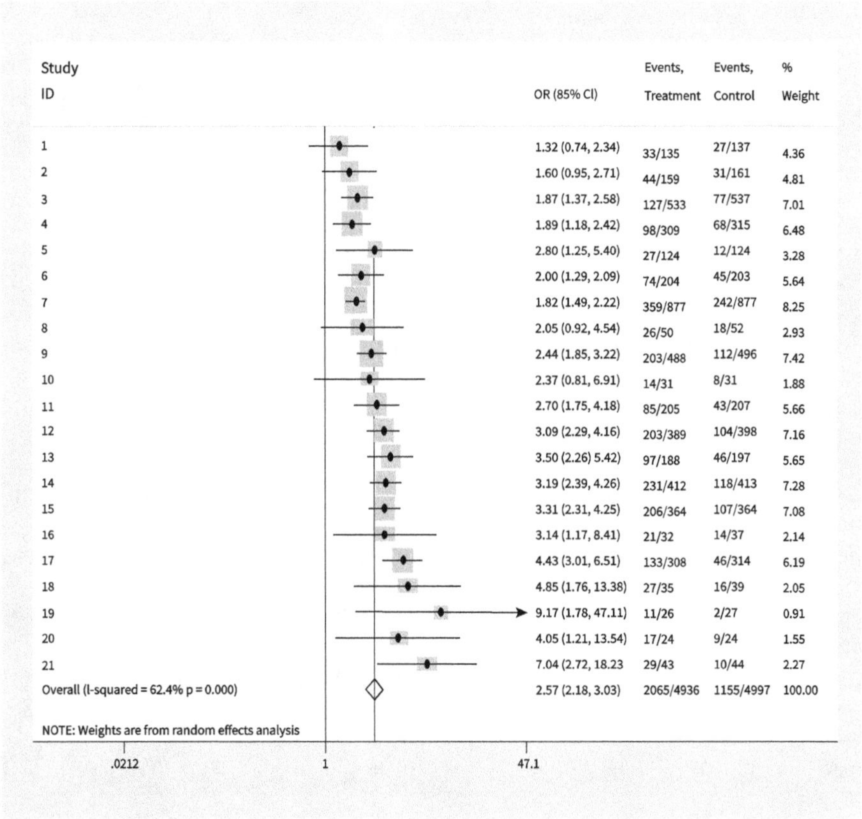

Study ID		OR (85% CI)	Events, Treatment	Events, Control	% Weight
1		1.32 (0.74, 2.34)	33/135	27/137	4.36
2		1.60 (0.95, 2.71)	44/159	31/161	4.81
3		1.87 (1.37, 2.58)	127/533	77/537	7.01
4		1.89 (1.18, 2.42)	98/309	68/315	6.48
5		2.80 (1.25, 5.40)	27/124	12/124	3.28
6		2.00 (1.29, 2.09)	74/204	45/203	5.64
7		1.82 (1.49, 2.22)	359/877	242/877	8.25
8		2.05 (0.92, 4.54)	26/50	18/52	2.93
9		2.44 (1.85, 3.22)	203/488	112/496	7.42
10		2.37 (0.81, 6.91)	14/31	8/31	1.88
11		2.70 (1.75, 4.18)	85/205	43/207	5.66
12		3.09 (2.29, 4.16)	203/389	104/398	7.16
13		3.50 (2.26) 5.42)	97/188	46/197	5.65
14		3.19 (2.39, 4.26)	231/412	118/413	7.28
15		3.31 (2.31, 4.25)	206/364	107/364	7.08
16		3.14 (1.17, 8.41)	21/32	14/37	2.14
17		4.43 (3.01, 6.51)	133/308	46/314	6.19
18		4.85 (1.76, 13.38)	27/35	16/39	2.05
19		9.17 (1.78, 47.11)	11/26	2/27	0.91
20		4.05 (1.21, 13.54)	17/24	9/24	1.55
21		7.04 (2.72, 18.23)	29/43	10/44	2.27
Overall (I-squared = 62.4% p = 0.000)		2.57 (2.18, 3.03)	2065/4936	1155/4997	100.00

NOTE: Weights are from random effects analysis

.0212   1   47.1

Figure 9.2 Forest Plot of Intervention Effects
ORs refer to odds ratios, or the odds of obtaining an 80% grade on the posttest compared to the pretest. From Koller and Stuart (2016).

diamond at the bottom of the forest plot on the second vertical line) indicated that students were, on average, 2.57 times more likely to receive an A grade at posttest compared to pretest, indicating a positive outcome overall.

Table 9.2 shows the results of the logistic regressions. As in Table 9.1, an odds ratio at or near 1 means there was no association between the studied variable and the outcome. If the 95% confidence interval for the odds ratio includes 1, it means the results are not statistically significant. Odds ratios less than 1 indicate lower success for a given variable, whereas odds ratios greater than 1 indicate a better outcome for a given variable. Table 9.2 shows males were 40% less likely than females to obtain an A grade at posttest, although males who self-reported a mental illness were 60% more likely to be successful. Self-disclosed mental illness was not significant for females. Baseline levels of social acceptance, improvements in attitudes, prior

Table 9.2 Mixed Effects Logistic Regression Results Examining Factors Associated With Greater Than 80% Correct on the Social Acceptance Scale

Variable	All Participants		Males		Females	
	Odds Ratio (95% CI)	*p* value	Odds Ratio (95% CI)	*p* value	Odds Ratio (95% CI)	*p* value
Grade						
• 9	Baseline	—	Baseline	—	Baseline	—
• 10	0.89 (0.68, 1.2)	.387	0.82 (0.54, 1.2)	.356	0.91 (0.65, 1.3)	.598
• 11	0.97 (0.76, 1.2)	.813	1.0 (0.72, 1.5)	.871	0.94 (0.69, 1.3)	.702
• 12	1.1 (0.86, 1.5)	.396	1.1 (0.73, 1.7)	.628	1.2 (0.83, 1.6)	.383
• Female	Baseline	—	—	—	—	—
• Male	0.62 (0.52, 0.75)	<.001				
Self-reported mental illness	1.1 (0.89, 1.4)	.360	1.6 (1.1, 2.2)	.<009	0.88 (0.66, 1.2)	.394
Attitude improvement score	1.3 (1.2, 1.3)	.360	1.3 (1.2, 1.4)	.<001	1.2 (1.2, 1.3)	.001
More class time	1.9 (1.5, 2.3)	.<001	1.2 (1.6, 3.0)	.<001	1.7 (1.4, 2.2)	.001
Enjoyed the presentation	1.7 (1.3, 2.2)	.<001	1.7 (1.2, 2.5)	.005	1.7 (1.2, 2.3)	.005
Think differently	1.2 (0.99, 1.5)	.057	1.2 (0.90, 1.7)	.197	1.2 (0.93, 1.6)	.145
More presentations like this	1.2 (0.99, 1.6)	.059	1.2 (0.86, 1.7)	.261	1.2 (0.88, 1.6)	.253
Pretest social acceptance score	0.78 (0.77, 0.79)	.<001	0.79 (0.76, 0.81)	.<001	0.78 (0.76, 0.80)	.<001
Prior contact	1.4 (1.1, 1.6)	.<001	1.5 (1.1, 2.0)	.009	1.3 (1.1, 1.7)	.<001

From Koller and Stuart (2016).

contact with someone with a mental illness, wanting more class time, and enjoying the presentation were associated with overall success. Grade, thinking differently about mental illnesses, and wanting more presentations were not significantly associated with outcomes.

Discussion

The contact-based interventions evaluated in this study generally improved social acceptance toward people with a mental illness. On average, students were 2.5 times more likely to report a nonstigmatizing response at posttest compared to the pretest. Considerable variability emerged across programs in terms of their attention to critical ingredients (Chen et al., 2016). These differences included the amount of ancillary literacy-based information provided, the extent to which teachers were involved, the infrastructure to support program activities, the skills of the speakers and the quality of their stories, and the provision of an environment that promoted student engagement and active discussion.

Successful antistigma strategies have the potential to substantially improve students' health status, healthy life expectancy, and quality of life (Stuart, 2006), and schools present ideal sites to implement these programs. Unfortunately, most school health and wellness programs do not routinely include antistigma interventions. Programs tend to be ad hoc, be implemented at the request of a specific teacher, and have minimal infrastructure and support. These results show that the implementation of antistigma programs can promote inclusion within high schools and reduce stigmatizing behaviors. The use of schools to conduct these programs is efficient because youth must attend in most countries, and the public health infrastructure to provide health promotion and prevention programs already exists. Antistigma programs can build on existing curricula or school activities. Schools also have the ability to offer a broad scope of companion interventions (Stuart et al., 2012). Consequently, school-based, contact-based educational strategies are an important public health resource that are highly recommended.

Key Considerations

- It is important for individuals who want to reduce stigma in secondary schools to adopt the most promising practices in the field. This chapter identifies contact-based education as a promising practice, capable of increasing self-reported social tolerance.
- Programs differ in how they implement antistigma interventions. Short, didactic programs are unlikely to bring about change, whereas more standardized and evidence-based approaches maximize the chance for transformative learning.

- Males may experience mental illness and stigma reduction programs differently than females. It is important to consider gender in the context of antistigma programming, and there is a need for more research into gender differences in stigma experiences and stigma reduction.
- Programs are strongly encouraged to use simple scales, such as those developed in this evaluation, to assess program effectiveness and to continue to build an evidence base that supports contact-based antistigma interventions.

References

Angermeyer, M. C., & Dietrich, M. C. (2006). Public beliefs about and attitudes towards people with mental illness: A review of population studies. *Acta Psychiatrica, 113*, 163–179.

Boak, A., Hamilton, H., Adlaf, E., Beitchman, J., Wolfe, D., & Mann, R. (2014). *The mental health and well-being of Ontario students 1991–2013: Detailed OSDUHS findings* (CAMH Research Document Series No. 38). Centre for Addiction and Mental Health.

Bowers, H., Manion, I., Papadopoulos, D., & Gauvreau, E. (2013). Stigma in school-based mental health: Perceptions of young people and service providers. *Child and Adolescent Mental Health, 18*(3), 165–170.

Boyd, J. E., Katz, E. P., Link, B. G., & Phelan, J. C. (2010). The relationship of multiple aspects of stigma and personal contact with someone hospitalized for mental illness, in a nationally representative sample. *Social Psychiatry and Psychiatric Epidemiology, 45*, 1063–1070.

Chandra, A., & Minkovitz, C. S. (2007). Factors that influence mental health stigma among 8th grade adolescents. *Journal of Youth and Adolescence, 36*, 763–774.

Chen, S.-P., Koller, M., Krupa, T., & Stuart, H. (2016). Contact in the classroom: Developing a program model for youth mental health contact-based anti-stigma education. *Community Mental Health Journal, 3*(281). https://doi.org/10.1007/s10597-015-9944-7

Comeau, J., Georgiades, K., Duncan, L., Wang, L., & Boyle, M. (2019). Changes in the prevalence of child and youth mental disorders and perceived need for professional help between 1983 and 2014: Evidence from the Ontario Child Health Study. *The Canadian Journal of Psychiatry, 64*(4), 256–264.

Corrigan, P. (2004). How stigma interferes with mental health care. *American Psychologist, 59*, 614–652.

Corrigan, P. W., Druss, B. G., & Perlick, D. A. (2014). The impact of mental illness stigma on seeking and participating in mental health care. *Psychological Science in the Public Interest, 15*(2), 30–70.

Corrigan, P., Morris, S., Michaels, P., Rafacz, J., & Rusch, N. (2012). Challenging the public stigma of mental illness: A meta-analysis of outcome studies. *Psychiatric Services, 63*(10), 963–973.

Gore, F. M., Bhloem, P. J., Patton, G., Ferguson, J., Joseph, V., Coffey, C., Sawyer, S. M., & Mathers, C. D. (2011). Global burden of disease in young people aged 10–24 years: A systematic analysis. *The Lancet, 377*(9783), 2093–2102.

Gulliver, A., Griffiths, K. M., & Christensen, H. (2010). Perceived barriers and facilitators to mental health help-seeking in young people: A systematic review. *BMC Psychiatry, 10*, 113. https://doi.org/10.1186/1471-244X-10-113

Health Canada. (2002). *A report on mental illnesses in Canada.* Health Canada.

Kessler, R., Berglund, P., Demler, O., Jin, R., Merikangas, K., & Walters, E. (2005). Lifetime prevalence and age-of-onset distributions of *DSM-IV* disorders in the National Comorbidity Survey Replication. *Archives of General Psychiatry, 62*(6), 593–602.

Koller, M., & Stuart, H. (2016). Reducing stigma in high school youth. *Acta Psychiatrica Scandinavica, 134* (Suppl. 446), 63–70.

Kolodziej, M. E., & Johnson, B. T. (1996). Interpersonal contact and acceptance of persons with psychiatric disorders: A research synthesis. *Journal of Consulting and Clinical Psychology, 64*, 1387–1396.

Pinfold, V., Stuart, H., Thornicroft, G., & Arboleda-Flórez, J. (2005). Working with young people: The impact of mental health awareness programs in schools in UK and Canada. *World Psychiatry, 4*, 48–52.

Polanczyk, G. V., Salum, G. A., Sugaya, L. L., & Rohde, L. L. (2015). Annual research Review: A meta-analysis of the worldwide prevalence of mental disorders in children and adolescents. *Journal of Child Psychology and Psychiatry, 56*(3), 345–365.

Rickwood, D., Cavanagh, S., Curtis, L., & Sakrouge, R. (2004). Educating young people about mental health and mental illness: Evaluating a school-based programme. *International Journal of Mental Health Promotion, 6*(4), 23–32. https://doi.org/10.1080/14623730.2004.9721941

Rüsch, N., Angermeyer, M. C., & Corrigan, P. W. (2005). Mental illness stigma: Concepts, consequences, and initiatives to reduce stigma. *European Psychiatry, 20*, 529–539.

Sakellari, E., Leino-Kilpi, H., & Kalokerinou-Anagnostopoulou, A. (2011). Educational interventions in secondary education aiming to affect pupils' attitudes towards mental illness: A review of the literature. *Journal of Psychiatric and Mental Health Nursing, 18*, 166–176. https://doi.org/10.1111/j.1365-2850.2010.01644.x

Schachter, H. M., Girardi, A., Ly, M., Lacroix, D., Lumb, A. B., van Berkom, J., & Gill, R. (2008). Effects of school-based interventions on mental health. *Child and Adolescent Psychiatry and Mental Health, 2*(18), Article 18. https://doi.org/10.1186/1753-2000-2-18

Smetanin, P., Stiff, D., Briante, C., Adair, C., Ahmad, S., & Khan, K. (2011). The life and economic impact of major mental illnesses in Canada: 2011 to 2041. RiskAnalytica.

Stuart, H. (2006). Psychosocial risk clustering in high school students. *Social Psychiatry and Psychiatric Epidemiology, 41*, 498–507.

Stuart, H., Arboleda-Florez, J., & Sartorius, N. (2012). *Paradigms lost: Fighting stigma and the lessons learned.* Oxford University Press.

Stuart, H., Chen, S.-P., Christie, R., Dobson, K., Kirsh, B., Knaak, S., Koller, M., Krupa, T., Lauria-Horner, B., Luong, D., Modgill, G., Patten, S. B., Pietrus, M., Szeto, A., & Whitley, R. (2014). Opening Minds in Canada: Background and rationale. *Canadian Journal of Psychiatry, 59*(10, Suppl. 1), S8–S12.

Waddell, C., Offord, D., Shepherd, C., Hua, J., & McEwan, K. (2002). Child psychiatric epidemiology and Canadian public policy-making: The state of the science and the art of the possible. *Canadian Journal of Psychiatry, 47*, 825–832.

Waddell, C., Shepherd, C., Chen, A., & Boyle, M. (2013). Creating comprehensive children's mental health indicators for British Columbia. *Journal of Community Mental Health, 31*(1), 9–27.

Wei, Y., Hayden, J. A., Kutcher, S., Zygmunt, A., & McGrath, P. (2013). The effectiveness of school mental health literacy programs to address knowledge, attitudes, and help seeking among youth. *Early Intervention in Psychiatry, 7*, 109–121. https://doi.org/10.1111/eip.12010

World Health Organization. (1996). *The health of youth: A cross-national survey.* WHO Regional Publications, European Series No 69.

World Health Organization.

10

Stigma Reduction in Postsecondary Settings

Moving From Individual Initiatives to Holistic Mental Health Approaches

Andrew C. H. Szeto and Brittany L. Lindsay

Mental health has been a growing discussion in the postsecondary (PS) community in the second decade of the 21st century. Not surprisingly, research has shown that North American PS students have many mental health concerns, including feelings of anxiety, anger, depression, exhaustion, hopelessness, loneliness, extreme stress, and thoughts of suicide or suicide behaviors (e.g., American College Health Association [ACHA], 2019; Cvetkovski et al., 2012; Eisenberg et al., 2007; Wiens et al., 2020). Addressing these concerns is a priority for PS institutions within North America and beyond. However, commensurate with this priority should be a focus on reducing the stigma of mental illness. Although many efforts are being made to reduce mental illness stigma on campuses, this is still a concern for PS institutions (see Linden et al., 2018), given that stigma does exist on campuses, is held by students, and has negative impacts (e.g., Lally et al., 2013; Martin, 2010; Pompeo-Fargnoli, 2020).

Research has identified several areas that make PS students especially vulnerable to these mental health concerns, such as financial burdens, academic pressure, an increased use of technology, and the drastic lifestyle change that often accompanies the transition from high school to PS (Eisenberg et al., 2007; Kruisselbrink Flatt, 2013). Students with mental health concerns, such as depression and anxiety, can have more academic issues (e.g., lower grade point averages, more missed classes, higher dropout rate), more physical health concerns, and an increased risk of substance use problems (Eisenberg, Golberstein, et al., 2009; Eisenberg et al., 2007; Walters et al., 2018). Some research has also demonstrated that mental health concerns experienced by American (Prince, 2015) and Canadian PS students have been increasing since 2010, particularly as indicated by Canadian data from the last three cycles of the National College Health Assessment (see ACHA, 2013, 2016, 2019; for a summary, see Linden et al., 2018). Wiens et al. (2020) also found some increases in prevalence in both mood disorders and anxiety disorders around roughly the same time frame (i.e., 2011 to 2017) for female students. These data, along with recent media attention on PS student mental health and student suicides, have brought about what some people consider a "mental health crisis" on PS campuses (e.g., Shackle, 2019; Swanbrow Becker, 2020).

Population-based probability sampling research (as opposed to convenience sample data such as the National College Health Assessment) provides nuance to what this mental health crisis may entail. This research suggests that PS students may have similar prevalence of mental illnesses as their same-aged peers (Blanco et al., 2008; Cvetkovski et al., 2012) or even a lower prevalence of some mental illnesses (Wiens et al., 2020). This latter finding may even suggest that PS context may be a protective factor for mental illnesses for this age group. Epidemiological data also show that within this age cohort (and in other age groups as well) there has been a stable prevalence of diagnosed mental illnesses from the 2000s to mid-2010s (Pies, 2016). Although PS students may experience a similar or lower prevalence of mental illnesses, another finding within this research indicates that PS students experience more (subclinical) distress or higher perceptions of stress compared to their same-aged cohorts (Cvetkovski et al., 2012; Wiens et al., 2020).

Beyond the previously cited research that discusses the prevalence of mental health problems in this PS population, the current mental health crisis experienced at PS institutions may also be a function of factors other than increases in students having a mental illness. For example, in interviews with counseling directors and staff, Watkins et al. (2012) found that there has been an increase in the severity and complexity of student mental health problems in recent years (see also Crozier & Willihnganz, 2005; Prince, 2015). In other words, students are accessing services for more clinically severe disorders (e.g., major depression) as opposed to developmental challenges (e.g., stress). Additionally, students are reporting more substance use to their service providers. On a related note, Watkins et al. (2012) found that PS students have more exposure to mental health services from their families and from receiving services prior to entering PS education, resulting in the need for transition and continuation of care and more complex models of service delivery at PS institutions. As a corollary, demand has increased for counseling services at PS institutions. For example, LeViness et al. (2019) reported data from the Association for University and College Counseling Center Directors annual survey, which found a 12% increase in both client and appointment numbers from 2018 to 2019. Although there is nuance to what the PS mental health crisis may entail, this crisis may be broadly characterized by an increased demand for PS mental health and counseling services as a function of increasing complexity and intensity of mental health concerns in their students, accompanied by increasing experiences of (subclinical) distress.

Varied factors may drive increased demand for PS mental health services and the general PS mental health crisis. In addition to those we have already cited, Kutcher (2018) suggested that factors such as low mental health literacy, an increasing perception that being unwell equates to negative emotions, and mislabeling everyday negative emotions as pathological may be tied to the increased scrutiny of mental health on PS campuses, particularly by the media. Kutcher also explains that technology has led to decreased social connection and increased loneliness, which is likely another contributing factor. Although Kutcher does not make an explicit link, some of these factors may be responsible for the increase in demand for campus mental health services.

Another factor that might be increasing the demand for PS mental health services is a potential improvement in public perceptions, or a reduction in stigma, of mental health problems. Research has demonstrated a link between increased help seeking and lower levels of mental illness stigma in both PS students (Eisenberg, Downs, et al., 2009; Lally et al., 2013) and the broader population (e.g., Clement et al., 2015). For example, in a sample of 5,555 students across 13 universities, Eisenberg, Downs, et al. (2009) found that a student's personal stigma negatively impacted their help-seeking behaviors, with certain characteristics (e.g., male, young, Asian, international, religious, lower socioeconomic status) making some students more vulnerable than others. This research suggests that those with higher stigma are less likely to engage in help-seeking behaviors; therefore, if help seeking is becoming more common in PS institutions, it could be a consequence of stigma reduction, as some have suggested (e.g., Linden et al., 2018; Wiens et al., 2020), although there is no current empirical evidence to support this. When considering that this mental health crisis may be a function of an increase in help-seeking behaviors for those who will benefit from services, stemming from a potential decrease in stigma, it can be argued that there may be a silver lining, because students are actively seeking help. However, one of the challenges for those who provide PS mental health services is how to meet this increased demand.

Given that this link between help seeking and stigma is widely known, many PS institutions have been diligent in trying to reduce the stigma of mental illnesses on campuses to increase help-seeking behaviors in their students. There are many approaches to reducing this stigma on campuses, from specific initiatives (e.g., mass media campaigns, stigma reduction intervention, peer support) to taking a more holistic approach (e.g., mental health strategies or frameworks) (cf., Centre for Innovation in Campus Mental Health, n.d.). Many, if not most, of the specific PS initiatives target interpersonal stigma reduction, or reducing public stigma (e.g., in students, faculty) toward those with mental illnesses, and do not address either intrapersonal (i.e., self-stigma) or structural (i.e., policies, procedures) stigma.

Intrapersonal stigma, or self-stigma, occurs when an individual or group internalizes the stigma of their mental illness (Corrigan & Watson, 2002). This form of stigma can lead to lower self-esteem, lower self-efficacy, and reduced likelihood of help seeking (Corrigan & Watson, 2002; Link et al., 2001). Despite its negative impact, PS initiatives have not focused on intrapersonal stigma reduction in their communities. Regarding structural stigma, recent research with over 60,000 students and over 75 U.S. PS institutions found that PS campus–level stigma was negatively associated with student suicide thoughts and self-harm (although not depression or anxiety), even when controlling for individual-level stigma (Gaddis et al., 2018). This research emphasizes the need for structural stigma reduction at a PS institutional level. This is particularly important because PS institutions have been recently criticized in the media for not addressing student suicides on their campuses (e.g., Goffin, 2017; Nassar, 2019), and Gaddis et al.'s (2018) results suggest structural stigma might be impacting those with suicide behaviors more than those with mental illnesses such as depression or anxiety.

Mental illness stigma reduction should continue to be a priority for PS campuses (Linden et al., 2018) and is critical in addressing the current mental health crisis on campuses. Although many PS institutions are addressing interpersonal stigma, their approaches need to expand. What follows is a broad review of mental illness stigma reduction on PS campus, both evidence-based and promising practices. Although only PS students have been mentioned thus far, the broader campus community, including staff and faculty, is discussed, particularly within the context of holistic mental health initiatives on PS campuses.

Reducing Stigma: What Can Help?

Mass Media Approaches

A review of experimental mass media intervention research (i.e., using mediums intended for broad distribution as opposed to face-to-face interactions) suggests that they may be effective at reducing prejudice (i.e., negative attitudes), but they are inconclusive regarding discrimination (Clement et al., 2015). In practice, mass media campaigns have been successful to some extent, but may reach limited audiences. For example, antistigma campaigns across several German cities yielded a total awareness rate of 6.9% for the campaigns, with the most acknowledged individual campaign at 3.8% (Gaebel et al., 2008). A more recent regional antistigma campaign using traditional media (i.e., television ads) with in-game promotion (i.e., professional hockey game) and social media coverage resulted in almost 25% awareness in its intended target age group of 13- to 25-year-olds (Livingston et al., 2013). Another regional, short-term antistigma campaign found similar results with a 23% awareness in its intended target age group of 25- to 45-year-olds during the campaign (Evans-Lacko et al., 2010). However, these authors found awareness dropped to 6% post campaign, which was similar to precampaign levels of 5%.

Mass media campaigns have also been implemented at PS institutions with some success. In Canada, the Bell Let's Talk Day (https://letstalk.bell.ca/en/) has been a ubiquitous mental health initiative and antistigma campaign that has occurred at the end of January each year since 2010. Bell Let's Talk focuses on four pillars: fight stigma, improve access to care, support research, and workplace leadership in mental health. According to Bell Canada (2020), in the 2020 iteration of the campaign, 227 PS institutions from every province and territory participated in Bell Let's Talk Day, with over 500 planned events and over 1.7 million participating students. For PS institutions, events for this day included social media promotion (e.g., #BellLetsTalk), writing messages of hope in talk bubbles, free branded swag giveaways (e.g., toques), and initiatives and partnerships with campus athletic teams.

PS institutions have also supported national initiatives or campaigns for increasing awareness and reducing mental illness stigma that have not specifically targeted PS institutions. For example, Not Myself Today is a workplace initiative that aims to create mental health conversations and shift the culture of mental health in workplaces (Canadian Mental Health Association, 2020). Organizations can sign up for the initiative and receive a digital and physical toolkit with materials that support planning, implementing, and evaluating the campaign within their organization. Although intended for the workplace, some PS institutions have made the program accessible for students, in addition to staff and faculty (e.g., Trent University, 2013). Another example is the Employer Pledge (Time to Change, n.d.), which is a specific initiative of the United Kingdom's Time to Change national campaign from 2011 to June 2020. Workplaces could pledge their commitment to the initiative and enact the Employer Action Plan. The Employee Action Plan encourages organizations to implement actions to reduce prejudice and discrimination related to mental illnesses among employees. At the time of the Employer Pledge retirement, over 1,500 organizations, including PS institutions, had signed on to this pledge. PS institutions that pledged included Oxford University (Time to Change, 2012), Sheffield United (Time to Change, 2012), and many others.

These mass media campaigns have more facets than just dissemination of awareness and antistigma messaging through mass media channels. Presumably, some of the activities and initiatives related to the umbrella campaign may use, for example, speakers with lived experience or other efficacious ways to reduce stigma. Broadly, these campaigns are impactful in the sense that they have engagement from many PS institutions and generate participation from the whole campus community. Even though some of these initiatives have been evaluated at the national level (e.g., Time to Change; see Henderson et al., 2016), it is unclear if these initiatives are effective on campuses. A related efficacy question is how long the impacts from these initiatives are sustained, because some are short-term or single-day events (e.g., Bell Let's Talk). Despite this lack of research, several factors may help support such an approach on campuses (as opposed to broad regional or national campaigns). First, PS campuses are smaller communities in both size and population, as opposed to a city or country with millions of individuals and broad regional expanses. Second, most campuses have a physical location where the campus community comes together within confined spaces during specific times. For example, high-foot-traffic areas (e.g., quads, cafeterias) may be conducive for campaign messaging. Third, there are generally multiple means to reach the campus community with messaging that is accessible to the entire community, such as through institutional communications channels (e.g., email, newsletter, website, social media). Regardless, PS institutions should make it a priority to reduce stigma on their campuses. As well, these initiatives should be evaluated for their effectiveness to ensure they reduce negative attitudes and/or prejudice toward people with mental illnesses. This evaluation must go beyond simply assessing awareness, uptake, or reach of the campaign.

Stigma Reduction Programming

Mental illness stigma reduction programs that are implemented at PS institutions vary in scope, format, and target group. This type of programming may specifically address mental illness stigma reduction or, more often than not, mental health literacy with embedded elements of stigma reduction. The format of programming also varies in terms of length (e.g., half-day workshop, 2-day workshop) and modality (e.g., face to face, online module). These programs may target students, staff and faculty, or both. Additionally, the stigma reduction component may also vary from providing knowledge to contact-based education via different forms, which can all be effective in stigma reduction (Corrigan et al., 2012). A recent systematic review of stigma reduction interventions at educational institutions found similar variety in terms of scope, format, target group, and stigma reduction mechanism (Waqas et al., 2020). This review also found that most interventions were successful at reducing negative attitudes and social distance, improving attitudes and beliefs, and increasing mental health knowledge and help seeking.

Mental Health First Aid

Mental Health First Aid (MHFA) is a program that "empower[s] and equip[s] individuals with the knowledge, skills and confidence needed to support a friend, family member or co-worker experiencing a mental health problem or experiencing a crisis such as being suicidal" (MHFA International, 2020). This program is being implemented in 24 countries and has had over 4 million participants (MHFA International, 2020). In Canada, MHFA is offered in various formats and course types, although there is no specific course for the PS community (Mental Health Commission of Canada, 2020). The program addresses stigma reduction, improving understanding of mental illnesses and their recognition, how to intervene and support individuals effectively, and mental health resources (Mental Health Commission of Canada, 2020). A recent systematic review found that MHFA did improve MHFA knowledge, mental illness recognition, beliefs about treatment, and both confidence and intentions to help someone, all with small to medium effect sizes (Morgan et al., 2018). However, Morgan et al. found that of all the measured outcomes, MHFA was least effective at reducing negative attitudes, with small effect sizes (i.e., Cohen's d ranging from 0.08 to 0.14). Similarly, Massey et al. (2014) found that at a Canadian university, negative attitudes did not differ between a group of student service professions that did and did not take MHFA. Several studies have examined MHFA in PS students demonstrating positive impact of the program on various outcome measures (e.g., Burns et al., 2017).

Starting the Conversation: Raising Our Awareness of Student Mental Health

Another intervention used at a PS institution is the Starting the Conversation: Raising Our Awareness of Student Mental Health program that was evaluated at Algonquin College in Canada (Stuart et al., 2014). This program is an online training program divided into three 20-minute modules with the aim of helping faculty members improve their attitudes toward and better support students with mental health problems and to help faculty members initiate conversations about help seeking and refer students to resources. The program uses video-based contact of young people with lived experience to highlight critical aspects of the program and to demonstrate the impact of mental illnesses on the student journey. Pre- and postevaluations indicated that the online program positively shifted attitudes such that 57.9% of participants at postprogram, compared to only 20.4% at preprogram, achieved an "A grade" on the 15-item stigma measure (i.e., 80% or more of the 15 items were answered with a nonstigmatizing response).

The Inquiring Mind Post-Secondary (TIM PS) is a program developed to reduce negative attitudes toward people with mental illnesses, promote positive mental health, and teach coping skills to increase resiliency in PS students (Szeto et al., 2020). This program was based on the Working Mind (Dobson et al., 2019) and the Working Mind for First Responders (Szeto et al., 2019). Although TIM PS is based on successful and efficacious programs (see Dobson et al., 2019; Szeto et al., 2019), the developers wanted to create a program that was meaningful for, and would resonate with, PS students. Therefore, to develop TIM PS, a group of PS stakeholders from the University of Calgary including students, student service professionals, and faculty members acted as an advisory group to guide the development process and offer suggestions and comments on program content.

The main key component of TIM PS is traditional video-based contact that is supported by research to reduce mental illness–related stereotypes, affective reactions, and behavioral intentions (e.g., Corrigan et al., 2012). Within the program, a series of videos follow a group of PS students with lived experience of mental illnesses discussing various topics, from signs and indicators of poor mental health to experiences of prejudice and discrimination to the definition of self-stigma. One of the most important aspects of the video is the incorporation of the recovery narrative that conveys the message of hope and that individuals can recover from a mental illness, although that journey may be difficult (see Knaak et al., 2014).

The other main components of TIM PS are not directly related to reducing negative attitudes, but may play an indirect role. For example, the mental health continuum model (Government of Canada, 2017; for an evaluation of the model see Chen et al., 2020) reconceptualizes mental health on a continuum of four colors (green, yellow, orange, and red), where positive functioning and positive mental health are at the left end of the continuum (i.e., green) and severe functional impairment is at the right end of the continuum (i.e., red). The mental health continuum model also contains a bidirectional arrow that indicates movement back and forth on the continuum and functioning along five domains (e.g., physical, thinking, and attitude). Depiction of mental illnesses as a continuum from mild to severe is related to less stigmatizing attitudes; it is believed that this type of conceptualization places everyone on the continuum, lessening the distinction between "us" (i.e., those without a mental illness) and "them" (i.e., those with a mental illness; Schomerus et al., 2016).

In an evaluation at 16 PS institutions in Canada, TIM PS had improvements from pre- to postworkshop on two primary outcomes (i.e., negative attitudes and resiliency skills; Szeto et al., 2020). At the follow-up 3-month point, the gains for these two outcomes were maintained, with some regression back toward baseline. Currently, TIM PS is being implemented in numerous PS institutions across Canada. The Working Mind program has also been implemented for staff and faculty at various Canadian PS institutions. Dobson et al.'s (2019) evaluation of this program demonstrates positive outcomes related to reducing stigmatizing attitudes and resiliency skills.

Holistic Mental Health and Well-Being Approaches

One of the emerging practices in the 2010s (particularly the last half) at PS institutions in Canada has been the development and implementation of mental health strategies. An environmental scan by the Best Practices in Canadian Higher Education (2019) identified several factors that drove the development and implementation of mental health strategies on Canadian campuses. These factors included (a) the high and increasing prevalence of mental health problems in National College Health Assessment data, (b) the recognition that PS institutions have a role to play in, and can positively impact, student mental health, (c) the recognition that PS students are at a transitional stage in their lives, (d) the suicide rate in the PS student age group, and (e) the need to address student diversity (including students with disabilities). Along with these drivers, the environmental scan also identified several important documents published in the 2010s that have informed and shaped the development and implementation of mental health strategies. Two particular noteworthy documents were *Post-Secondary Student Mental Health: Guide to a Systemic Approach* (Canadian Association of College & University Student Services [CACUSS] and Canadian Mental Health Association [CMHA], 2013) and the *Okanagan Charter: An International Charter for Health Promoting Universities and Colleges* (2015). The former document describes how to develop a holistic framework to address and foster positive mental health in PS students. Of note, *Post-Secondary Student Mental Health: Guide to a Systemic Approach* describes a framework with seven key components that PS institutions should address in their mental health strategies (see Figure 2 in CACUSS and CMHA, 2013, p. 9). The *Okanagan Charter* (2015), the latter document, takes a complementary holistic approach with two calls to action for institutions: institutions should (a) embed health into all aspects of their campus culture (i.e., administration, operations, and academic mandates), including physical spaces, polices, and programs and services; and (b) work at collaborating both at a local and at a global level to promote and lead in health promotion.

Many PS institutions across Canada have adopted similar frameworks that are consistent with these two documents. Although specific initiatives targeting mental illness stigma reduction are an important activity that PS institutions should continue to do (Linden et al., 2018), stigma reduction has been embedded within the systematic and holistic approaches being implemented as a part of the mental health and well-being strategies across Canadian PS institutions. For example, the University of British Columbia has committed to the *Okanagan Charter*, has created a Wellbeing Strategic Framework, and is working to embed well-being in many aspects of their campus, such as policies and practices (https://wellbeing.ubc.ca/). Similarly, the University of Calgary's Campus Mental Health Strategy (https://www.ucalgary.ca/mentalhealth) has committed to creating a community of caring by targeting six strategic focus areas, from upstream mental health promotion and awareness, to mental health service delivery, programming, and resources, to organizational aspects that impact mental health (e.g., policies, physical environments).

The importance of campuses developing and implementing strategies that are consistent with a holistic mental health approach is twofold regarding mental illness stigma reduction. First, campuses are directly addressing stigma on their campus through direct stigma reduction activities (e.g., Bell Let's Talk Day, TIM PS), alongside initiatives that increase mental health awareness or mental health literacy. Second, embedded within the systematic and holistic approach is a call to address mental health at the cultural and organizational level, such as examining policies, processes, and procedures through a mental health lens or creating an inclusive campus climate (CACUSS and CMHS, 2013; *Okanagan Charter*, 2015). Addressing mental health at this level effectively contributes to reducing mental illness–related structural stigma, or "rules, policies, and procedures of social institutions that arbitrarily restrict the rights and opportunities of people living with mental health and substance use issues" (Livingston, 2020, p. 4). As well, addressing public stigma at the interpersonal level is not sufficient, because structural stigma also negatively affects PS students (see Gaddis et al., 2018).

One promising practice for addressing structural stigma at PS institutions is reviewing and developing policies through a mental health lens. Olding and Yip (2014) conducted an environmental scan of policy practices and approaches at PS institutions in Canada (and the United Kingdom). One of their conclusions was that Canadian PS institutions had mental health–related policies at the individual level that addressed issues such as academic accommodations; however, general policies that have more broad implications for student mental health have not been "mainstreamed" through a mental health lens. One emerging practice identified by Olding and Yip (2014) was to create a formal mechanism to examine the mental health impacts of policies at PS institutions. The Canadian Standards Association's (CSA; 2020a) *Mental Health for Post-Secondary Students* (i.e., the Post-Secondary Standard) also recommends that PS institutions develop a mechanism to review policies through a mental health lens. Additionally, the *Post-Secondary Standard Compendium* (CSA, 2020b) has a specific chapter giving guidance on how PS institutions may conduct policy reviews through a mental health lens. It is unclear at this point how many PS institutions have this type of mechanism or whether evaluations of its impacts exist. The University of Calgary, as a recommendation in their Campus Mental Health Strategy (Recommendation 5.3), has created a dedicated committee to review policies through a mental health lens and reviewed at least 18 university policies since its creation in 2016.

Another promising practice that targets the structural level at PS institutions is to examine mental health and well-being within the context of the teaching and learning environment (see CACUSS and CMHA, 2013; CSA, 2020a). For example, Simon Fraser University's Wellbeing in Learning Environments project (https://www.sfu.ca/healthycampuscommunity/learningenvironments.html) emphasizes fostering mental health and well-being in various learning contexts. One of this project's tools is a guide that identifies 10 factors (i.e., social connection, optimal challenge, civic engagement, instructor support, inclusivity, personal development, services and supports, positive classroom culture, flexibility, real-life learning) that can positively impact well-being in learning environments (Simon Fraser University, 2020). Adopting a universal design for learning in the classroom environment has also been recommend as a way to support well-being and improve student learning outcomes (see CSA, 2020b; La et al., 2018; Simon Fraser University, 2020). This approach tries to reduce barriers and improve student engagement by considering the varying needs of the learners during course design and curriculum development and in the classroom environment (La et al., 2018).

Embedding concepts of mental health and well-being in the curriculum or in courses may be an important next step for PS institutions to change mental health culture and create learning environments that support mental health and well-being. This emerging practice may take various forms: inserting a mental health statement or resources in the course syllabus (e.g., see section 5.1e, https://www.ucalgary.ca/pubs/calendar/current/e-1.html), incorporating mental health and well-being into course design (e.g., Dyjur et al., 2017), creating for-credit courses around positive psychology (in addition to courses on mental illness or abnormal psychology; e.g., https://www.tru.ca/distance/courses/psyc3991.html), or creating full programs or certificates on mental health and well-being. One example is the Embedded Certificate in Mental Wellbeing and Resilience that is offered by the University of Calgary for undergraduate students (https://www.ucalgary.ca/mentalhealth/education/certificate), the first of its kind in Canada. This certificate's three core courses teach students (a) to better support themselves through optimal coping and increasing resilience, (b) to better support others' well-being, and (c) to cultivate future mental health and well-being champions for the workplace and community.

The Stigma of Suicide

Research suggests that negative attitudes toward suicide have decreased from 1988 to 2007 (Witte et al., 2010). Although 93% of American PS students surveyed in 2006 indicated they would be willing to be friends with someone who has attempted suicide in the past year (if they met and liked them), only half indicated they would date the person, indicating negative attitudes do still exist (Lester & Walker, 2006). Additionally, research has indicated a variety of negative stereotypes toward suicide-attempt survivors, including ideas of attention seeking, malingering (e.g., over-emphasizing struggles), and incompetence (Sheehan et al., 2017). Given these results, along with increases in suicide ideation and attempts in students (e.g., ACHA, 2013, 2019), PS institutions have participated in various suicide awareness and prevention initiatives. One large initiative in Canada for suicide awareness, prevention, and hope is Mysterious Barricades (https://www.mysteriousbarricades.org/). This cross-Canada concert during World Suicide Prevention Week unites people across the nation, opening the door to tough conversations through music. Free concerts are held across Canada, some at PS institutions, which are then available to stream online. Many PS campuses also offer training to their staff, faculty, and students in hopes of increasing awareness and understanding about suicide and providing knowledge and tools for individuals to help those with suicide behaviors. The QPR Gatekeeper Training (https://qprinstitute.com/individual-training), for example, is a 60-minute training that teaches participants how to question, persuade, and refer someone who may be suicidal. Applied Suicide Intervention Skills Training (https://www.suicideinfo.ca/workshop/asist/) is an interactive 2-day course that trains participants to intervene with an individual who is having suicidal thoughts, including recognition and creating a plan for their immediate safety. Both these programs have demonstrated success in supporting those who may be at risk of suicide in PS settings (e.g., Mitchell et al., 2013; Shannonhouse et al., 2017). However, it is unclear if the programs positively impact public attitudes toward suicide.

To address negative perceptions toward suicide, and suicide more generally, some campuses have implemented Zero Suicide, an international initiative for suicide prevention and care that was originally developed in a healthcare setting (http://zerosuicide.edc.org/about). This initiative has seven main pillars: lead culture change; train workforce; identify, engage, treat, and transition those at risk; and improve policies and procedures. The Zero Suicide framework has been endorsed by various PS institutions in the United Kingdom and some universities in North America. For example, Georgia Tech has created Tech Ends Suicide Together, a bold plan to eliminate suicide on their campus, along with resources to help other campuses implement the framework of Zero Suicide (https://endsuicide.gatech.edu/). Within Canadian PS institutions, the University of Calgary has also adopted the Zero Suicide framework for their campus and convened an advisory committee to implement the framework (https://www.ucalgary.ca/wellness-services/suicide-awareness-and-prevention-framework). Although not directly tied to Zero Suicide, the University of Alberta has developed a suicide prevention framework that address suicide on their campus through five categories: (a) policy and implementation; (b) education, awareness, and communication; (c) services and supports; (d) a welcoming, connected, and supportive community; and (e) supports following a campus death (University of Alberta, 2020).

Last, because of the recent criticism that PS institutions have received about not acknowledging suicides on campus (e.g., Goffin, 2017; Nassar, 2019), research at the University of Calgary (Lindsay, 2020) investigated whether media articles that acknowledge a student suicide can be used to decrease negative perceptions of suicide on campus. This research found that students who read articles that respectfully acknowledged a student suicide on campus, along with suicide information (e.g., correct terminology, discuss struggle, emphasize recovery and resources such as the recommendations from *Mindset; The Canadian Journal Forum on Violence and Trauma*, 2014) from a variety of sources (an expert, a friend of the student who died, or a suicide survivor), showed fewer stereotypes toward suicide survivors than students who received a control article about student heath. These results suggest that these types of mass media interventions could be effective as a strategy in addressing the concerns about PS silence on this issue, as well as the negative perceptions of suicide more generally in the PS community.

Key Considerations/Recommendations for Implementation

Stigma reduction and mental health and well-being have been priorities for PS institutions since around 2010. The PS community, as a whole, has been progressive in the development and implementation of holistic frameworks to address mental health on campuses. The following recommendations will sustain the current momentum and promote innovation in the PS community.

- PS institutions have implemented various stigma reduction initiatives that address public stigma or stigma at the interpersonal level and should continue to address this type of stigma (Linden et al., 2018). However, stigma at the structural and intrapersonal (i.e., self-stigma) levels has not been addressed adequately, particularly the latter.
- Taking a holistic mental health approach (e.g., mental health strategy) reduces stigma at the structural level, such as policies. In addition, this type of approach will also address mental health promotion and prevention and improve mental health services and resources.
- PS institutions in the process of developing a holistic mental health approach for their campus should use the *Post-Secondary Student Mental Health: Guide to a Systemic Approach* (CACUSS and CMHA, 2013), the *Okanagan Charter* (2015), and the *Post-Secondary Standard* (CSA, 2020a) as guiding documents in their development process.

- A holistic approach for mental health and well-being requires the inclusion of the whole campus community of students, staff, and faculty (see Best Practices in Canadian Higher Education, 2019). This approach can take the form of a mental health strategy or adoption of the *Post-Secondary Standard* (for students) and the *Workplace Standard* (for faculty and staff).
- Although holistic approaches are recommended and should be an effective approach, they should be evaluated to see if they are having the intended effect. Currently, only a few PS institutions have explored evaluation of these holistic approaches.
- Stigma reduction initiatives, whether using mass media campaigns or programs, should continue to be evaluated for their effectiveness and efficacy. In particular, more evidence is needed to support the implementation of mass media campaigns at PS institutions specifically.
- More research is needed to ascertain the effectiveness of various stigma reduction initiatives in groups that are a part of the campus community. Targeted initiatives (e.g., for graduate students, international students, faculty), whether they are programming or messaging, seem to be more effective than general initiatives.
- Stigma reduction initiatives need to be evaluated with more scientific rigor (e.g., using more rigorous designs, such as random control trials). As well, more research is needed to identify the critical components of stigma reduction programming using experimental designs, because current evaluations are "black box" evaluations that assess a program as a whole.
- Suicide is an important topic for PS institutions. PS institutions should take steps to reduce the stigma associated with self-injury and suicide, in addition to increasing awareness and preventing suicides in their campus community.

References

American College Health Association. (2013). *American College Health Association–National College Health Assessment II: Canadian Reference Group Executive Summary Spring 2013*.

American College Health Association. (2016). *American College Health Association–National College Health Assessment II: Canadian Consortium Executive Summary Spring 2016*.

American College Health Association. (2019). *American College Health Association–National College Health Assessment II: Canadian Consortium Executive Summary Spring 2019*.

Bell Canada. (2020). *Canadian students making every action count for campus mental health as partners in the 2020 Bell Let's Talk Day campaign*. https://letstalk.bell.ca/en/news/1224/canadian-students-making-every-action-count-for-campus-mental-health-as-partners-in-the-2020-bell-let-s-talk-day-campaign

Best Practices in Canadian Higher Education. (2019). *An environmental scan of Canadian campus mental health strategies*.

Blanco, C., Okuda, M., Wright, C., Hasin, D. S., Grant, B. F., Liu, S. M., & Olfson, M. (2008). Mental health of college students and their non-college-attending peers: Results from the national epidemiological study on alcohol and related conditions. *Archives of General Psychiatry, 65*(12), 1429–1437. https://doi.org/10.1001/archpsyc.65.12.1429

Burns, S., Crawford, G., Hallett, J., Hunt, K., Chih, H. J., & Tilley, P. M. (2017). What's wrong with John? A randomised controlled trial of Mental Health First Aid (MHFA) training with nursing students. *BMC Psychiatry, 17*(1), 111.

Canadian Association of College & University Student Services and Canadian Mental Health Association. (2013). *Post-secondary student mental health: Guide to a systemic approach.*

Canadian Mental Health Association. (2020). *Not Myself Today: Mental health is everyone's business.* https://www.notmyselftoday.ca/

Canadian Standards Association. (2020a). *Mental health for post-secondary students.* CAN/CSA Z2003:20.

Canadian Standards Association. (2020b). *Standards compendium.*

Centre for Innovation in Campus Mental Health. (n.d.) *Peer support on campus: What, how, who and where?* https://campusmentalhealth.ca/toolkits/campus-peer-support/the-case-for-peer-support-on-campus/peer-support-on-campus/

Chen, S. P., Chang, W. P., & Stuart, H. (2020). Self-reflection and screening mental health on Canadian campuses: Validation of the mental health continuum model. *BMC Psychology, 8*(1), 1–8.

Clement, S., Schauman, O., Graham, T., Maggioni, F., Evans-Lacko, S., Bezborodovs, N., Morgan, C., Rüsch, N., Brown, J. S. L., & Thornicroft, G. (2015). What is the impact of mental health-related stigma on help-seeking? A systematic review of quantitative and qualitative studies. *Psychological Medicine, 45*(1), 11–27. https://doi.org/10.1017/S0033291714000129

Corrigan, P. W., Morris, S. B., Michaels, P. J., Rafacz, J. D., & Rusch, N. (2012). Challenging the public stigma of mental illness: A meta-analysis of outcome studies. *Psychiatry Services, 63*(10), 963–973. https://doi.org/10.1176/appi.ps.201100529

Corrigan, P. W., & Watson, A. C. (2002). The paradox of self-stigma and mental illness. *Clinical Psychology: Science and Practice, 9*, 35–53. https://doi.org/10.1093/clipsy.9.1.35

Crozier, S., & Willihnganz, N. (2005). *Canadian Counselling Centre survey.* CUCCA.

Cvetkovski, S., Reavley, N. J., & Jorm, A. F. (2012). The prevalence and correlates of psychological distress in Australian tertiary students compared to their community peers. *Australian and New Zealand Journal of Psychiatry, 46*(5), 457–467. https://doi.org/10.1177/0004867411435290

Dobson, K. S., Szeto, A. C. H., & Knaak, S. (2019). The Working Mind: A meta-analysis of a workplace mental health and stigma reduction program. *Canadian Journal of Psychiatry, 64*(Suppl. 1), 39S–47S. https://doi.org/10.1177/0706743719842559

Dyjur, P., Lindstrom, G., Arguera, N., & Bair, H. (2017). Using mental health and wellness as a framework for course design. *Papers on Postsecondary Learning and Teaching, 2*, 1–9.

Eisenberg, D., Downs, M. F., Golberstein, E., & Zivin, K. (2009). Stigma and help seeking for mental health among college students. *Medical Care Research and Review, 66*(5), 522–541. https://doi.org/10.1177/1077558709335173

Eisenberg, D., Gollust, S. E., Golberstein, E., & Hefner, J. L. (2007). Prevalence and correlates of depression, anxiety, and suicidality among university students. *American Journal of Orthopsychiatry, 77*(4), 534–542. https://doi.org/10.1037/0002-9432.77.4.534.

Eisenberg, D., Golberstein, E., & Hunt, J. (2009). Mental health and academic success in college. *The B.E. Journal of Economic Analysis & Policy, 9*(1), 1–37. https://doi.org/10.2202/1935-1682.2191

Evans-Lacko, S., London, J., Little, K., Henderson, C., & Thornicroft, G. (2010). Evaluation of a brief anti-stigma campaign in Cambridge: Do short-term campaigns work? *BMC Public Health, 10*, 339. https://doi.org/10.1186/1471-2458-10-339

Gaddis, S. M., Ramirez, D., & Hernandez, E. L. (2018). Contextualizing public stigma: Endorsed mental health treatment stigma on college and university campuses. *Social Science & Medicine, 197*, 183–191.

Gaebel, W., Zäske, H., Baumann, A. E., Klosterkötter, J., Maier, W., Decker, P., & Möller, H.-J. (2008). Evaluation of the German WPA program against stigma and discrimination because of schizophrenia—Open the Doors: Results from representative telephone surveys before and after three years of anti-stigma interventions. *Schizophrenia Research, 98*, 184–193.

Goffin, P. (2017, August 12). How many Ontario post-secondary students die by suicide each year? No one knows for sure. *The Star.* https://www.thestar.com/news/gta/2017/08/12/how-many-ontario-post-secondary-students-die-by-suicide-each-year-no-one-knows-for-sure.html

Government of Canada. (2017, July 27). *The military mental health continuum model.* http://www.dnd.ca/en/caf-community-health-services-r2mr-deployment/mental-health-continuum-model.page

Henderson, C., Stuart, H., & Hansson, L. (2016). Lessons from the results of three national antistigma programmes. *Acta Psychiatrica Scandinavica, 134*(Suppl. 446), 3.

Knaak, S., Modgill, G., & Patten, S. B. (2014). Key ingredients of anti-stigma programs from health care providers: A data synthesis of evaluative studies. *The Canadian Journal of Psychiatry, 59*(Suppl. 1), S19–S26. https://doi.org/10.1177/070674371405901s06

Kruisselbrink Flatt, A. (2013). A suffering generation: Six factors contributing to the mental health crisis in North American higher education. *College Quarterly, 16*(1), n1.

Kutcher, S. (2018, March 26). *Is my child depressed? Being moody isn't a mental illness?* The Conversation. https://theconversation.com/is-my-child-depressed-being-moody-isnt-a-mental-illness-92789

La, H., Dyjur, P., & Bair, H. (2018). *Universal design for learning in higher education. Taylor Institute for Teaching and Learning.* University of Calgary.

Lally, J., Conghaile, A., Quigley, S., Bainbridge, E., & McDonald, C. (2013). Stigma of mental illness and help-seeking intention in university students. *The Psychiatrist, 37*(8), 253–260. https://doi.org/10.1192/pb.bp.112.041483

Lester, D., & Walker, R. L. (2006). The stigma for attempting suicide and the loss to suicide prevention efforts. *Journal of Crisis Intervention and Suicide Prevention, 27*(3), 147–148. https://doi.org/10.1027/0227-5910.27.3.147

LeViness, P., Gorman, K., Braun, L., Koenig, L., & Bershad, C. (2019). *The Association for University and College Counselling Centre Directors Annual Survey: 2019.* Association for University and College Counselling Centre Directors. https://www.aucccd.org/assets/documents/Survey/2019%20AUCCCD%20Survey-2020-05-31-PUBLIC.pdf

Linden, B., Stuart, H., & Gray, S. (2018). *Scoping review of the current literature around Post-secondary mental health and wellness.* Mental Health Commission of Canada. https://doi.org/10.13140/RG.2.2.17337.62566

Lindsay, B. L. (2020). *Investigating the influence of media articles on the stigma of suicide and other campus-related factors after a suicide on campus* [Unpublished master's thesis]. University of Calgary.

Link, B. G., Struening, E. L., Neese-Todd, S., Asmussen, S., & Phelan, J. C. (2001). The consequences of stigma for the self-esteem of people with mental illnesses. *Psychiatric Services, 52*(12), 1621–1626. https://doi.org/10.1176/appi.ps.52.12.1621

Livingston, J. D. (2020). *Structural stigma in health-care contexts for people with mental health and substance use issues: A literature review.* Mental Health Commission of Canada.

Livingston, J. D., Tugwell, A., Korf-Uzan, K., Cianfrone, M., & Coniglio, C. (2013). Evaluation of a campaign to improve awareness and attitudes of young people towards mental health issues. *Social Psychiatry and Psychiatric Epidemiology, 48*(6), 965–973.

Martin, J. M. (2010). Stigma and student mental health in higher education. *Higher Education Research & Development, 29*(3), 259–274. https://doi.org/10.1080/07294360903470969

Massey, J., Brooks, M., & Burrow, J. (2014). Evaluating the effectiveness of Mental Health First Aid training among student affairs staff at a Canadian university. *Journal of Student Affairs Research and Practice, 51*(3), 323–336.

Mental Health Commission of Canada. (2020). *Courses*. https://www.mhfa.ca/en/course-types

MHFA International. (2020). *What is Mental Health First Aid?* https://mhfainternational.org/

Mitchell, S. L., Kader, M., Darrow, S. A., Haggerty, M. Z., & Keating, N. L. (2013). Evaluating question, persuade, refer (QPR) suicide prevention training in a college setting. *Journal of College Student Psychotherapy, 27*(2), 138–148.

Morgan, A. J., Ross, A., & Reavley, N. J. (2018). Systematic review and meta-analysis of Mental Health First Aid training: Effects on knowledge, stigma, and helping behaviour. *PLoS One, 13*(5), e0197102.

Nassar, S. (2019, March 18). *"It doesn't feel human": Students angry U of T not acknowledging campus suicides*. CBC. https://www.cbc.ca/news/canada/toronto/university-toronto-suicide-campus-1.5061809

Okanagan Charter: An International Charter for Health Promoting Universities and Colleges. (2015). https://www.acha.org/documents/general/Okanagan_Charter_Oct_6_2015.pdf

Olding, M., & Yip, A. (2014). *Policy approaches to post-secondary student mental health*. OCAD University & Ryerson University Campus Mental Health Partnership Project.

Pies, R. W. (2016). The astonishing non-epidemic of mental illness. *Psychiatric Times, 33*(11). https://www.psychiatrictimes.com/view/astonishing-non-epidemic-mental-illness

Pompeo-Fargnoli, A. (2020). Mental health stigma among college students: Misperceptions of perceived and personal stigmas. *Journal of American College Health*, 1–10. https://doi.org/10.1080/07448481.2020.1784904

Prince, J. P. (2015). University student counseling and mental health in the United States: Trends and challenges. *Mental Health & Prevention, 3*(1-2), 5–10.

Schomerus, G., Angermeyer, M. C., Baumeister, S. E., Stolzenburg, S., Link, B. G., & Phelan, J. C. (2016). An online intervention using information on the mental health-mental illness continuum to reduce stigma. *European Psychiatry, 32*, 21–27.

Shackle, S. (2019). The way universities are run is making us ill': inside the student mental health crisis. The Guardian, September 27, 2019, retrieved June 22, 2021 from https://www.theguardian.com/society/2019/sep/27/anxiety-mental-breakdowns-depression-uk-students

Shannonhouse, L., Lin, Y. W. D., Shaw, K., Wanna, R., & Porter, M. (2017). Suicide intervention training for college staff: Program evaluation and intervention skill measurement. *Journal of American College Health, 65*(7), 450–456.

Sheehan, L. L., Corrigan, P. W., & Al-Khouja, M. A. (2017). Stakeholder perspectives on the stigma of suicide attempt survivors. *Journal of Crisis Intervention and Suicide Prevention, 38*(2), 73–81. https://doi.org/10.1027/0227-5910/a000413

Simon Fraser University. (2020). *Well-being in learning environments*. https://www.sfu.ca/content/dam/sfu/healthycampuscommunity/PDF/WLE/Creating%20Conditions%20for%20Well-being%20in%20Learning%20Environments.pdf

Stuart, H., Koller, M., & West Armstrong, A. (2014). *Opening Minds in a post-secondary environment: Results of an online contact-based anti-stigma intervention for college staff—starting the conversation*. Mental Health Commission of Canada.

Swanbrow Becker, M. (2020). *The mental health crisis on campus and how colleges can fix it*. The Conversation. https://theconversation.com/the-mental-health-crisis-on-campus-and-how-colleges-can-fix-it-127875

Szeto, A. C. H., Dobson, K. S., & Knaak, S. (2019). The Road to Mental Readiness for First Responders: A meta-analysis of program outcomes. *Canadian Journal of Psychiatry, 64*(Suppl. 1), 18S–29S. https://doi.org/10.1177/0706743719842562

Szeto, A. C. H., Henderson, L., Lindsay, B., Knaak, S., & Dobson, K. S. (2020). *Increasing resiliency and reducing mental illness stigma in post-secondary students: A meta-analytic evaluation of the Inquiring Mind Program* [Manuscript in preparation] Department of Psychology, University of Calgary, Canada.

Time to Change. (n.d.). *Employer pledge.* https://www.time-to-change.org.uk/get-involved/get-your-workplace-involved/employer-pledge

Time to Change. (2012) *Oxford University and Sheffield United sign the Time to Change pledge.* https://www.time-to-change.org.uk/news/oxford-university-and-sheffield-united-sign-time-change-pledge

Trent University. (2013). *Trent University launches Not Myself Today mental health campaign.* https://www.trentu.ca/humanresources/news-events/4421

University of Alberta. (2020). *Suicide prevention framework.* https://www.ualberta.ca/campus-life/suicide-prevention.html.

Walters, K. S., Bulmer, S., Troiano, P., Obiaka, U., & Bonhomme, R. (2018). Substance use, anxiety, and depressive symptoms among college students. *Journal of Child & Adolescent Substance Abuse, 27*, 1–9. https://doi.org/10.1080/1067828X.2017.1420507

Watkins, D. C., Hunt, J. B., & Eisenberg, D. (2012). Increased demand for mental health services on college campuses: Perspectives from administrators. *Qualitative Social Work, 11*(3), 319–337. https://doi.org/10.1177/1473325011401468

Waqas, A., Malik, S., Fida, A., Abbas, N., Mian, N., Miryala, S., Amray, A. N., Shah, Z., & Naveed, S. (2020). Interventions to reduce stigma related to mental illnesses in educational institutes: A systematic review. *The Psychiatric Quarterly, 91*(3), 887–903. https://doi.org/10.1007/s11126-020-09751-4

Wiens, K., Bhattarai, A., Dores, A., Pedram, P., Williams, J. V., Bulloch, A. G., & Patton, S. B. (2020). Mental health among Canadian postsecondary students: A mental health crisis? *The Canadian Journal of Psychiatry, 65*(1), 30–35. https://doi.org/10.1177/0706743719874178

Witte, T. K., Smith, A. R., & Joiner, T. E. (2010). Reason for cautious optimism? Two studies suggesting reduced stigma against suicide. *Journal of Clinical Psychology, 66*(6), 611–626. https://doi.org/10.1002/jclp.20691

11

Stigma Reduction in the General Workplace

Dorothy Luong and Bonnie Kirsh

Mental illnesses affect one in four people at some point in their lives (World Health Organization, 2001), so it is not surprising that it is a leading contributor to the overall economic costs affecting employers. Poor mental health in employees often results in lost productivity in the forms of absenteeism, presenteeism, turnover, and premature withdrawal from work (Dewa et al., 2007; D. Lim et al., 2000; K. L. Lim et al., 2008). These indirect costs of mental illnesses have been estimated to be more than double the amount associated with direct costs (i.e., costs associated with medication, physician visits, hospitalization). For example, of the US$2.5 trillion total global estimated costs of mental illnesses in 2010, US$1.7 trillion was attributed to indirect costs, while US$0.8 trillion was attributed to direct costs (David et al., 2012). At an organizational level, short-term and long-term disability claims related to mental illnesses can add up to significant financial losses for businesses (Sainsbury Centre for Mental Health, 2007). These types of claims have been found to be longer in duration and more costly than non–mental health related claims (Dewa et al., 2010). On a global level, the total economic costs of mental illnesses were estimated to be US$2.5 trillion in 2010 (David et al., 2012) and are expected to double by 2030 (Trautmann et al., 2016).

Given the awareness of the relationship between financial strain and mental illnesses in the working population, the workplace has increasingly become a site of interest for addressing mental wellness (Corbière et al., 2009; Graveling et al., 2008). However, the capacity of the workplace to effectively do so may be compromised by the stigma accompanying mental illness in the workplace. Research shows that people with mental illness often encounter discriminatory hiring practices and beliefs (Stefan, 2002; Stuart, 2006) and are disadvantaged by workplace policies related to absenteeism. They often experience difficulty receiving appropriate accommodations (Corrigan et al., 2004; Lysaght & Krupa, 2011) and face negative attitudes and experience social distancing from coworkers who are unwilling to work closely with or socialize with them (Pescosolido et al., 2010; Stuart, 2004). Consequently, workplace stigma restricts help-seeking behaviors, resulting in an underutilization of workplace healthcare services. There is evidence that individuals are reluctant to use employee health benefits for mental health–related concerns, particularly during early stages of illness when prevention efforts would be beneficial (Rüsch & Thornicroft, 2014), fearing that potential disclosure or awareness of the use of mental health services would lead to negative opinions from management and impact career opportunities (Corrigan et al., 2014; Walton, 2003). As a result, employees delay seeking support and allow their illness/symptoms to progress to stages where more significant and costly interventions are needed. Thus, although businesses are recognizing the need to address workplace mental health through interventions promoting employee mental health, it is pertinent to the facilitation and uptake of these interventions that workplace stigma be addressed.

The need for contextually specific antistigma initiatives, such as those targeting the workplace, is clear. While mass public mental illness antistigma initiatives have emerged in recent years (Corrigan & Gelb, 2006; Crisp, 2004; Evans-Lacko et al., 2010; Gaebel et al., 2008), these "campaigns" have typically demonstrated low amounts of increases in public awareness, limited sustained effectiveness, and lack of transferability of positive messaging to different contexts (Szeto & Dobson, 2010). Targeted, context-specific interventions were thus seen to hold greater promise for combatting stigma; along with the development and implementation of such programs comes the need for systematic evaluation of their effectiveness.

Because of the unique ways that stigma manifests itself in the workplace, intervention work in this context requires a critical understanding of how stigma presents itself in the workplace and how the workplace may perpetuate stigma. A conceptual model of workplace stigma (see Figure 11.1), developed by Krupa et al. (2009), provides a framework for this. The key components of the model include the consequences of stigma, the assumptions that underlie the expressions of stigma, the salience and intensity of those assumptions, and the outside influences that perpetuate these assumptions. The model suggests that fundamental negative beliefs and stereotypes about people with mental illness influence discriminatory behaviors in the workplace and that stigma varies across workplace situations and persons. Accordingly, it is critical to the effectiveness of antistigma interventions to identify the key assumptions that exist in the workplace, as well as where and how they emerge, and to directly challenge them. The more relevant, or tailored, antistigma messages can be based on existing assumptions in the particular workplace, the more salience they will hold. The model also suggests that overarching organizational culture and policies are at play in the workplace and that an analysis of these factors significantly contributes to the understanding of the work context and its relationship to stigma, the processes involved in program implementation, and the interpretation of program evaluation results.

Although there has been growing interest in the evaluation of workplace antistigma initiatives in recent years, the number of published high-quality, rigorous evaluations conducted in diverse working populations remains limited (Hanisch et al., 2016). In this chapter, we highlight the efforts of the Mental Health Commission of Canada's

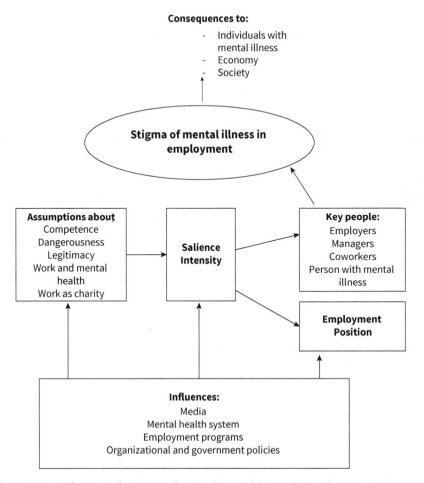

Figure 11.1 A Theoretical Framework to Understand Stigma in Employment

Reprinted from *Work, 33*, Krupa, T., Kirsh, B., Cockburn, L. and Gewurtz, R., Understanding the stigma of mental illness in employment, 413–425, Copyright (2009), with permission from IOS Press.

Opening Minds (OM) initiative to advance and evaluate antistigma interventions in the general workplace and introduce the methods, knowledge, tools, and expertise developed in conducting this work. We describe the steps taken in the implementation of our evidence-based approach to stigma reduction and the development of two new outcome measures to assess stigmatizing attitudes, highlight a variety of early projects, and introduce the adaptation and implementation of the Working Mind. Insights and tools related to our experiences with engaging employers and the process of implementing and evaluating programs are provided throughout to serve as consideration points for those wishing to further contribute to workplace antistigma initiatives.

The Opening Minds Initiative in the Workplace

Although OM was established in 2007 by the Mental; Health Commission of Canada (MHCC; 2012), the workplace was the last of OM's four targeted areas of focus to initiate (the others being healthcare providers, youth, and the media). The workplace team was formalized in 2010 and foundational work began with an examination of the literature on workplace antistigma interventions. The literature was scant at this early time, making a systematic review impossible. Thus, a more general review (Szeto & Dobson, 2010) was conducted to explore the various types and formats of workplace antistigma programs in existence across the globe. A scoping review (Malachowski & Kirsh, 2013) was also conducted to identify and describe principles and characteristics of existing workplace antistigma programs. While the reviews identified multiple programs with the potential to reduce various components of stigma, scientific rigor in the evaluation and implementation of these programs was lacking. In particular, standardized interventions and validated tools for evaluating the effectiveness of stigma reduction were deemed to be essential but absent.

The Opening Minds Scales for Assessing Workplace Stigma

The OM workplace team set out to address the evaluation gap by creating two new scales in order to standardize the measurement approach for conducting evaluations:

1. The Opening Minds Scale for Workplace Attitudes (see Chapter 5) is a 22-item measure that assesses stigmatizing attitudes, beliefs, and behaviors in the workplace. This measure was used in evaluations where interventions targeted general or front-line employees. While it was initially validated on a student sample, further validation work is underway in both an employed community sample and other workplace samples.
2. Recognizing that supervisors hold unique roles in influencing how mental illnesses and workers with a mental illness can be understood and treated in the workplace, the Opening Minds Scale for Supervisor Workplace Attitudes (see Appendix 11.1) was developed to assess stigmatizing attitudes, beliefs, and behaviors specific to the supervisor role. This 11-item measure was used when evaluating programs targeted at supervisors and was derived from various market research studies (Fine-Davis et al., 2005; Millward Brown IMS, 2007; Shaw Trust, 2006). Psychometric evaluation of this scale is in progress.

These scales formed the basis for all evaluation work and were coupled with other outcome measures as appropriate, depending on the program and objectives of the program and/or workplace (e.g., mental health literacy, well-being, intervention usage). Qualitative inquiry was also incorporated into evaluations wherever possible to examine the experience of antistigma programs in greater depth and detail. Interviews and/or focus groups were conducted with antistigma program participants and program facilitators to gain further theoretical understanding of the process of building successful antistigma programs in the workplace. Together, the two approaches (qualitative and quantitative) led to the identification of best practices and processes in antistigma program implementation.

Engaging Employers

While these program evaluation tools were being developed, strategies for engaging employers were under way. Medium and large organizations across a range of occupational categories with the structural capacity to implement initiatives were targeted. The goal was to connect organizations with appropriate programs (programs with contact-based components; i.e., involving people who have personal experience with mental illness sharing their personal stories) for implementation while forging partnerships to evaluate these programs. Engaging numerous employers to implement a variety of programs and conducting evaluations using the standardized measures would facilitate the systematic evaluation of program outcomes, as well as provide insight into best practices and essential components of workplace-based antistigma interventions.

Developing partnerships with employers was often a lengthy and slow process, with many organizations resistant to formally commit to program implementation and evaluation. Despite attempts to facilitate implementation by offering programs at cost, ensuring assistance with logistical concerns, and proposing the evaluation component as a complimentary service, uptake was still slow. One of the biggest barriers was a lack of awareness or buy-in of the benefits of reducing stigma or increasing awareness of mental health in the workplace. In the same way that stigma can affect individual uptake of mental health services, some organizations believed that implementation of antistigma programs would imply that there was a problem within the organization. Another barrier was the catch-22 situation that the programs to be evaluated lacked efficacy data. While some workplaces were willing to discuss workplace mental health and mental illness stigma reduction, they were resistant to implement programs that lacked evidence or that were not specifically endorsed by OM or other experts. In other cases, although they were willing to consider some form of programming, they were resistant to the idea of evaluation, viewing it as formal documentation of what may be wrong in their workplace. Organizations also expressed reluctance to engage in evaluation activities because of the added time constraints and additional time away from workers' workplace duties.

Relationship building began with face-to-face meetings between OM researchers and/or the OM director with the specific workplace. Successful partnerships were generally established when key employees within the organization, who understood the importance and effects of mental health and mental illness in the workplace, were engaged. These individuals were usually at the managerial level and acted as the "champion" liaison for the partnership within the company. In most cases, while these individuals were enthusiastic about partnering with OM, approval from senior executives to proceed with a partnership agreement or the delivery of an intervention or an evaluation was still needed. At this stage, the largest factor that affected program and evaluation uptake by a company or organization was the extent to which the senior managers or executives acknowledged the potential impact of the stigma of mental illness in the workplace and/or endorsed psychological health and safety in their workplace. Lack of buy-in at this level was what generally stalled or slowed discussions. Another key finding was that while general approval was needed from senior executives, there was a need for specific endorsement of a given antistigma initiative, or messaging that the programming was valued and participation in the program was expected. Taking the time to develop and obtain executive-level endorsement greatly facilitated the partnership between employers, researchers, and programs and the implementation and evaluation activities that followed.

The process from implementation to evaluation of a program was often more time-consuming than anticipated. Several levels of approval within the organization or multiple meetings with various levels of leadership were required. Approvals were often delayed because of competing priorities, reduced activities during certain times of the year (e.g., summer months, holiday seasons), and organizational change and restructuring. On several occasions, certain organizations had expressed interest in partnering with OM, but subsequent changes to the organization or leadership affected the priority of workplace mental health. Similarly, turnover of the mental health champion at an organization led to stalled or delayed proceedings because new liaisons needed to be engaged. Additionally, the evaluation work required ethics clearance, and in some cases the organization's internal ethics board and the researchers' university-based research ethics boards were needed. This process lengthened timelines for the projects.

The knowledge of barriers and facilitators gleaned from OM's work may help others mitigate the navigation challenges related to developing collaborations with employers. To this end, the lessons and learnings from OM's work in engaging organizations have been compiled in a checklist (see Appendix 11.2). Others wishing to engage with employers in program implementation and evaluation efforts can use this checklist as a guide in their process. While not all barriers are under the control of researchers, an awareness of them, as well as the factors that enable relationship development, can have an important impact on successfully engaging workplaces, their uptake of antistigma programming, and facilitating ensuing implementation and evaluation activities.

Collaborative Evaluation Frameworks

In the OM workforce team's work, once a partnership was established and an intervention was selected for implementation, a formal evaluation framework was drawn up in consultation with the employer and/or program. This type of collaboration in research is often described in the literature as "integrated knowledge translation." Incorporating integrated knowledge translation during the research process was shown to increase the accessibility, relevance, and endurance of research outcomes (Oborn et al., 2013). *Accessibility* refers to the ability of knowledge users to understand and apply the research (Oborn et al., 2013); *relevance* refers to the applicability of the research questions to current concerns and increases the likelihood of incorporating findings into practice and policy (Graham & Tetroe, 2009; Grimshaw et al., 2012; Keown et al., 2008; Kothari & Wathen, 2013; Oborn et al., 2013); and *endurance* refers to sustainability of changes associated with the research findings because of the long-term partnerships that are formed (Oborn et al., 2013). The use of this type of collaborative framework presented an opportunity for OM researchers to facilitate the relevant development of antistigma programs and the implementation of these programs in workplaces. The design of the framework ensured that the evaluation was guided by objectives and processes appropriate and fitting to each program and workplace context, maximizing the value of the evaluation for all stakeholders and the potential transition between research findings and real-life application. The framework also allowed employers to better understand the purpose of the evaluation by clearly outlining the reasons for the program implementation, allowing them to see how the program met those needs and understand how outcome measures would assess changes related to those needs. The specific procedures for conducting the evaluation were also outlined in this stage, and concerns related to privacy and confidentiality that were often raised in the engagement process were able to be addressed.

The evaluation framework created was based on components recommended in various program evaluation models (Payne, 1994). A copy of the framework with guidelines on how to use it can be found in Appendix 11.3. The framework begins by identifying the evaluation objectives and main evaluation question. Next, what the program will impact and how it will do so are outlined. Then, outcome measures, what they evaluate, and when they will be administered are determined. The structure of the program implementation plan is also highlighted in this framework, the procedures for the evaluation are listed, and, finally, organizations are asked if they would like an individualized report or summary of the evaluation outcomes. While the framework was customized accordingly for programs and employers, there was some standardization in evaluation methodology. For example, all antistigma programs evaluated were assumed to have an impact on stigmatizing attitudes, knowledge, and behavioral intent; these components were evaluated using the Opening Minds Scale for Workplace Attitudes and/or the Opening Minds Scale for Supervisor Workplace Attitudes. The administration of measures usually consisted of a pre, post, and 3-month follow-up design. Although this design format was not necessarily the first choice of design for researchers, the flexibility of the format compared to something such as a randomized controlled design allowed for the evaluation to better fit into the organization's processes and timelines of their implementation plans. Measures for pre and post were employed directly before and after participating in the program and generally yielded high participation levels. However, high attrition levels were found at the follow-up period, where participants were not incentivized or required to complete measures.

Consulting with employers on the framework, and in particular the evaluation procedures, provided an opportunity to negotiate the needs and goals of the evaluation and the goals and needs of the organization. While this often resulted in compromise over some aspects of the evaluation (such as the research design), it also offered an opportunity to highlight how findings may be relevant for the organization, advocate for as many best practices of an evaluation as possible, and troubleshoot ways to facilitate the evaluation process within each workplace. Involving organizations in the research process in this way is a critical aspect for conducting partnership work. Giving organizations the space for feedback in the research process will often result in a better understanding of the general need for evaluation work and how the evaluation can be used for their needs. This investment can lead to a prioritization of the evaluation and facilitates a way to optimize strategies for conducting it.

Opening Minds Workforce Team's Early Evaluation Work

With the slow start to engaging employers in program implementation and evaluation, the early evaluation experiences of the OM workplace group varied in terms of effectiveness and types of programs used by different organizations, as well as the ability of researchers to conduct evaluations using standardized methods.

In one early case in an industrial company (Szeto et al., 2019), a needs assessment using focus groups and an employee survey found that workers were not experiencing any particular concerns in terms of distress or experiences of stigma. Based on these results, leadership did not plan further activities and the partnership ended there.

In another collaboration, evaluation results showed an increase in stigma after program participation (Szeto et al., 2019). In this instance, the mental health awareness program was implemented by an oil and gas company and consisted of a presentation of a worker's past and continuing struggles with mental illnesses. While this program used contact-based education, an important antistigma program component (Corrigan et al., 2014; Malachowski & Kirsh, 2013), the presentation lacked emphasis on other important elements needed for effective antistigma programs, such as descriptions of recovery, help seeking, or adaptive coping (Knaak et al., 2014).

In another example of an early collaboration, a large telecommunications company had implemented a multicomponent set of interventions to enhance employee well-being, with each component being voluntary (Stuart et al., 2014). The implementation of this program, however, began before OM was engaged for the evaluation component. While this collaboration presented an opportunity to investigate workplace stigma within the context of a voluntary and unstandardized program, it did not allow for the pre–post–follow-up design that OM workplace researchers were trying to standardize across evaluations. A qualitative component to the evaluation was done, and process-oriented results indicated that the voluntary nature of the program allowed less than full participation. Meanwhile, a content-oriented finding called for programs to attend to the specific mental health issues that arise in particular workplace contexts. In this case, call center workers indicated that shift work, difficult customers, and work targets were issues unique to them that needed to be addressed in programming.

A final example of an early collaboration was with a large municipal government. In this instance, the organization received an individualized version of a program developed by a mental health agency. This organization used a top-down approach to implementation, with all supervisors receiving training first, followed by employees receiving a modified version of the program. Support from the organization's senior leaders facilitated the implementation and evaluation of the program, with some caveats. In particular, when conducting the evaluation of the program delivered to employees, the number of items in the Opening Minds Scale for Workplace Attitudes was reduced so that the time to complete the evaluation was proportionate to the amount of time needed for participation in the program (a relatively short program, at only 1 hour in length). This evaluation found a reduction in stigmatizing attitudes in both supervisors and employees after participating in their respective programs. Additional qualitative work (Kirsh et al., 2018) with supervisors in this organization allowed OM researchers to further explore stakeholder perceptions of distinct factors that influence stigma. Interviews exploring supervisors' experiences and perceptions of mental illness and stigma in the workplace revealed that mental health problems in the workplace manifest in various ways and that there are a range of responses to these problems by supervisors. The interviews also revealed the importance and relevance of workplace mental health training as it pertains to the role of supervisors. Overall, findings suggested that workplace antistigma initiatives require targeted messages and strategies for supervisors and that they differ from those required by employees.

These early findings of the OM workplace group, particularly around the importance of contact-based education, targeted workplace-specific context messaging, and targeted stakeholder messaging, played a salient role in the work that followed around the adaptation of a new workplace antistigma initiative.

The Working Mind

After several small-scale evaluations of various programs, OM became aware of the work of the Canadian Department of National Defence (and their program, the Road to Mental Readiness. This program was developed for mental health resiliency training in the Canadian military and included some elements of stigma reduction and mental health literacy. OM first adapted this program for use in first responder groups (see Chapter 12) by demilitarizing the content, adding a dedicated module for stigma, and incorporating contact-based education through videotaped content of a person with lived experience. In late 2012, the program was further adapted for the general workplace and retitled the Working Mind (TWM). Two versions of TWM were created to reflect OM's earlier findings that supervisors hold unique roles in navigating mental illness in the workplace. The version for front-line office workers is half a day in length. The longer, full-day version for managers and leaders builds on the half-day version and includes content that highlights supervisors' extended roles in assessing, supporting, and managing mental health and illness–related issues in the workplace.

Both versions of the program incorporate three core elements of Road to Mental Readiness pertaining to mental health literacy and knowledge, coping skills, and antistigma (Szeto et al., 2019):

1. The mental health continuum model: This nondiagnostic tool teaches people to view mental health on a continuum (see Figure 11.2). Signs and indicators of good to poor mental health are categorized into a four-color continuum: green (healthy), yellow (reacting), orange (injured), and red (ill), and people are taught to look for signs and indicators in themselves (and others) for each color. This model teaches that everyone is somewhere on the continuum at any given time, that a person's position on the continuum is not static, and that a person may experience signs and symptoms that place them on multiple parts of the continuum. The model also proposes appropriate actions at various stages of the continuum to either stay mentally healthy or take action when signs and indicators of concern are identified.

The Working Mind - Mental Health Continuum Model

HEALTHY	REACTING	INJURED	ILL
Normal fluctuations in mood	Nervousness, irritability, sadness	Anxiety, anger pervasive sadness, hopelessness	Excessive anxiety, easily enraged, depressed
Normal sleep patterns	Trouble sleeping	Restless or disturbed sleep	Unable to fall or stay asleep or sleeping too much
Physically well, full of energy	Tired/low energy, muscle tension, headaches	Fatigue, aches and pains	Exhaustion, physical illness
Consistent performance	Procrastination	Decreased performance	Unable to perform duties
Socially active	Decreased social activity	Social avoidance or withdrawal	Isolation, avoiding social events
No trouble/impact due to substance use	Limited to some trouble/impact due to substance use	Increased trouble/impact due to substance use	Dependence
			Suicidal thoughts and/or intentions

Multiple versions of the Mental Health Continuum Model can be found on the world wide web. This version is available from the Mental Health Commission of Canada (2017) and should be used only in concert with other program aspects.

Figure 11.2 The Mental Health Continuum Model

2. The Big 4 skills: Four coping strategies are taught within the programs. They include SMART goal setting, mental rehearsal, positive self-talk, and diaphragmatic breathing. These strategies incorporate several aspects of cognitive behavioral therapy and have been used widely in sports psychology to help athletes manage and increase performance in stressful situations.
3. Contact-based education: Video clips from actual employees are presented throughout the program to reflect and add relevance to the material presented and to allow participants the opportunity to identify with the scenarios presented.

The program uses trained facilitators, workshop manuals, discussion exercises, and personal goal-setting exercises as part of the program delivery. The preferred method for delivery is a "train-the-trainer" model, wherein employers select individuals within their organization to become facilitators. These individuals receive an intensive week-long training, which includes experiencing the program, learning the manuals and materials, and practicing the delivery of the program. Facilitators are evaluated at the end of the week before receiving approval to deliver the program. This train-the-trainer method is ideal for implementation, in that it results in facilitators from the specific organization where the program will be implemented, provides the organization with internal experts, and facilitates program sustainability. Using facilitators from within the organization also increases the likelihood that these individuals will be able to deliver the program within the contextual lens of the organization, helping increase the relevancy of the program messaging. If organizations do not have the capacity to send individuals for training or prefer otherwise, external facilitators can be sent in to deliver the programs.

With the development of TWM, interest in the implementation and evaluation work with OM grew. Organizations were receptive to the evidence-based and evidence-informed approach to the development of the program. Additionally, with the publication of the National Canadian Standard for Psychological Health and Safety in the Workplace (2012), organizations were increasingly interested in applying concrete actions to address workplace mental health concerns. To that end, TWM was implemented and evaluated in eight sites across Canada and a meta-analysis was conducted (Dobson et al., 2019). The program was associated with moderate reductions in stigma. Specifically, reductions were found on the overall Opening Minds Scale for Workplace Attitudes, as well as the five subscales capturing the following dimensions of stigma: the desire to avoid, perceptions of dangerousness and unpredictability, negative attitudes about mental illness in the workplace, negative attitudes toward helping people with a mental illness, and beliefs about responsibility for having a mental illness. Findings also suggested that the program was associated with increased self-reported resilience and increased coping abilities. Standardization of the program resulted in a high fidelity of program delivery, and the program appeared to be applicable across diverse workplace audiences and sectors. The delivery of TWM has now reached over 40,000 employees within government, postsecondary institutions, and the private sector. New work associated with TWM is now concentrating on booster sessions and exploring more sustainable and accessible forms of program delivery.

Conclusions

While the momentum of the workplace OM initiative was considerably delayed compared to the three other OM target groups, the early work and findings were foundational to later success and overall advancement and insight of work in this field. Findings around successful engagement of workplaces to optimize evaluation in these types of setting were determined, two new tools to evaluate stigmatizing attitudes in the workplace were created, and a well-established workplace antistigma program was created and widely disseminated across a variety of workplace settings across Canada.

Key Considerations

Key considerations from this work include the following:

Conceptual Frameworks for Understanding Stigma in the Workplace

- Stigma has unique and various ways of manifesting in the workplace because of the many horizontal and vertical relationships within organizations.
- Intervention work in this context requires a critical understanding of how stigma presents itself in the workplace.
- Conceptual frameworks (see Figure 11.1) can help programs and employers understand where and how stigma is presenting in the workplace in order to target antistigma messaging.

The Need for Standardized Interventions and Validated Tools for Evaluating the Effectiveness of Stigma Reduction in the Workplace

- Systematic evaluation of the effectiveness of antistigma programming in the workplace requires the use of standardized tools, as well as standardized programs, so that consistency in approach can be achieved and comparisons can be made.
- Organizations are more receptive to implementing programs that are standardized or have been developed using an evidence-based approach.
- The Opening Minds Scale for Workplace Attitudes and the Opening Minds Scale for Supervisor Workplace Attitudes are two outcome measures that have been developed and can be used to measure stigmatizing attitudes in the workplace.

- TWM offers a solution for standardized antistigma programming in the general workplace.

The Need for Workplace Antistigma Messaging to Be Contextually Specific

- While standardization is important, the unique nature of workplaces require context-specific messaging.
- Employers and programs should consider the additional training needs of leadership compared to front-line workers when selecting or developing programs to implement.
- Programs should consider ways to incorporate mental health issues specific to particular workplace contexts, such as through customization of components of a standardized program (e.g., group discussions, contact-based education), in order to increase the salience of antistigma messaging.

Contact-Based Education

- While contact-based education is an important antistigma program component, it is pertinent that messaging include elements of recovery and help seeking.
- Impassioned stories of past and continuing struggles with mental illness, alone, may increase stigma instead.

Developing Partnerships With Employers Is a Process

- Partnering with workplaces will take time.
- Leadership-level understanding of the importance and impact of mental health in the workplace is essential for successful program and evaluation implementation.

Collaborative Frameworks Facilitate Relevant Development, Implementation, and Evaluation of Antistigma Programs

- Involving programs and employers in the research process increases the understanding and relevance of the evaluation and optimizes the ability to conduct research in the workplace setting,
- Collaboration and ongoing relationships can also help with the sustainability of antistigma programming in the workplace.

Future Directions for Evaluation Efforts in the Workplace

- Organizations are resistant to employing randomized-controlled trials, but using a collaborative framework in the evaluation design may help negotiate for this in future settings.
- Strategies for optimizing the ability to measure long-term changes are needed (i.e., ways to increase completion of outcome measures at follow-up), and longer follow-up intervals may be considered.
- Other strategies to evaluate long-term effectiveness of programs should also be considered (e.g., use of employee health benefits, improved corporate culture, respect in the workplace).

References

Corbière, M., Shen, J., Rouleau, M., & Dewa, C. S. (2009). A systematic review of preventive interventions regarding mental health issues in organizations. *Work, 33*, 81–116. https://doi.org/10.3233/WOR-2009-0846

Corrigan, P., & Gelb, B. (2006). Three programs that use mass approaches to challenge the stigma of mental illness. *Psychiatric Services, 57*(3), 393–398. https://doi.org/10.1176/appi.ps.57.3.393

Corrigan, P. W., Druss, B. G., & Perlick, D. A. (2014). The impact of mental illness stigma on seeking and participating in mental health care. *Psychological Science in the Public Interest, 15*(2), 37–70. https://doi.org/10.1177/1529100614531398

Corrigan, P. W., Markowitz, F. E., & Watson, A. C. (2004). Structural levels of mental illness stigma and discrimination. *Schizophrenia Bulletin, 30*(3), 481–491. https://doi.org/10.1093/oxfordjournals.schbul.a007096

Crisp, A. (2004). The college's anti-stigma campaign, 1998–2003: A shortened version of the concluding report. *Psychiatric Bulletin, 28*, 133–136. https://doi.org/10.1192/pb.28.4.133

Bloom, D. E., Cafiero, E., Jané-Lopis, E., Abrahams-Gessel, S., Bloom, L. R., Fathima, S., Feigl, A. B., Gaziano, T., Hamandi, A., Mowafi, M., O'Farrell, D., Ozaltin, E., Pandya, A., Prettner, K., Rosenberg, L., Seligman, B., Stein, A. Z., Weinstein, C., & Weiss, J. (2012). *The global economic burden of noncommunicable diseases*. Ideas. https://ideas.repec.org/p/gdm/wpaper/8712.html

Dewa, C. S., Chau, N., & Dermer, S. (2010). Examining the comparative incidence and costs of physical and mental health-related disabilities in an employed population. *Journal of Occupational and Environmental Medicine, 52*(7), 758–762. https://journals.lww.com/joem/Fulltext/2010/07000/Examining_the_Comparative_Incidence_and_Costs_of.14.aspx

Dewa, C. S., McDaid, D., & Ettner, S. L. (2007). An international perspective on worker mental health problems: Who bears the burden and how are costs addressed? *The Canadian Journal of Psychiatry, 52*(6), 346–356. https://doi.org/10.1177/070674370705200603

Dobson, K. S., Szeto, A., & Knaak, S. (2019). The Working Mind: A meta-analysis of a workplace mental health and stigma reduction program. *Canadian Journal of Psychiatry. Revue canadienne de psychiatrie, 64*(1 Suppl.), 39S–47S. https://doi.org/10.1177/0706743719842559

Evans-Lacko, S., London, J., Little, K., Henderson, C., & Thornicroft, G. (2010). Evaluation of a brief anti-stigma campaign in Cambridge: Do short-term campaigns work? *BMC Public Health, 10*(1), 339. https://doi.org/10.1186/1471-2458-10-339

Fine-Davis, M., McCarthy, M., Edge, G., & O'Dwyer, C. (2005). *Mental health and employment: Promoting social inclusion in the workplace.* National Flexiwork Partnership Work–Life Balance Project/EQUAL Community Initiative. Centre for Gender and Women's Studies Trinity College.

Gaebel, W., Zäske, H., Baumann, A., Klosterkötter, J., Maier, W., Decker, P., & Möller, H.-J. (2008). Evaluation of the German WPA "Program against stigma and discrimination because of schizophrenia—Open the Doors": Results from representative telephone surveys before and after three years of antistigma interventions. *Schizophrenia Research, 98*, 184–193. https://doi.org/10.1016/j.schres.2007.09.013

Goetzel, R. Z., Long, S. R., Ozminkowski, R. J., Hawkins, K., Wang, S., & Lynch, W. (2004). Health, absence, disability, and presenteeism cost estimates of certain physical and mental health conditions affecting U.S. employers. *Journal of Occupational and Environmental Medicine, 46*(4), 398–412. https://journals.lww.com/joem/Fulltext/2004/04000/Health,_Absence,_Disability,_and_Presenteeism_Cost.13.aspx

Graham, I. D., & Tetroe, J. M. (2009). Getting evidence into policy and practice: Perspective of a health research funder. *Journal of the Canadian Academy of Child and Adolescent Psychiatry, 18*(1), 46–50.

Graveling, R., Crawford, J., Cowie, H., Amati, C., & Vohra, S. (2008). *A review of workplace interventions that promote mental wellbeing in the workplace.* Institute of Occupational Medicine.

Grimshaw, J. M., Eccles, M. P., Lavis, J. N., Hill, S. J., & Squires, J. E. (2012). Knowledge translation of research findings. *Implementation Science, 7*, Article 50. https://doi.org/10.1186/1748-5908-7-50

Hanisch, S. E., Twomey, C. D., Szeto, A. C. H., Birner, U. W., Nowak, D., & Sabariego, C. (2016). The effectiveness of interventions targeting the stigma of mental illness at the workplace: A systematic review. *BMC Psychiatry, 16*, 1. https://doi.org/10.1186/s1288-015-0706-4

Keown, K., Van Eerd, D., & Irvin, E. (2008). Stakeholder engagement opportunities in systematic reviews: Knowledge transfer for policy and practice. *Journal of Continuing Education in the Health Professions, 28*(2), 67–72. https://doi.org/10.1002/chp.159

Kirsh, B., Krupa, T., & Luong, D. (2018). How do supervisors perceive and manage employee mental health issues in their workplaces? *Work, 59*, 547–555. https://doi.org/10.3233/WOR-182698

Knaak, S., Modgill, G., & Patten, S. B. (2014). Key ingredients of anti-stigma programs for health care providers: A data synthesis of evaluative studies. *Canadian Journal of Psychiatry. Revue canadienne de psychiatrie, 59*(10, Suppl. 1), S19–S26. https://doi.org/10.1177/070674371405901s06

Kothari, A., & Wathen, C. N. (2013). A critical second look at integrated knowledge translation. *Health Policy, 109*(2), 187–191. https://doi.org/10.1016/j.healthpol.2012.11.004

Krupa, T., Kirsh, B., Cockburn, L., & Gewurtz, R. (2009). Understanding the stigma of mental illness in employment. *Work (Reading, Mass.), 33*, 413–425. https://doi.org/10.3233/WOR-2009-0890

Lim, D., Sanderson, K., & Andrews, G. (2000). Lost productivity among full-time workers with mental disorders. *The Journal of Mental Health Policy and Economics, 3*, 139–146. https://doi.org/10.1002/mhp.93

Lim, K. L., Jacobs, P., Ohinmaa, A., Schopflocher, D., & Dewa, C. (2008). A new population-based measure of the economic burden of mental illness in Canada. *Chronic Diseases in Canada, 28*, 92–98.

Lysaght, R., & Krupa, T. (2011). *Employers' PERSPECTIVES on intermittent work capacity—What can qualitative research tell us?* (HRSDC Contract No. 7616-09-0016/00). Skill Development Canada.

Malachowski, C., & Kirsh, B. (2013). Workplace antistigma initiatives: A scoping study. *Psychiatric Services, 64*(7), 694–702. https://doi.org/10.1176/appi.ps.201200409

Mental Health Commission of Canada. (2012). *Changing directions, changing lives: The mental health strategy for Canada*. Mental Health Commission of Canada. http://strategy.mentalhealthcommission.ca/pdf/strategy-text-en.pdf

Millward Brown IMS. (2007). *Mental health in the workplace: National economic and social forum*. [http://www.files.nesc.ie/nesf_archive/nesf_research_series/nesf_rs_04.pdf

Oborn, E., Barrett, M., Prince, K., & Racko, G. (2013). Balancing exploration and exploitation in transferring research into practice: A comparison of five knowledge translation entity archetypes. *Implementation Science, 8*, 104. https://doi.org/10.1186/1748-5908-8-104

Payne, D. A. (1994). *Designing educational project and program evaluations: A practical overview based on research and experience*. Kluwer Academic.

Pescosolido, B. A., Martin, J. K., Long, J. S., Medina, T. R., Phelan, J. C., & Link, B. G. (2010). "A disease like any other"? A decade of change in public reactions to schizophrenia, depression, and alcohol dependence. *The American Journal of Psychiatry, 167*(11), 1321–1330. https://doi.org/10.1176/appi.ajp.2010.09121743

Rüsch, N., & Thornicroft, G. (2014). Does stigma impair prevention of mental disorders? *British Journal of Psychiatry, 204*(4), 249–251. https://doi.org/10.1192/bjp.bp.113.131961

The Sainsbury Centre for Mental Health. (2007). *Mental health at work: Developing the business case*. https://www.centreformentalhealth.org.uk/sites/ default/files/2018-09/mental_health_at_work.pdf

Shaw Trust. (2006). *Mental health: The last workplace taboo*. http://www.tacklementalhealth.org.uk/assets/documents/ mental_health_report_2010.pdf

Stefan, S. (2002). *Hollow promises: Employment discrimination against people with mental disabilities*. American Psychological Association.

Stuart, H. (2004). Stigma and work. *HealthcarePapers, 5*, 100–111. https://doi.org/10.12927/hcpap.16829

Stuart, H. (2006). Mental illness and employment discrimination. *Current Opinion in Psychiatry, 19*(5), 522–526. https://journals.lww.com/co-psychiatry/Fulltext/2006/09000/Mental_illness_and_employment_discrimination.14.aspx

Stuart, H., Chen, S.-P., Christie, R., Dobson, K., Kirsh, B., Knaak, S., Koller, M., Krupa, T., Lauria-Horner, B., Luong, D., Modgill, G., Patten, S. B., Pietrus, M., Szeto, A., & Whitley, R. (2014). Opening Minds in Canada: Targeting change. *Canadian Journal of Psychiatry. Revue canadienne de psychiatrie, 59*(10, Suppl. 1), S13–S18. https://doi.org/10.1177/070674371405901s05

Szeto, A., Dobson, K. S., Luong, D., Krupa, T., & Kirsh, B. (2019). Workplace antistigma programs at the Mental Health Commission of Canada: Part 1. Processes and projects. *Canadian Journal of Psychiatry. Revue canadienne de psychiatrie, 64*(1 Suppl.), 5S–12S. https://doi.org/10.1177/0706743719842557

Szeto, A. C. H., & Dobson, K. S. (2010). Reducing the stigma of mental disorders at work: A review of current workplace anti-stigma intervention programs. *Applied and Preventive Psychology, 14*(1), 41–56. https://doi.org/10.1016/j.appsy.2011.11.002

Trautmann, S., Rehm, J., & Wittchen, H.-U. (2016). The economic costs of mental disorders: Do our societies react appropriately to the burden of mental disorders? *EMBO Reports, 17*(9), 1245–1249. https://doi.org/10.15252/embr.201642951

Walton, L. (2003). Exploration of the attitudes of employees towards the provision of counselling within a profit-making organisation. *Counselling and Psychotherapy Research, 3*(1), 65–71. https://doi.org/10.1080/14733140312331384658

World Health Organization. (2001). *The world health report: 2001: Mental health: New understanding, new hope*.

12

Reducing the Stigma of Mental Illness in First Responders

Beth Milliard

The first responder profession, defined here as including police officers, firefighters, and emergency medical services, attracts individuals who want to help others. In the community's eyes, first responders are often seen as brave, fearless, and, in some cases, superhuman because someone who chooses to be a first responder after knowing the risks associated with the profession is truly altruistic. However, for some first responders, the toll of the profession can be physically demanding and emotionally draining and can lead to a range of mental health problems. While a common belief is that first responders predominantly experience post–traumatic stress disorder (PTSD), this is not the most prevalent condition. In addition to PTSD, first responders also suffer from anxiety and depression, which can sometimes lead to a substance use disorder (Heffren & Hausdorf, 2016).

Mental health issues may not be solely a product of the traumatic incidents seen by first responders. Their jobs are complex, with a myriad of organizational, operational, and personal stressors that can lead to mental health challenges. In general, first responders are aware of the nature of the job and are very resilient. However, first responders are often affected by cumulative stress that builds up over the years. Cumulative stress is ongoing stress that builds layer upon layer, like a brick wall, until eventually the layers of that wall crack. When the layers crack, it is a warning sign that first responders need to seek help. However, in most cases the warnings signs are not addressed. Instead of seeking professional help, first responders often try to deal with the stress themselves. There are many reasons why first responders do not get help, but the most prominent one is the stigma associated with mental illness and how people with mental health issues are treated.

This chapter discusses the stigma associated with mental health issues by first responders. Stigma is defined as the negative attitudes and/or discrimination toward someone based on that person being diagnosed with a mental illness. Self-stigma involves the thoughts someone feels when they have a mental health diagnosis and becomes aware of public stigma, agrees with and internalizes those thoughts, and applies them to oneself. This chapter also describes programs and initiatives that address mental wellness and stigma reduction in the first responder community.

Why Does Stigma Persist?

While mental health education and awareness have made huge strides in the second decade of the 21st century, stigma is alive and well for first responders. A large percentage of the research regarding help seeking and first responders points to the stigma associated with mental illness. It remains taboo for first responders to openly talk about their depression or that they experience anxiety that sometimes causes panic attacks. *Stigma* (plural, stigmata) is a "Greek word that in its origins referred to a kind of tattoo mark that was cut or burned into the skin of criminals, slaves, or traitors in order to visibly identify them as blemished or morally polluted persons" (Encyclopedia.com, 2019, para. 1). Further, these individuals were to be ignored and were treated as outcasts in public places. The word stigma was then later applied to other personal attributes that are considered shameful. For first responders this means suffering in silence and trying to self-manage or live in denial for fear of being labeled or branded by supervisors, coworkers, and even family as weak, lazy, or unable to do their job.

Karaffa and Tochkov (2013) observed that the stigma associated with seeking out mental health services among police officers is correlated. For example, Karaffa et al. (2015) reported that police officers often underestimate their coworkers' willingness to seek mental health services for a variety of mental health issues. The difference in stigma among police officers and the general public regarding the discussion or reporting of mental health issues is potentially a result of the nature of police work as a career. For instance, an officer who seeks help for a mental health–related issue may lose out on a promotion, be forced into administrative duty, or have their firearm confiscated, which may also mean a loss of status (Crowe et al., 2015). Watson and Andrews (2018) found that the greatest barrier to officers reaching out for help is the potential harm it may cause to their career, as well as a fear that their coworkers will lose confidence, and therefore trust, in them. This is also tied in to organizational stigma. White et al.'s (2015) research with juvenile probation officers indicated that those who suffered burnout as a result of their profession also stigmatized mental health treatment and support.

Crowe et al. (2015) found that disbelief, discrimination, and shame were prevalent among the general population and first responders when self-reporting on mental health issues and that people do not come forward out of fear that others will think they are "faking it" because mental illnesses cannot be seen. For first responders,

> seeking help for mental health issues may lead others to perceive them as not pulling their weight, dodging calls, or not being a team player. Significantly, first responders associated shame with admitting that they are suffering and need help, and they associated discrimination with a fear of being treated differently by co-workers. (Milliard, 2020, p. 32)

These fears are justified because mental health issues are often perceived as representing weakness and unreliability, which is antithetical to a culture that covets strength, steadfastness, and commitment to performing one's duty (Bullock & Garland, 2017). These stereotypes can cause first responders to lose status among their coworkers and have their abilities to do the job called into question, which can be detrimental.

It is unfortunate that police are the first responders for the majority of mental health–related calls in Ontario, Canada, because this call pattern can result in the person being apprehended under the provincial Mental Health Act. Because people with mental health issues may be stereotyped as being violent and dangerous (Iacobucci, 2014), mental health issues are often associated with criminality, which results in the police being called to deal with these situations (Marzano et al., 2016). Again, these beliefs and attitudes also feed into the stigma around mental health–related issues that prevent police officers from seeking help. Only recently has mental health training and education outlining the differences between mental health issues, mental illnesses, and mental disorders for first responders been explored.

Self-stigma develops when people start to believe the negative viewpoints of others in relation to mental health and then project those views and opinions onto themselves. Self-stigma is even more problematic than public stigma. It is important to recognize and educate people about self-stigma because it is a huge barrier to care. Specifically, in the first responder community, it is harder to come forward when working in an environment that is full of judgment or if it is perceived that there is a lack of support from coworkers and supervisors.

Approaches to Mental Wellness and Stigma Reduction Based on Evidence

Over the years, first responders have looked for ways to improve mental wellness and help alleviate the stigma associated with mental illness. The next sections review some of the ways that this issue has been addressed through the following: choosing a mental health champion(s) (MHC), the implementation of Project Safeguard, creation of peer support, equine therapy, introducing and following up with the Working Mind for First Responders and Family program, and the HEROES project and the warr;or21 program. All of these programs have been studied and each provides evidence-based results that, if implemented properly, will help alleviate the stigma associated with mental health problems and mental illness diagnosis among first responders.

Creating Mental Health Champions

One of the key elements of organizational change for most first responder groups is to select one or more mental health champions (MHCs). MHCs are not only educated about the signs and symptoms of mental health, but also able to support and instruct others through their passion and their own lived experience. Mental health education is different from the other courses that first responders attend; it is much more than standing in front of a class and teaching from a deck of presentation slides. Instead, MHCs need to "sell" the importance of mental health and how it involves every facet of the lives of first responders and the public that they serve.

The greatest motivation for first responders is to help people, so it is not uncommon for people to want to be MHCs, especially when this role provides the opportunity to help the people with whom they work. In my experience as a police officer and creating and implementing a peer support program at my organization, MHCs should have some type of lived experience related to mental health, which can include both direct and indirect experience. Direct experience means that the person has lived through a mental illness or has indirect experience with a mental health issue with a family member or coworker or through their profession. When looking at the scope of the lived experience as a first responder, it would be difficult to find someone who does not fit this criterion. However, the key is how they manage their direct or indirect experiences and their level of resiliency. It also means that MHCs are self-aware, they are able to manage their emotions, and they are able to identify where they fall on the mental health continuum. The mental health continuum uses a

"color-coded (green, yellow, orange, red) figure, to increase mental health literacy; a bidirectional arrow in the MHCM captures movement along the continuum, indicating that there is always the possibility for a return to full health and functioning; behavioral indicators under each color category in the MHCM familiarize first responders with basic mental health and mental illness concepts." (Fikretoglu, Liu, Nazarov, Blacker, 2019, p. 3)

When looking at the mental health continuum model, many first responders speak about physical issues and injuries without even knowing that they could be related to mental health concerns. Specifically, first responders dismiss their symptoms of lack of interest, irritability, isolation, headaches, and stomach issues as a result of working shift work. Therefore, to yield optimal success, self-awareness is a key component of a MHC.

MHCs are not required to have a degree in psychology, but they must know the general signs and symptoms of good, declining, and poor mental health. MHCs will possess the drive and passion to push the envelope and think outside the box, especially in first responder organizations where stigma is still prevalent. MHCs are responsible for setting the foundation and encouraging conversation when it comes understanding and supporting others with mental health issues. Last, MHCs should ensure that they do their homework by researching new training and technology and creating important contacts and partnerships to encourage employees' psychological wellness.

Another area where people can become MHCs is when key leaders in an organization talk about the importance of mental health or even share their own stories. For example, the International Association of Chiefs of Police (2014) report explains, "Hearing from the chief personally and candidly carries a tremendous amount of weight. In particular, police chiefs or others who have triumphed over their own mental health issues should champion this subject and share their own success stories" (para. 5).

MHCs in first responder organizations must ensure they are creating external partnerships that will help provide options for members because mental health issues are complex and require more than one solution. Because of the stigma, first responders often try to manage their symptoms on their own, and by the time they finally come forward and ask for help, their level of treatment is more complicated. The role of the MHCs is to create those key relationships in the community, which includes mental health professionals, inpatient and outpatient treatment centers, addiction facilities and groups, faith-based healing, and other supports, which could include equine therapy, group counseling, and peer support.

According to the Government of Canada (2019), MHCs must be the face of the vision, engage unions and employees at all levels, and raise awareness of the importance of psychological health and safety. Together with other organizational leaders, MHCs are responsible to

> develop and ensure the sustainability of a psychologically healthy and safe workplace, establish key objectives toward continual improvement of psychological health and safety in the workplace; and ensure that psychological health and safety are part of all organizational decision-making processes. (Government of Canada, 2019, para. 4)

Organizations need to choose MHCs who are passionate and credible. As such, the process of picking a MHC must be methodical and strategic, especially when first starting up any mental health program, initiative, or unit in an organization. As with any company starting a new venture, it is important to ensure that key people occupy these critical positions. If an organization does not carefully select its MHCs, the credibility of the program or the intentions of the organization can be damaged. For example, if the effort is to provide a quick fix or to prove that the organization is doing "something," a single person is often assigned to oversee this set of activities or the huge undertaking is given to person at a high management/leadership level who is already overtaxed. The proper selection of champions and ensuring they have the resources to fulfill the role they take on are critical.

Project Safeguard

Project Safeguard originated in the FBI in the early 1980s as a program to psychologically assess and support undercover officers (Krause, 2009). The premise of the program is that an employer could potentially be putting employees in positions that could make them psychologically vulnerable. Although this could be said about all aspects of the first responder profession, there are roles specific to policing that put individuals at risk of psychological harm more than other positions.

One of the units that has gained the most attention since the beginning of the 21st century has been the Internet Child Exploitation Unit (Milliard, 2010). Originally, investigations involving children fell under child abuse or crimes against children. However, with the rapid increase of technology, explicit photos of young children that were once developed at a local camera shop quickly changed to images of children exposed in video and on the Dark Web. As a result, many new laws regarding crimes such as luring and child exploitation have been created, and more police officers are required to conduct these horrific investigations.

Research conducted specifically with the York Regional Police Internet Child Exploitation Unit in 2010 indicated that all of the officers involved were affected by the nature of their work (Milliard, 2010). In addition to the time spent reviewing and cataloging images and videos, investigators mentioned other hazardous aspects of their work that could affect them physically or mentally. Specifically, they spoke about the moral injury of conducting these types of investigations. Moral injury is a type of response that may emerge after engaging in or witnessing behaviors that are contrary to an individual's values and moral beliefs. Situations that result in moral injury include investigations of children who were physically and sexually abused over many years. In such cases, police officers may feel moral injury if they cannot locate the victim, learn that the suspect is related to the victim or is a person who is in a position of trust or authority, or finally arrest a suspect but discover that when the case gets to court, the accused person is only given probation or the charges are withdrawn (Milliard, 2010).

Because of these factors, a high percentage of investigators experience compassion fatigue, anxiety, depression, or PTSD. Police organizations have started using safeguard measures to ensure the suitability and longevity of investigators in these units. As one example, Project Safeguard starts with a psychological assessment to establish a baseline for the member. This assessment is followed by an interview with a clinical psychologist to help to ensure the candidate's psychological fitness for high-stress jobs and to ensure they are not entering a stressful position if they are already struggling with mental health issues. As we have stated, police officers may not be aware they are having issues or dismiss their concerns because they are in denial. The initial assessment allows the psychologist to explain the findings and educate the members on the nature of the job. It is also a time to talk about the physiology of stress and to explore the officer's level of support, their resilience, and their motivations for entering high-risk units.

Project Safeguard has been instrumental in breaking down the resistance to speaking with a mental health professional. Similar to seeking regular medical and dental check-ups, Project Safeguard opened the door to allowing police officers to speak to a psychologist as part of their job assignment. In my organization, police officers explained that Project Safeguard is just a requirement of the job assignment; for the majority of police officers, having this support and knowing they could speak to a psychologist at any time before their yearly follow-up makes a huge difference in how officers deal with the stressors of their job.

Peer Support

A large percentage of first responders are reluctant to admit they need mental health support. As a result, many are forced to suffer in silence, which, in the extreme, may even lead them take their own lives. Stuart's (2017) research supports the importance of including "anti-stigma training as a means of creating a supportive work environment, improving the psychological health and wellness of police officers, and promoting help seeking" (p. 22), and the creation of peer support programs is a strategy that has been adopted by first responder organizations to break down the stigma associated with mental health–related issues. For example, first responders in Ontario, Canada, have created peer support teams to provide their members with mental health support in the last decade.

Peer support programs provide first responders with an opportunity to share their experiences with other first responders, which is important because first responders are perhaps best able to relate to their colleagues' experiences. Peer support has been widely accepted as a confidential outlet for first responders to speak free from judgment and a means of sharing private information. It is critical to promote the idea that first responders are not alone and that there is no shame attached to help seeking. The premise of peer support is coworkers or colleagues talking about aspects of the job, family, or other issues that may affect their well-being. However, peer support in first responder organizations has proven to be crucial because of the stigma associated with mental health concerns. First responders often talk to coworkers before reaching out to a psychologist because they may feel comfortable and more at ease sharing with people who have similar experiences and understand the nature of the job and the culture. The main goals of peer support are to provide an empathic, listening ear; to provide low-level psychological intervention; to identify peers who may be at risk to themselves or others; and to facilitate a conduit for professional help (Milliard, 2020, p. 1).

Peer support has been implemented in first responder organizations in the United States and abroad for decades. The main objective of a peer support program is to resolve employee and workplace problems before they escalate to crisis levels by providing an extra network of support in the workplace (Wallace, 2016). However, peer support programs have only really taken off in police services in Canada since 2016. One of the main reasons for this change is that two Ontario ombudsman's investigations for police and emergency medical services mentioned the importance of the creation and maintenance of peer support programs for first responders. A study was conducted on the effectiveness of peer support in police organizations on the overall mental health of police officers (Milliard, 2020). The results indicated that peer support is more than just a conversation. The two most prevalent findings were that peer support increased mental health literacy and decreased the attitudinal stigma associated with mental illness. For example, police officers explained that by sharing their mental health concerns with someone who understood and could relate, the officers were able to reach out for help from a mental health professional without feeling ashamed and judged.

Mental health literacy is the ability to understand the difference between mental health disorders and mental health issues, the importance of early treatment, the definition of stigma and how it relates to mental health, and how to develop competencies to improve mental health (Kutcher et al., 2016). Mental health literacy among police officers had been improved through education about the differences between good, declining, and poor mental health; education about the differences between mental health issues and mental disorders; and the various sources of stress for police officers. This education is important because there is a misconception that most police stress comes from attending traumatic incidents. All participants agreed that mental health education, which includes resources and support for members after traumatic incidents, was minimal and support and resources for their families were nonexistent prior to the establishment of the peer support program (Milliard, 2020).

The stigma associated with mental health is alive and well throughout society, but it is even more prevalent for first responders. People do not want to come forward for fear of being labeled. However, many participants reported that the creation of peer support programs was effective in decreasing the stigma surrounding mental health and making officers feel more comfortable seeking help (Milliard, 2020). In addition, stigma reduction in peer support programs included the degree to which peer support team members were seen as credible and trustworthy within the organization. For example, the idea of peer support is strengthened by the peers' perceived credibility as a result of their lived experience, which in turn makes them trustworthy, and hence, peers are more likely to reach out for help. Indeed, the information gathered through the interviews indicated that one cannot provide high-quality peer support to a member who has been involved in a police shooting if they have not gone through the same experience themselves (Milliard, 2020).

Peer support should be supplementary to other educational or awareness programs at any first responder organization. In addition, peer supporters must be carefully selected and should adhere to Project Safeguard or a similar psychological assessment component and additional follow-up. Peer supporters must be credible and, most of all, must have some direct or indirect lived experience. Peer support is not a substitute for professional mental health treatment, and although the International Association of Chiefs of Police and the Mental Health Commission of Canada provide guidelines for peer support, official standards have yet to be developed. Therefore, having a MHC that can navigate and take a leadership role in creating and maintaining a peer support program is important to its success.

The Working Mind for First Responders

In 2013, the Mental Health Commission of Canada teamed up with the Calgary Police Service and took the Road to Mental Readiness course, which was originally developed for the Department of Defense and recreated for police (Szeto et al., 2019). The course was piloted in Ontario in 2014 at York Regional Police and subsequently adopted at the Ontario Police College for new recruits; it was then expanded across all first responder communities. The Mental Health Commission of Canada changed the name from Road to Mental Readiness to the Working Mind for First Responders in 2019. Although some of the work cited here was done prior to the name change, this chapter refers to the Working Mind for First Responders for the sake of consistency.

The results indicated that the Working Mind for First Responders was "effective at reducing the stigma of mental illness and increasing resiliency skills after program implementation in participants across 16 different sites and in 5 different first-responder groups" (Szeto et al., 2019, p. 3). Two of the main objectives of the course are stigma reduction and reduced barriers to care. First responders talk about the nature of stigma, why it exists in first responder organizations, and what organizations can do to help alleviate it. When York Regional Police rolled out the mandatory training in 2015, they received permission from the Mental Health Commission of Canada to create their own member videos. Eleven members (sworn and civilian) told their stories regarding a mental health issue and what they did to get through their experience. These videos were pivotal in breaking down the stigma because they showed that mental health can affect anyone at any time and that support at work and at home can make a real difference in recovery.

Evidence-based and results-driven training is often missing in first responder training. Training may be implemented with good intentions but have limited follow through. When the Working Mind for First Responders program was rolled out across Canada, its effectiveness was studied by researchers at the University of Calgary. The results indicated that the program was successful in achieving its main course objectives. Participants reported "fewer stigmatizing attitudes towards those with mental health illnesses and felt more prepared to handle stressful and traumatic events in their workplace" (Szeto et al., 2019, p. 9).

In addition to reducing stigmatizing attitudes, the program also yielded statistically significant increases in self-reported resiliency. For example,

> well over half (59.2%) of the respondents reported at follow-up that they had actively used the skills learned in the program. Of those, 62.4% said they had used at least one of the "Big 4" coping skills before the 3-month follow-up. Furthermore, 14% of the follow-up respondents had used what they learned in the program to support someone else's mental health, and 6.3% had sought professional help or helped a co-worker seek help because of the program. (Szeto et al., 2019, p. 10)

In addition to reducing negative attitudes and improving resiliency, the programs also helped generate conversation, potentially promoting a shift in the organizational culture if other key factors were in place. These factors included "organizational readiness, strong leadership support and support from organizational champions, ensuring good group dynamics, credibility of the trainers, implementing widely and thoroughly, and implementing [the program] as one piece of a larger puzzle" (Knaak et al., 2019, p. 36).

Finally, in addition to teaching members in the first responder organization, it is also important to include family members. Family members are essentially the "first responders to the first responders." Issues may arise when first responders shut down and isolate themselves from loved ones. Family members who are not educated on the signs and symptoms of mental health problems may dismiss these key indicators or think they are indicative of bad behavior. To address this concern, the Mental Health Commission of Canada also created a family version of the Working Mind for First Responders program. This 2.5-hour educational resource is offered to family members who are 18 years old and older. The main objectives are to "identify how workplace stigma cultures can impact family mental health, apply the mental health continuum model and to use the mental health continuum model to open a constructive dialogue about mental health with family members" (Mental Health Commission of Canada, 2019, para. 3).

Equine-Assisted Therapy

One way to alleviate the stigma related to first responders and seeking help for mental health issues is to look at other forms of therapy. According to Romaniuk et al. (2018), there has been a "growing interest in adjunct therapy interventions which can be considered a part of the various interventions that may be useful in the management of mental health issues such as PTSD which is equine assisted therapy" (p. 2). Equine-assisted therapy (EAT) has been used with diverse clients, including victims of violence, troubled teenagers, and children with autism. EAT incorporates horses into the therapeutic process as people engage in activities such as grooming, feeding, and leading a horse while being supervised by a mental health professional.

The goals of EAT include the development of emotional awareness skills, social skills, impulse control, confidence, trust and empathy, and problem-solving skills. According to Gehrke et al. (2018), early research in equine-assisted interventions for PTSD showed a marked improvement in each of the symptom domains, including relationship skills, self-regulation, and a decrease in hyperarousal. Based on such results, since the second decade of the 21st century EAT has become an option for military members and their families and, more recently, for first responders with PTSD, operational stress injuries, and other mental health–related issues. Research has found that EAT uses mainstream psychological theories to explain the horse–human bond that can produce effects through mind, body, emotional, and/or spiritual healing. In particular, "the basic premises suggested that moving beyond the self connects an individual to expansive and more meaningful life experiences. These life experiences may include working with non-humans to assist healing and growth of an individual in EAT" (Wara-Goss, 2020, p. 78). Further, studies have shown that analyses of a couples EAT program for veterans indicated that "symptoms of depression, stress, and PTSD significantly reduced by the conclusion of the program and this reduction remained three months later" (Romaniuk et al., 2018, pp. 9 and 10). The analysis also demonstrated "a gradual reduction in anxiety symptoms from pre-intervention resulting in a significant reduction at the three month follow-up point and participants' self-reported happiness and quality of life significantly increased from the beginning to the conclusion of the program" (Romaniuk et al., 2018, p. 10).

Can Praxis is an EAT program that has been successful with military, police, emergency personnel, and fire services since 2013 (Can Praxis, 2019). Can Praxis is a national mental health provider offering intensive treatment programs for Canadian veterans and first responders (serving and retired) living with an operational stress injury, such as PTSD. Can Praxis consists of three phases, and after the initial program, a social network is set up with participants to ensure ongoing support after returning home. The injured person's spouse/partner/family member is included in the program because operational stress injuries have a profound impact on the entire family. In addition to working with horses, the 3-day retreat includes classroom education on communication skills for both the member and a loved one.

According to Can Praxis (2019), horses are incorporated into their programs because they understand us and can teach us about ourselves. They are experts at reading body language and pick up on all the nonverbal cues we bring to every interaction. Horses

> understand chain-of-command and are hyper-aware, always looking for an exit. As "flight" animals, they react to the body language of humans in their proximity. Our facilitators offer a translation of the horses' behaviour when interacting with participants individually, as a means to increase the level of self-awareness. (Can Praxis, 2019, para. 5)

The HEROES Project

No antistigma education or mental health program can be implemented in first responder organizations without acknowledging the issue of suicide. The rate of suicide among first responders has increased exponentially in recent years, and although definitive statistics are hard to obtain, research on first responder suicide in 2017 in the United States suggested that police officers and firefighters are more likely to die by suicide than in the line of duty (Heyman et al., 2018). Suicide prevention research strongly encourages measures to decrease mental disorders and to enhance psychological resilience to effectively inoculate the brain against the devastating effects of trauma (Rabon et al., 2019).

One broad-based training program introduced in the United States is the HEROES Project. The HEROES Project is a 6-week online course "that combines the therapeutic tools of clinical and organizational psychology and provides first responders access to a self-driven well being program" (Thornton et al., 2020, p. 155). The theme for each of the six sessions corresponds to the letters in the title: hope, efficacy, resilience, optimism, empathy, and socialization, and the course utilizes active-learning techniques and provides participants with a number of strategies (Thornton et al., 2020).

The HEROES Project sampled first responders (police and firefighters) from the U.S. Midwest to participate in the project. The results showed that participants with higher distress and lower psychological resources before the training benefited most from the HEROES Project, but that "the training significantly improved psychological capital and reduced stress, depression, anxiety, and trauma symptoms for all participants" (Thornton et al., 2019, p. 2). Most important,

> the psychological skills training program endured through the two-year assessment point and there was some indication that participants continued to improve past the conclusion of the program and that the skills developed during the six-week training were utilized long after participants ended the program. (Thornton et al., 2020, p. 12)

Warr;or21

The warr;or21 program is a "21-day set of various practices developed based on previous research that seeks to achieve positive outcomes of increasing first responders' inner strength, enhancing their resiliency, and in turn, increasing their positive mental health" (Thompson & Drew, 2020, p. 3). The program emphasizes four pillars of resilience: awareness, wellness, purpose, and positivity. These pillars of resilience are based on neuroscience and include the following:

> awareness: understanding the basics of psychology and its impact on the first responder's daily life, as well as controlled breathing practices; wellness: mental and physical health, as both are profoundly connected to each other in relation to developing inner strength and overall positive mental health, purpose: possessing specific goals for the self and goals that serve a greater good and positivity: having a positive outlook and relationships, having realistic optimism, and expressing gratitude. (Thompson et al., 2020, p. 4)

The results of the warr;or21 program have been reported to be very positive. A large percentage of participants reported it had met or exceeded their expectations and would recommend the course to others. The specific activities, including breathing and gratitude exercises, were reported to be useful for participants. Perhaps most important, "the majority of participants indicated that they intended to keep using the strategies that they had learned during the program and that the program has most impact on feelings of calmness and gratitude" (Thompson et al., 2020, p. 15).

Replication of the program's results and longer term evaluations are clearly warranted based on the positive early reports.

Conclusions

Mental health awareness, training, and education for first responders has come a long way in the early 21st century. Unfortunately, a stigma still exists among first responders, which prevents them from seeking help. Fearing how they will be treated if they come forward, they often choose to manage their mental health issues themselves. Fortunately, many supports and programs have been implemented across first responder organizations. The stigma among first responders will not go away overnight, but if organizations continue to make mental health a priority and implement proactive mental health programs and leadership training, stigma can be reduced. The MHCs in each organization will be called on to discern what is best for their members, because no single approach will fit all groups. Antistigma programming and education will depend on the size of the organization, geographical location, budget, and availability of resources. Last, mental health programmers will have to be creative and may need to lean on neighboring first responder organizations or external partnerships to promote or implement novel mental health programs.

Key Considerations

Some key recommendations for first responder organizations derive from the information presented in this chapter. These ideas are supplemented by ideas based on the author's 20 years of experience as a first responder:

- Mandatory mental health education: There is an abundance of training and recertification training for first responders. Education and training for mental health should be included in the list of yearly or biyearly mandatory training. Training should include resiliency skills, the mental health continuum, stigma reduction, and suicide prevention and awareness.
- Creation of an internal policy on mental health: First responder organizations should create a policy related to mental health. This policy should set the tone and solidify the chief and organization's stance on mental health and its importance.
- Creation of a robust peer support program: First responder organizations are encouraged to develop peer support programs, with credible peers with indirect and direct experience, to assist other first responders as early as possible with any concerns.
- Introducing mental health professionals into first responder organizations: A great way for first responders to understand the role of mental health

professionals, and how they can help first responders, is to bring mental health professionals to education and training programs, send them on ride-alongs, and have them assist after traumatic events.

- Picking MHCs: First responder organizations need people in the organization to ensure mental health programming, initiatives, and supports are implemented. Depending on the size and nature of the organization, the required resources must be provided to enhance to the mental wellness of first responders.
- Encourage seeing a mental health professional early: One of the ways to minimize the stigma associated with mental illness is to see a mental health professional when a first responder is in good mental health. Similar to the promotion of dental or physical hygiene, first responders should be encouraged to see a mental health professional early and throughout their career to stay mentally well across its many stages.

References

Blumberg, D., Girominin, L., Papazogou, K., & Thornton, R. (2019). Impact of the HEROES project on first responders' wellbeing. *Journal of Community Safety and Well-Being, 5*(1). https://doi.org/10.35502/jcswb.116

Bullock, K., & Garland, J. (2017). Police officers, mental (ill-) health and spoiled identity. *Criminology & Criminal Justice, 18*(2), 173–189. https://doi.org/10.1177/1748895817695856

Can Praxis. (2019). *Can Praxis—Veterans, PTSD, horses*. https://crackmacs.ca/guest-blog-posts/can-praxis/

Crowe, A., Glass, S., Lancaster, M., Raines, J., & Waggy, M. (2015). Mental illness stigma among first responders and the general population. *Journal of Military and Government Counseling, 3*(3), 132–228. http://acegonline.org/wp-content/uploads/2013/02/JMGC-Vol-3-Is-3.pdf#page=5

Encylopedia.com. (2020). Stigma. https://www.encyclopedia.com/plants-and-animals/botany/botany-general/stigma

Fikretoglu, D., Liu, A., Nazarov, A., & Blacker, K. (2019). A group randomized control trial to test the efficacy of the Road to Mental Readiness (R2MR) program among Canadian military recruits. *BMC Psychiatry, 19*, 326. https://doi.org/10.1186/s12888-019-2287-0

Gehrke, E. K., Tontz, P., Bhawal, R., Schiltz, P., Mendez, S., & Myers, M. P. (2018). A mixed-method analysis of an equine complementary therapy program to heal combat veterans. *Journal of Complementary Medicine and Alternative Healthcare, 8*(3), 555739.

Government of Canada. (2019). *Role and definition of a workplace mental health champion*. https://www.canada.ca/en/government/publicservice/wellness-inclusion-diversity-public-service/health-wellness-public-servants/mental-health-workplace/resources-organizations/role-definition-workplace-mental-health-champions.html

Heffren, C. D., & Hausdorf, P. A. (2016). Post-traumatic effects in policing: Perceptions, stigmas and help seeking behaviours. *Police Practice and Research, 17*(5), 420–433. https://doi.org/10.1080/15614263.2014.958488

Heyman, M., Dill, J., & Douglas, R. (2018). *The Ruderman white paper on mental health and suicide of first responders*. Ruderman Family Foundation. https://rudermanfoundation.org/white_papers/police-officers-and-firefighters-are-more-likely-to-die-by-suicide-than-in-line-of-duty/.

Iacobucci, F. (2014). *Police encounters with people in crisis: An independent review for the Toronto Police Service.* https://www.torontopolice.on.ca/publications/files/reports/police_encounters_with_people_in_crisis_2014.pdf

InternationalAssociationofChiefsofPolice.(2014).*IACPNationalSymposiumonLawEnforcement Officer Suicide and Mental Health: Breaking the silence on law enforcement suicides.* Office of Community Oriented Policing Services. https://www.theiacp.org/resources/document/iacp-national-symposium-on-law-enforcement-officer-suicide-and-mental-health

Karaffa, K., Openshaw, L., Koch, J., Clark, H., Harr, C., & Stewart, C. (2015). Perceived impact of police work on marital relationships. *The Family Journal, 23*(2), 120–131. https://doi.org/10.1177/1066480714564381

Karaffa, K. M., & Tochkov, K. (2013). Attitudes toward seeking mental health treatment among law enforcement officers. *Applied Psychology in Criminal Justice, 9*(2), 75–99.

Knaak, S., Luong, D., McLean, R., Szeto, A., & Dobson, K. (2019). Implementation, uptake, and culture change: Results of a key informant study of a workplace mental health training program in police organizations in Canada. *The Canadian Journal of Psychiatry, 1–9.* https://doi.org/10.1177/0706743719842565

Krause, M. (2009). History and evolution of the FBI's undercover safeguard program. *Consulting Psychology Journal: Practice and Research, 61*(1), 5–13. https://doi.org/10.1037/a0015280

Kutcher, S., Wei, Y., & Coniglio, C. (2016). Mental health literacy: Past, present, and future. *The Canadian Journal of Psychiatry, 61*(3), 154–158. https://doi.org/10.1177/0706743715616609.

Marzano, L., Smith, M., Long, M., Kisby, C., & Hawton, K. (2016). Police and suicide prevention: Evaluation of a training program. *Crisis: The Journal of Crisis Intervention and Suicide Prevention, 37*(3), 194–204. https://doi-org.ezp.waldenulibrary.org/10.1027/0227-5910/a000381

Mental Health Commission of Canada. (2019). *The Working Mind First Responders family package.* https://theworkingmind.ca/working-mind-first-responders-family-package

Milliard, B. (2010). *Project S.A.F.E.T.Y.: A leadership strategy for promoting the psychological well-being of police officers* [Unpublished master's thesis]. University of Guelph.

Milliard, B. (2020). Utilization and impact of peer-support programs on police officers' mental health. *Frontiers in Psychology, 11,* 1686. https://doi.org/10.3389/fpsyg.2020.01686

Rabon, J. K., Hirsch, J. K., & Chang, E. C. (2019). Positive psychology and suicide prevention: An introduction and overview of the literature. In J. Hirsch, E. Chang, & J. K. Rabon (Eds.), *A positive psychological approach to suicide. Advances in mental health and addiction* (pp. 1–15) Springer. https://doi.org/10.1007/978-3-030-03225-8_1

Romaniuk, M., Evans, J., & Kidd, C. (2018). Evaluation of an equine-assisted therapy program for veterans who identify as "wounded, injured or ill" and their partners. *PLoS ONE, 13*(9), e0203943. https://doi.org/10.1371/journal.pone.0203943

Stuart, H. (2017). Mental illness stigma expressed by police to police. *The Israel Journal of Psychiatry and Related Sciences, 54*(1), 18–23. https://cdn.doctorsonly.co.il/2017/08/04_Mental-Illness-Stigma.pdf

Szeto, A., Dobson, K., & Knaak, S. (2019). The Road to Mental Readiness for first responders: A meta-analysis of program outcomes. *The Canadian Journal of Psychiatry. Revue canadienne de psychiatrie, 64*(1 Suppl.), 18S–29S. https://doi.org/10.1177/0706743719842562

Thompson, J., & Drew, J. (2020). Warr;or21: A 21-day program to enhance first responder resilience and mental health. *Frontiers of Psychology, 11,* 02078. https://doi.org/10.3389/fpsyg.2020.02078

Thornton, A. R., Blumberg, D. M., Papazoglou, K., & Gironimi, L. (2020). The HEROES Project: Building mental resilience in first responders. In C. A. Bowers, D. C. Beidel, & M. R. Marks (Eds.). *Mental Health Intervention and Treatment of First Responders and Emergency Workers.* Hershey, Pennsylvania, IGI Global. (pp. 154–168).

Wallace, J. R. (2016). Field test of a peer support pilot project serving federal employees deployed to a major disaster. *Social Work and Christianity, 43*, 127–141.

Wara-Goss, R. (2020). *Horses healing the wounded warrior: A qualitative inquiry of equine-facilitated psychotherapy in treating posttraumatic stress disorder for female veterans* [PhD dissertation, California Institute of Integral Studies]. https://habricentral.org/resources/69100/download/Rebecca_Wara-Goss_Dissertation_HORSES_HEALING_THE_WOUNDED_WARRIOR_2020.pdf

Watson, L., & Andrews, L. (2018). The effect of a trauma risk management (TRiM) program on stigma and barriers to help-seeking in the police. *International Journal of Stress Management, 25*(4), 348–356. https://doi.org/10.1037/str0000071

White, L. M., Aalsma, M. C., Holloway, E. D., Adams, E. L., & Salyers, M. P. (2015). Job-related burnout among juvenile probation officers: Implications for mental health stigma and competency. *Psychological Services, 12*(3), 291–302. https://doi-org.ezp.waldenulibrary.org/10.1037/ser0000031

13

Stigma Reduction for Healthcare Workers

Bianca Lauria-Horner

According to the World Health Organization (WHO), mental illness is becoming the number one cause of years lived with disability worldwide (Murray et al., 2015). The direct and indirect cost of mental illness was estimated at US$2.5 trillion in 2010, and the World Economic Forum expects this amount will double by 2030 (Trautmann et al., 2016). Depression, one of the most prevalent and costly conditions in our society, affects over 400 million people globally and ranks as the single largest contributor to global disability, at 7.5% of all years lived with disability in 2015 (World Health Organization, 2017). When mental illness co-occurs with other chronic medical conditions, there is a higher morbidity and cost to the healthcare system (Naylor, 2013; Statistics Canada, 2015).

In recent years, the integration of mental health in primary care has become an area of focus. According to the WHO (2008), "Primary healthcare providers are often the first point of contact," and while a certain percentage of the population could benefit from specialized treatment, the vast majority can be handled early and effectively in this setting. By increasing quality of care capacity at the primary care level, persons with lived experiences (PWLE) can receive prompt and effective evidence-based interventions where they have established trust (Mickus et al., 2000). Healthcare providers (HCPs) become part of the care network, reducing the number of referrals to specialty services and wait times to obtain care, even as they promote cost-effective, person-centered care (Crowley et al., 2015; Kauye et al., 2014).

Numerous training programs have been developed to improve the detection and management of mental illness. Despite these efforts, most educational programs do not translate into changes in practice or impact HCPs' attitudes toward mental illness (Kalet et al., 2010; Sikorski et al., 2012). Mental illnesses are frequently underrecognized, and even when a diagnosis is made, less than 20% of PWLE receive adequate treatment (Mulsant et al., 2003). For example, family physicians commonly prescribe antidepressants (Kendrick et al., 2005) that are not necessarily associated with improved long-term outcomes in mild/moderate cases (Fournier et al., 2010; Kirsch et al., 2008). Cognitive behavior therapy in these clients may have an enduring effect with lower rates of relapse, and many patients prefer nondrug options (van Schaik et al., 2004). Where clinically appropriate, client choice of evidence-based options improves outcomes (Sherbourne et al., 2001). These facts underscore that barriers in increasing mental health care capacity in primary care are not solely related to HCP knowledge deficits, but result from complex interdependent factors.

HCP mental health–related stigma is an important factor and is of particular concern because it undermines successful treatment outcomes. Stigma usually stems from lack of knowledge (ignorance, misinformation) and is described as a process involving prejudices (negative attitudes, beliefs, fear) and discrimination (actions, policies, directives aimed at PWLE) associated with social exclusion, missed opportunities, and lower self-esteem (Dudley, 2000; Goffman, 1964). Research suggests that as students, HCPs embark on their career holding the same stereotypical beliefs as the general public (Emrich et al., 2003). As healthcare professionals, despite being more knowledgeable about mental illnesses and supportive of PWLE civil rights, they continue to hold these stigmatized beliefs (Pellegrini, 2014). There is ample evidence of manifestations of stigma in healthcare settings, from provision of substandard or no care to unfair or demeaning treatment (e.g., pressuring ambivalent clients into or being made to wait longer for treatment) (Knaak, Mantler, et al., 2017; Rao et al., 2009). HCPs are commonly less optimistic about treatment adherence and outcomes (prognostic negativity) (Caldwell & Jorm, 2001; Henderson et al., 2014), refer more frequently to specialty services, and tend to attribute physical illnesses to a mental health diagnosis (diagnostic overshadowing), increasing morbidity and mortality for both mental and physical illness (Corrigan et al., 2014; Jones et al., 2008). The culture of medicine further exacerbates the problem because it encourages an image of invincibility, emphasizes professional competence and outstanding performance (Adshead, 2005), and determines HCPs' own experience with emotional problems (willingness to disclosure, help seeking), which in turn affects their interactions with PWLE. When pressures of a busy practice, compassion fatigue, and burnout are added, the HCP preference may be clinical distancing.

Stigma also resonates through healthcare facilities into policies and procedures that guide mental health care. For this reason, a central target for health policy makers in reducing the global mental health care service gap is to tackle stigma among HCPs. To do so, it is essential to understand this multifaceted problem from a complex adaptive system perspective with multiple interdependencies. Here we present some examples of common factors that affect HCP stigma.

HCP Lack of Perceived Need for Stigma Reduction Training

Contact-based education is a well-established best practice to reduce stigma and break down stereotypes. However, HCPs do not recognize a need in stigma reduction training because they report being in frequent contact with PWLE. Even so, the majority of experiences are disproportionate in that clients are frequently distressed or in an acutely unwell phase of illness rather than experiencing a first person's account of coping with the illness and recovery journey. HCPs may not be aware how their own prejudices (Rössler, 2016), stigmatizing language ("crazy," "frequent flyers"), or seeing the illness, not the person (e.g., the bipolar, the psychotic) can be harmful and considered offensive (Horsfall et al., 2010). Contact-based education is different from regular patient care in that (a) providers hear a recovery-oriented story, (b) the journey is directed by the PWLE instead of the provider, (c) the speaker is of equal status with the provider, and (d) the speaker is the teacher, the provider, and the learner (Patten et al., 2012).

Comfort and Confidence Managing Mental Health

Many primary care providers extend care to a large number of domains with competing training demands. These demands can lead to a lack of educational exposure to mental health training. If providers feel unprepared, there can be a sense of helplessness, associated anxiety, and less confidence that they can realistically help clients recover and contribute to society, reinforcing a pattern to avoid (Brown et al., 2003), especially if specialty backup proves to be difficult or nonexistent. Providers also report anxiety about proper communication with clients (Loeb et al., 2012; MacCarthy et al., 2013).

Time Constraints

HCP often cite lack of time as a main barrier. For example, primary care physicians often deal with several medical problems per visit, but the daily case load can severely limit each client's time to 10–15 minutes compared to the psychiatrist's hour (Loeb et al., 2012; Nease et al., 2006). Studies show an inverse relationship between time available and desire to avoid, although this relationship seems to dissipate with older age and years of work experience (Henderson et al., 2014).

Complexity and Level of Responsibility

HCPs' interactions with PWLE are different than those of the general population because they often extend care to complex clients, often with two or more chronic and interacting physical and/or mental conditions. The complexity of presentation (acute or active symptoms, client communication barriers, seriousness of the condition) is also significant. In this context, there is a heightened sense of responsibility and anxiety about whether they are "missing something." Furthermore, providers may find it difficult to encourage acutely unwell ambivalent clients to embark on interventions.

Diagnostic Challenges

Mental health is often intertwined with physical health. When patients consult their doctor, they generally do not describe symptoms of "psychiatric illness," but issues such as sleep problems, fatigue, or gradual decline in functioning at work, which can mislead assessment and potential diagnosis (Haftgoli et al., 2010). When clients report vague physical symptoms, detection is 22% compared to 77% with psychological symptom presentation (Kirmayer et al., 1993). Given these diagnostic issues, an overwhelming number of psychiatric problems are missed with delayed treatment, resulting in increased likelihood of more severe disability.

Systems Support Factors

There are many policy, structural, or legislative barriers to provide care, such as an insufficient number mental health specialists, ineffective interdisciplinary teams, and inefficient or inadequate reimbursement, all of which conspire to create a sense of HCP isolation and frustration and translate into long wait times for clients, poor continuity of care, and overburdened mental health systems. Studies suggest that colocated collaborative care models improve chronic disease care and decrease stigmatization by reducing unwanted disclosure (Institute of Medicine, 2006; Loeb et al., 2012).

Client Factors

Client factors such as client beliefs, fears, guilt, dominant cultural beliefs, and self-blame surrounding mental illness may engender feelings of vulnerability or lead to postponed contact with professionals (Nyblade et al., 2019; Stuart & Sartorius, 2017). Lack of knowledge or awareness of what they are experiencing, reluctance to disclose, awareness of HCPs' time pressures, adherence issues (e.g., motivational issues; therapeutic ambivalence; structural barriers accessing care such as transportation, costly uninsured services, lack of community services) are also important (Pereira et al., 2011; Unützer et al., 2006). Stigma-reduction programs should tackle as many stigma-related client concerns as possible for optimal effectiveness (see Figure 13.1 for common concerns).

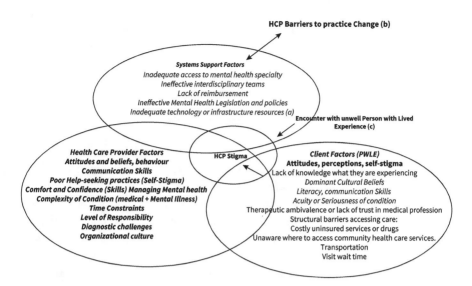

Figure 13.1 Common HCP Mental Health Stigma-Drivers Conceptual Model

(a) HCP stigma toward PWLE—resonates through healthcare facilities into policies and procedures that guide mental healthcare, which can reinforce HCP stigma toward PWLE.

(b) Mitigate as feasibly as possible HCP barriers to practice change in antistigma programming (see Key Recommendations)—because barriers are both fueled by and reinforce HCP stigma.

(c) Encounters with PWLE when distressed or in acutely unwell phase of illness—rather than experiencing a first person's account of coping with the illness and recovery journey—contribute to negative or pessimistic views of recovery. This not only reinforces HCP stigma toward PWLE, clinical distancing, and barrier to practice change, but also can contribute to HCP implicit and explicates harmful behaviors assisting in clients' self-blame, self-stigma, and vulnerabilities.

Opening Minds Research Targeting Healthcare Providers

Process Model for Successful Antistigma Programs for Healthcare Providers

The Mental Health Commission of Canada (MHCC) initiated Opening Minds (OM) with a mandate to reduce mental health–related stigma. Through a qualitative grounded theory methodology based on core guiding principles to tackle HCP stigma, a team of OM academic researchers developed a process model to design and deliver antistigma programs for healthcare professionals. A four-stage process has been proposed: (a) set up for success, which occurs at the planning stage. Considerations include the involvement of key stakeholders such as leaders, consumers, and target audience and discussions about sustainability; (b) build the program using six key ingredients: personal testimony, social contact, enthusiastic facilitator modeling person-first behavior, recovery-oriented stories, stigma aware-ness and myth-busting, and skills building to increase confidence; (c) use best prac-tices in participatory learning; and (d) work toward culture change to maximize sustainability (Knaak & Patten, 2016).

The British Columbia Adult Mental Health Practice Support Program

OM identified the British Columbia Adult Mental Health Practice Support Program (AMHPSP), designed by the General Practice Services Committee in efforts to reform and revitalize primary care, as a promising antistigma program for HCP. A Vancouver Island shared-care team hypothesized that practitioners felt ill-equipped managing mental illness, leading to anxiety in client interactions, given the difficulties accessing timely mental health services. The program enhanced PCPs' and their office team's comfort and capacity to work with PWLE with mild/moderate depression and anx-iety disorders. The skills were general in nature and key for effective chronic illness care, however, such as improved communication skills and engagement of patients in recovery efforts (Turner et al., 2015). Active listening and hearing client's experiences were the cornerstones of the program.

The program consists of three half-day interactive workshops that introduce learn-ers to an organized approach from a problem and strength-based assessment to the development of an action plan. Providers and clients use the plan to negotiate user-friendly cognitive behavior therapy–based self-management options tailored to client needs. These options include the Cognitive Behavioral Interpersonal Skills workbook (CBIS); the BounceBack program, a telephone-guided mental health coaching ser-vice, and an antidepressant skills workbook. BounceBack can be an appealing form of support to some because it operates at arm's length of HCPs while providing essential information on diagnosis and care course trajectory.

Several management aspects have been integrated into the program. Contact-based education occurs through first-voice advocates who share their stories and recovery journey. Workshops are interspersed with 6- to 8-week action periods during which learners practice what they learned. During action periods, providers flexibly use a wealth of tools and strategies accessible electronically via a stepped-care approach algorithm that is conducive to complex client care management. The algorithms were developed for application within HCP time constraints, to a reflect a "real-world" sce-nario (Greenhalgh et al., 2004; Plsek, 2003). A practice support coordinator offers on-site guidance on office redesign and strategies that enhance implementation of tools and skills. Continuing medical education initiatives offer distinct, finite oppor-tunities to train for necessary skill sets, married with strategies that enable or rein-force program materials both immediately and repetitively within the scope of their practice. The protocols, prompts, and support help to guide, test, reflect on, and adapt new learnings in practices (plan–do–study–act model), because these strategies have maximal impact on practice behavior changes and patient outcomes (Davis et al., 1995; Miller et al., 1998). With a top-down and bottom-up approach, the AMHPSP incorporates the fundamentals of the four-stage process model. Qualitative evaluations of the program showed positive impact on several key outcomes (MacCarthy et al., 2013; Weinerman et al., 2011).

Based on the early success described previously, the Nova Scotia Department of Health and Wellness and the MHCC sponsored a 2013 demonstration trial of the AMHPSP to evaluate its effectiveness on key outcomes through a cluster randomized controlled trial. The intention was that if the program was effective, there could be a broader adoption of the program across the country. As described in Stage 1 of the process model, the engagement of Nova Scotia regional and provincial mental health programs funders and policy makers proved to be invaluable. Physicians expressed concerns about the lack of reimbursement for program-required tasks (e.g., exceeding the number of billable counseling visits approved by the Medical Services Insurance Program, which would trigger audits and potential clawbacks). The Department of Health and Wellness created new service fee codes through a participation grant and made use of two existing fee codes to compensate for these tasks as a temporary measure until such time as research results would become available. Participating physicians were exempt from restrictions during and after the demonstration if claim criteria were met.

Program sustainability discussions also occurred at the outset of the planning phase. HCPs raised concerns such as time constraints and lack of awareness or availability of community support resources and provided recommendations to sustain practice changes. Trainers created and adapted patient-specific weekly electronic and hard-copy information gathering tools for screening, diagnosis, and management, from which providers could review client progress. Trainers also invited specialists and allied health professionals to the workshops for networking opportunities and incorporated a presentation on local community resources.

The research team led the demonstration from 2014 to 2016. The aims of this study were broad and included whether training family physicians in the AMHPSP would lead to greater improvements in perceived confidence, comfort, and skills in providing care for PWLE and changes to social distance and stigmatization, patient depression scores, occupational/general functioning, quality of life, and physicians' antidepressant prescribing compared to the control group (see Appendix 13.1 for outcome measures).

Outcomes of the AMHSPP Project

One hundred ten primary care physicians were randomly assigned to intervention or control groups (Beaulieu et al., 2017). Most analyses consisted of between-group independent samples comparisons (such as t tests) to examine potential group differences.

Table 13.1 *Preplanned Primary Opening Minds Stigma Scale for Health Care Providers Analysis Adjusted for Practice Size*

Stigma Dimension	t test ($df = 70$), p
Total scale (15 item)	$-1.91, p = .06$
Attitudes subscale	$-0.68, p = .50$
Disclosure/help seeking	$-0.36, p = .72$
Social distance	$-2.17, p = .03$

As shown in Table 13.1, a significant reduction was observed in the intervention group physicians' preference for social distance ($t(70) = -2.17$, $p = .03$), an important dimension of stigma. Perceived global comfort, confidence, and skills in managing depression and other related mental health conditions was statistically significant between groups, $t(69) = 6.14$, $p < .001$, and reflected a large effect size (Cohen's $d = 1.48$). The independent evaluation of measures for confidence along the care pathway (e.g., screening, diagnosis, management, awareness of community resources, use of strategies and tools) improved significantly in all measures in intervention group participants except confidence to treat other mental health disorders. Finally, there was a significant correlation between increases in levels of confidence and comfort and improvements in overall stigma (Spearman's coefficient = .28; $z = 2.14$; $p = .03$).

As a second evaluation of changes in stigma, the minimum detectable change statistic (Kassam et al., 2012) was used to calculate the number of Opening Minds Stigma Scale for Health Care Providers (OMS-HC) scale units of change required to say with confidence that there was a "real" or true change. The calculated minimum detectable change for the scale is 6.51, and an improvement of more than 6.5 points from pre- to posttraining was detected in 23.7% of participants compared to only 8.8% for the control group.

In addition to stigma reduction, patient outcomes were also positive. The study showed a significant improvement in symptom ratings for depression. PHQ-9 scores diminished in both groups in the first 3 months (see Figure 13.2), but then scores continued to improve only in the intervention group from 3 to 6 months. In the intervention group, antidepressant prescribing was significantly lower at any time during the 6-month study period and was lower by 49% at 6 months. In other words, improvement of depression scores occurred despite fewer prescriptions. Between-group changes in functioning or quality of life were not significantly different, but these outcomes are known to take longer to improve (Hofmann et al., 2017). Seventy-one percent of intervention patients used program tools and strategies, with BounceBack having the highest use (51% of intervention patients) (Lauria-Horner et al., 2018).

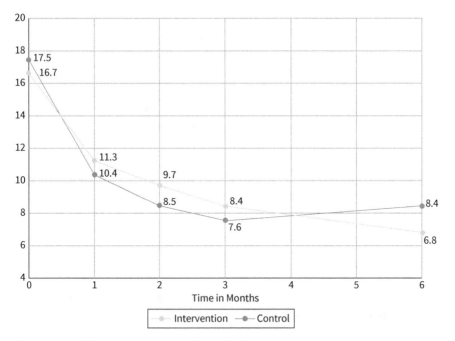

Figure 13.2 PHQ-9 Scores at Each Follow-Up Time Point: Intervention and Control Groups

Dissemination of the Program

Given the favorable study results, the program was transitioned on a provincial scale in Nova Scotia and disseminated to Newfoundland and Prince Edward Island. A qualitative evaluation in Newfoundland and Prince Edward Island showed similar positive findings for changes in stigma and confidence posttraining. In Newfoundland, the largest observed improvement in OMS-HC total scale as well as the three subscales was for the "negative attitudes" subscale, with an effect size of 0.25 (small to moderate effect; relative improvement 6.8%), consistent with first responder stigma-reduction programs (Knaak, Szeto, et al., 2017; Szeto et al., 2019). The number of participants who reached a "threshold of success" (at least 12 of 15 [80%] nonstigmatizing answers on the OMS-HC scale) increased from 54% to 63% postprogram. The perceived global confidence to manage mental illnesses (very confident) increased from 8.3% to 29.2%. Over one-third of participants agreed or strongly agreed they prescribed antidepressant less frequently, and 92% agreed or strongly agreed clients were partners in their mental healthcare. In Prince Edward Island, there were stigma reductions on the total OMS-HC scale and subscales with a large effect size (Cohen's $d = 1.09–1.26$), although providers did not shift their own willingness to disclose/seek help for a mental illness (Cohen's $d = 0.17$). Participants also indicated strong, notable improvements in confidence postprogram, with 100% feeling confident or very confident in nearly all assessed skills and knowledge areas. As noted, qualitative interviews were also conducted. The following are participants' feedback in two areas:

Feedback about the value of the program:

- "Doing more treatment for anxiety and depression in office."
- "I improved my knowledge to mental health conditions and gave me tools to use when discussing non-pharmacological Tx approach."

Reported feedback from PWLE:

- "Patients have a better understanding of health problems, more trust, feeling supported."
- "Positive. They appreciate being given information at office."
- "Enjoy patient centred approach."

Partnership With the Suriname Pan American Health Organization of the World Health Organization

The MHCC has a series of international partners, including the Pan American Health Organization of the World Health Organization (PAHO/WHO). PAHO/WHO adopted a plan of action to guide mental health interventions in the Americas from 2015 to 2020 (Cayon, 2015). Suriname is a member country of PAHO/WHO, where a small percentage of PWLE receive basic treatment and the number of suicides more than doubled between 2000 and 2009, placing suicide in the top 10 causes of death in the country. In November 2018, the MHCC in collaboration with Suriname Ministry of Health team leaders delivered a 3-day workshop that combined two complementary antistigma programs, Understanding Stigma and Cognitive Behavioural Interpersonal Skills for HCP (see Appendix 13.2), in Paramaribo to promote the human rights of PWLE (see https://www.facebook.com/pahowho). Thirty-nine PCP from across the country, representing a wide range of fields and backgrounds, attended. Attendees represented regional health services (family physicians, nurse practitioners, psychologists and psychologist professors, medical students, hospitalists, and hospital personnel), medical mission physicians and coordinators, the psychiatric center (director of the psychiatric center), Bureau of Public Health staff, and pedagogy professionals from the Department of Non-Communicable Diseases.

As with other work of the MHCC, comprehensive evaluations were conducted. In this case, evaluations looked at the change from pre- to posttraining and at 6 months' follow-up. Stigma was examined with the overall OMS-HC scale. Mean scores changed from pre- to posttests, 2.39 and 2.02, respectively, a 15.5% relative improvement representing a moderate effect (Cohen's $d = 0.65$). The largest improvement

Table 13.2 *Pre- to Follow-up Mean Scores and Effect Sizes: Opening Minds Stigma Scale for Health Care Providers (OMS-HC)*

OMS-HC	Pretest Mean (SD)	Posttest Mean (SD)	Follow-up Mean (SD)	Pre- to Follow-up Effect Size (Cohen's d)
Total scale	2.39 (.52)	2.01 (.61)	1.97 (.42)	0.86
Negative attitudes	2.22 (.64)	1.92 (.77)	1.75 (.52)	0.78
Willingness to disclose/seek help for a mental illness	2.95 (.57)	2.67 (.60)	2.33 (.68)	1.02
Preference for social distance	2.31 (.60)	1.87 (.63)	1.97 (.26)	0.66

Note: $n = 28$ for pre- and posttest; $n = 14$ for follow-up.

among the three OMS-HC subscales was for "preference for social distance," with an effect size of 0.72. At 6 months' follow-up, the overall total OMS-HC mean scores further improved from baseline with an average mean of 1.97 (Cohen's $d = 0.86$, a strong effect). When subscales were analyzed, further improvements were observed for the dimensions of attitudes ($M = 1.75$) and health providers' own willingness to disclose/seek help ($M = 2.33$), with strong effect sizes of 0.78 and 1.02, respectively. The effect size for preference for social distance remained in the moderate range (see Table 13.2). The "threshold of success" analysis showed a postprogram increase from 24.9% to 57.2%. All participants either agreed (64.3%) or strongly agreed (35.7%) that the program would be useful in their jobs, and 93% reported an increased in confidence working with PWLE. Overall, the results of this study were more positive than previous evaluations of either program alone.

As in the evaluations conducted in Canada, qualitative inquiries were made of participants' perceptions of the program and its benefits. The following are illustrative quotes that reflect these issues:

Activities/ parts of the program most affected your perception or understanding of mental illness?

- "The testimonials of people living with a mental illness most affected my perception. There is still a lot of taboo in my work area (e.g., cultural influence) on mental illness and I think that testimonials can help raise awareness that people can live a productive life even when they have such a challenge."
- "I would previously find myself angry at patients for various reasons such as not following through recommendations, now I understand."
- "I would dismiss a patient with mental illness, now I realize this was not the best approach."

Do you feel your behavior toward people with mental illness will be different than what it would have been before this program?

- "I now realize that if people are treated and guided properly, the person can function well in society."
- "Yes, be more patient and listen more. Why? Because sometimes the person doesn't need my advice but just someone that listens, really listens."
- "Yes, because you learn that some progress is made step by step and you should be patient with that encouraging the client, asking what helps and what is possible or what they want to try. Next to it the monitoring/follow up is important."

Suggested areas of improvement

- "The information given (delivered) in Dutch." (Suriname is a former Dutch colony.)
- "I would appreciate a follow up program."

The positive results seen in Suriname are encouraging and suggest that the program model can be applied to other countries. Further dissemination and evaluation are strongly encouraged.

Key Considerations/Recommendations for Implementation

HCPs are in an ideal position to affect social change; however, they need support to do so. Core barriers to HCP mental health practice and attitudinal changes center around two main challenges. First, providers need an increased capacity to provide mental health care. Second, factors that impede HCPs' motivation to change, such as the acceptability and feasibility to take on mental health services, need to be identified and overcome. The following is by no means an exhaustive list, but it provides important takeaway points for future work.

1. As noted previously, there is a need to strengthen HCPs' capacity to provide care for people with mental health and/or addiction challenges. This work needs to focus on programs that build skills and reduce stigma. To be effective, these programs must address HCPs' anxiety and sense of helplessness by providing up-to-date information to regain the confidence that they can realistically help clients recover and contribute to society. Experiences with positive client outcomes reduce a preference for clinical distancing. These programs further should increase HCPs' capacity and skill set to manage mental health in the context of complex patients through practical, time-efficient tools and strategies, feasibly applicable in a "real-world" context, leveraging technology to train and provide care (e.g., electronic access to data collection and time-efficient tools and management strategies, ability to integrate structured assessment scales/ tools in electronic medical records).

2. There should be a focus on programs that combine systematic delivery of mental health care education with practice support suited to retain new learning and desired changes in practice. Such programs should encourage provider–client shared responsibility in decision-making, client engagement in the recovery process through enhanced self-management skills, office staff training, practice support coordinator–supported action periods to facilitate implementation of new learning, continuous reflection, and tailoring of interventions to reflect emerging needs and knowledge. In settings where practice support programs may not be feasible (e.g., short-term workshops, residency programs), complementary programs such as Understanding Stigma and CBIS training may be attractive options.

3. It is critical to address HCPs' personal beliefs and attitudes about stigma and the damage it causes to the hopes and lives of clients. The reduction of negative attitudes and improved comfort and skills can mutually reinforce each other. This work requires clarity about how contact-based education is different from clinical practice exposure. Stigma reduction programs are needed that incorporate tools and strategies to improve communication skills. Working with clients as partners, listening, acknowledging concerns, working with their strengths, negotiate advantages and disadvantages of interventions, and conveying hope and recovery promote constructive working relationships, reduce client reluctance to disclose, and help to avoid them spiraling down into self-stigma, self-blame, shame, and treatment aversion. Negative organizational cultures need to be addressed by increasing awareness of how HCPs' own beliefs and attitudes toward mental illness—in addition to setting the stage for how they interact with and support clients—determine their own experience with emotional problems (willingness to disclosure, help seeking), creating a significant detriment to their health and workplace environment. Stigma reduction programs and booster training need to be provided to all HCP categories and health personnel who manage or work with PWLE, including office staff, emergency departments, and mental health care helpline personnel to better understand challenges PWLE face and facilitate more humane exchanges. The four-stage process model is a valuable guide for this purpose.

4. As much as possible, it is critical to address the lack of systems supports for mental health management, such as antidiscrimination policies and structural or legislative barriers. The ongoing inclusion of national and provincial leaders responsible for mental health care reform will help to maximize effectiveness and support for long-term sustainability. It is important to restructure service delivery, redistribute funding from physical to mental health care, and better coordinate mental health care services (e.g., billing services, policy to encourage evidence-based management of mental illness, technological support such as electronic medical records, adequate visit time for complex patients). Collaborative care models are encouraged where mental health support is physically or virtually colocated with primary care.

5. Client factors that curtail mental health services utilization or postpone treatment must be recognized and addressed. It is important to include clients in antistigma programs from the outset to gain insight into challenges they face and coordinate stigma reduction initiatives as part of a larger comprehensive community effort (Nyblade et al., 2019).

6. Ongoing research and evaluation are required in several domains. Long-term studies are needed to discern if the AMHPSP, perhaps in concert with booster sessions, can further reduce HCP mental health–related stigma or if other clinical outcomes can be improved. Randomized clinical trials are needed to rigorously evaluate changes in stigma for complementary combined Understanding Stigma and CBIS programs in other countries. Finally, it is important to further evaluate the factors that influence program outcomes, such as age, years of work experience, and decreased willingness to avoid.

The introduction of new knowledge into a provider's armamentarium only becomes part of the practice of "good medicine" if health professionals can implement a systemic, comprehensive, and sequential approach to its adoption. Stigma reduction efforts must be viewed from a complex systems perspective, and there must be ample opportunity for reflective adaptation. The marriage of skills-building strategies for HCPs with client engagement in the reform process offers a highly useful synergy. Where better to learn the skills than in a trusted, safe place such as primary care? This change, however, requires a paradigm shift in models of care and a stepping-stone toward collaborative care that strengthens patient-centered healthcare, in which the client is a partner and reclaims a sense of control in their journey. Programs that can influence practitioners, systems, and clients can create a sustainable and scalable response. The recognition of this reality can promote the effective integration of training programs in primary care and help to restructure services to deliver comprehensive, cost-effective, and patient-centered care proportional to the need.

References

Adshead, G. (2005). Healing ourselves: Ethical issues in the care of sick doctors. *Advances in Psychiatric Treatment, 11*(5), 330–337. https://doi.org/10.1192/apt.11.5.330

Beaulieu, T., Patten, S., Knaak, S., Weinerman, R., Campbell, H., & Lauria-Horner, B. (2017). Impact of skill-based approaches in reducing stigma in primary care physicians: Results from a double-blind, parallel-cluster, randomized controlled trial. *Canadian Journal of Psychiatry. Revue canadienne de psychiatrie, 62*(5), 327–335. https://doi.org/10.1177/0706743716686919

Bounce Back: Reclaim your health. (n.d.). Retrieved June 22, 2021, from https://bouncebackbc.ca/

Brown, L., Macintyre, K., & Trujillo, L. (2003). Interventions to reduce HIV/AIDS stigma: What have we learned? *AIDS Education and Prevention: Official Publication of the International Society for AIDS Education, 15*(1), 49–69. https://doi.org/10.1521/aeap.15.1.49.23844

Cognitive behavioural interpersonal skills manual. (2015, July). https://gpscbc.ca/sites/default/files/CBIS%20Manual-Electronic%20Copy%20-%20v2%20Oct%2022,%202015.pdf

Caldwell, T. M., & Jorm, A. F. (2001). Mental health nurses' beliefs about likely outcomes for people with schizophrenia or depression: A comparison with the public and other healthcare professionals. *Australian and New Zealand Journal of Mental Health Nursing, 10*(1), 42–54. https://doi.org/10.1046/j.1440-0979.2001.00190.x

Cayon, A. (2015, October 6). *PAHO/WHO | Plan of action on mental health 2015–2020.* Pan American Health Organization/World Health Organization.

Corrigan, P. W., Mittal, D., Reaves, C. M., Haynes, T. F., Han, X., Morris, S., & Sullivan, G. (2014). Mental health stigma and primary health care decisions. *Psychiatry Research, 218*(1), 35–38. https://doi.org/10.1016/j.psychres.2014.04.028

Crowley, R. A., Kirschner, N., & Crowley, R. A. (2015). The integration of care for mental health, substance abuse, and other behavioral health conditions into primary care: Executive summary of an American College of Physicians position paper. *Annals of Internal Medicine, 163*(4), 298–299. https://doi.org/10.7326/M15-0510

Davis, D. A., Thomson, M. A., Oxman, A. D., & Haynes, R. B. (1995). Changing physician performance: A systematic review of the effect of continuing medical education strategies. *JAMA, 274*(9), 700–705. https://doi.org/10.1001/jama.1995.03530090032018

Dudley, J. R. (2000). Confronting stigma within the services system. *Social Work, 45*(5), 449–455. https://doi.org/10.1093/sw/45.5.449

Emrich, K., Thompson, T. C., & Moore, G. (2003). Positive attitude: An essential element for effective care of people with mental illnesses. *Journal of Psychosocial Nursing & Mental Health Services; Thorofare, 41*(5), 18–25.

Fournier, J. C., DeRubeis, R. J., Hollon, S. D., Dimidjian, S., Amsterdam, J. D., Shelton, R. C., & Fawcett, J. (2010). Antidepressant drug effects and depression severity: A patient-level meta-analysis. *JAMA, 303*(1), 47–53. https://doi.org/10.1001/jama.2009.1943

Goffman, E. (1964). *Stigma: Notes on the management of spoiled identity.* By Erving Goffman. Englewood Cliffs, New Jersey: Prentice-Hall, 1963. *Social Forces, 43*(1), 127–128. https://doi.org/10.1093/sf/43.1.127

Greenhalgh, T., Robert, G., Macfarlane, F., Bate, P., & Kyriakidou, O. (2004). Diffusion of innovations in service organizations: Systematic review and recommendations. *The Milbank Quarterly, 82*(4), 581–629. https://doi.org/10.1111/j.0887-378X.2004.00325.x

Haftgoli, N., Favrat, B., Verdon, F., Vaucher, P., Bischoff, T., Burnand, B., & Herzig, L. (2010). Patients presenting with somatic complaints in general practice: Depression, anxiety and somatoform disorders are frequent and associated with psychosocial stressors. *BMC Family Practice, 11*, 67. https://doi.org/10.1186/1471-2296-11-67

Healthy Minds Cooperative (n.d.). http://www.healthyminds.ca

Henderson, C., Noblett, J., Parke, H., Clement, S., Caffrey, A., Gale-Grant, O., Schulze, B., Druss, B., & Thornicroft, G. (2014). Mental health-related stigma in health care and mental health-care settings. *The Lancet Psychiatry, 1*(6), 467–482. https://doi.org/10.1016/S2215-0366(14)00023-6

Hofmann, S. G., Curtiss, J., Carpenter, J. K., & Kind, S. (2017). Effect of treatments for depression on quality of life: A meta-analysis. *Cognitive Behaviour Therapy, 46*(4), 265–286. https://doi.org/10.1080/16506073.2017.1304445

Horsfall, J., Cleary, M., & Hunt, G. E. (2010). Stigma in mental health: Clients and professionals. *Issues in Mental Health Nursing, 31*(7), 450–455. https://doi.org/10.3109/01612840903537167

Institute of Medicine (U.S.). Committee on Crossing the Quality Chasm Adaptation to Mental Health and Addictive Disorders. (2006). *Improving the quality of health care for mental and substance-use conditions.* National Academies Press. http://ezproxy.msvu.ca/login?url=http://search.ebscohost.com/login.aspx?direct=true&scope=site&db=nlebk&db=nlabk&AN=156233

Jones, S., Howard, L., & Thornicroft, G. (2008). "Diagnostic overshadowing": Worse physical health care for people with mental illness. *Acta Psychiatrica Scandinavica, 118*(3), 169–171. https://doi.org/10.1111/j.1600-0447.2008.01211.x

Kalet, A. L., Gillespie, C. C., Schwartz, M. D., Holmboe, E. S., Ark, T. K., Jay, M., Paik, S., Truncali, A., Hyland Bruno, J., Zabar, S. R., & Gourevitch, M. N. (2010). New measures to establish the evidence base for medical education: Identifying educationally sensitive patient outcomes. *Academic Medicine, 85*(5), 844–851. https://doi.org/10.1097/ACM.0b013e3181d734a5

Kassam, A., Papish, A., Modgill, G., & Patten, S. (2012). The development and psychometric properties of a new scale to measure mental illness related stigma by health care providers: The Opening Minds Scale for Health Care Providers (OMS-HC). *BMC Psychiatry, 12*(1), 62. https://doi.org/10.1186/1471-244X-12-62

Kauye, F., Jenkins, R., & Rahman, A. (2014). Training primary health care workers in mental health and its impact on diagnoses of common mental disorders in primary care of a developing country, Malawi: A cluster-randomized controlled trial. *Psychological Medicine, 44*(3), 657–666. https://doi.org/10.1017/S0033291713001141

Kendrick, T., King, F., Albertella, L., & Smith, P. W. (2005). GP treatment decisions for patients with depression: An observational study. *The British Journal of General Practice, 55*(513), 280–286.

Kirmayer, L. J., Robbins, J. M., Dworkind, M., & Yaffe, M. J. (1993). Somatization and the recognition of depression and anxiety in primary care. *The American Journal of Psychiatry, 150*(5), 734–741. https://doi.org/10.1176/ajp.150.5.734

Kirsch, I., Deacon, B. J., Huedo-Medina, T. B., Scoboria, A., Moore, T. J., & Johnson, B. T. (2008). Initial severity and antidepressant benefits: A meta-analysis of data submitted to the Food and Drug Administration. *PLoS Medicine, 5*(2). https://doi.org/10.1371/journal.pmed.0050045

Knaak, S., Mantler, E., & Szeto, A. (2017). Mental illness-related stigma in healthcare. *Healthcare Management Forum, 30*(2), 111–116. https://doi.org/10.1177/0840470416679413

Knaak, S., & Patten, S. (2016). A grounded theory model for reducing stigma in health professionals in Canada. *Acta Psychiatrica Scandinavica, 134*(S446), 53–62. https://doi.org/10.1111/acps.12612

Knaak, S., Szeto, A. C. H., Kassam, A., Hamer, A., Modgill, G., & Patten, S. (2017). Understanding stigma: A pooled analysis of a national program aimed at health care providers to reduce stigma towards patients with a mental illness. *Journal of Mental Health and Addiction Nursing, 1*(1), e19–e29. https://doi.org/10.22374/jmhan.v1i1.19

Lauria-Horner, B., Beaulieu, T., Knaak, S., Weinerman, R., Campbell, H., & Patten, S. (2018). Controlled trial of the impact of a BC adult mental health practice support program (AMHPSP) on primary health care professionals' management of depression. *BMC Family Practice, 19*(1), 183. https://doi.org/10.1186/s12875-018-0862-y

Loeb, D. F., Bayliss, E. A., Binswanger, I. A., Candrian, C., & deGruy, F. V. (2012). Primary care physician perceptions on caring for complex patients with medical and mental illness. *Journal of General Internal Medicine, 27*(8), 945–952. https://doi.org/10.1007/s11606-012-2005-9

MacCarthy, D., Weinerman, R., Kallstrom, L., Kadlec, H., Hollander, M. J., & Patten, S. (2013). Mental health practice and attitudes of family physicians can be changed! *The Permanente Journal, 17*(3), 14–17. https://doi.org/10.7812/TPP/13-033

Mickus, M., Colenda, C. C., & Hogan, A. J. (2000). Knowledge of mental health benefits and preferences for type of mental health providers among the general public. *Psychiatric Services (Washington, D.C.), 51*(2), 199–202. https://doi.org/10.1176/appi.ps.51.2.199

Miller, W. L., Crabtree, B. F., McDaniel, R., & Stange, K. C. (1998). Understanding change in primary care practice using complexity theory. *The Journal of Family Practice, 46*(5), 369–376.

Mulsant, B. H., Whyte, E., Lenze, E. J., Lotrich, F., Karp, J. F., Pollock, B. G., & Reynolds, C. F. (2003). Achieving long-term optimal outcomes in geriatric depression and anxiety. *CNS Spectrums, 8*(12, Suppl. 3), 27–34. https://doi.org/10.1017/s1092852900008257

Murray, C. J. L., Barber, R. M., Foreman, K. J., Ozgoren, A. A., Abd-Allah, F., & Abera, S. F. (2015). Global, regional, and national disability-adjusted life years (DALYs) for 306 diseases and injuries and healthy life expectancy (HALE) for 188 countries, 1990–2013: Quantifying the epidemiological transition. *The Lancet, 386*, 2145–91.

Naylor, C. (2013). SP0115 The link between long-term conditions and mental health. *Annals of the Rheumatic Diseases, 71*(Suppl. 3), 28–29. https://doi.org/10.1136/annrheumdis-2012-eular.1590

Nease, D. E., Klinkman, M. S., & Aikens, J. E. (2006). Depression case finding in primary care: A method for the mandates. *International Journal of Psychiatry in Medicine; London, 36*(2), 141–151.

Nyblade, L., Stockton, M. A., Giger, K., Bond, V., Ekstrand, M. L., Lean, R. M., Mitchell, E. M. H., Nelson, L. R. E., Sapag, J. C., Siraprapasiri, T., Turan, J., & Wouters, E. (2019). Stigma in health facilities: Why it matters and how we can change it. *BMC Medicine, 17*. https://doi.org/10.1186/s12916-019-1256-2

Patten, S. B., Remillard, A., Phillips, L., Modgill, G., Szeto, A. C., Kassam, A., & Gardner, D. M. (2012). Effectiveness of contact-based education for reducing mental illness–related stigma in pharmacy students. *BMC Medical Education, 12*(1), 120. https://doi.org/10.1186/1472-6920-12-120

Pellegrini, C. (2014). Mental illness stigma in health care settings a barrier to care. *CMAJ: Canadian Medical Association Journal, 186*(1), E17. https://doi.org/10.1503/cmaj.109-4668

Pereira, B., Andrew, G., Pednekar, S., Kirkwood, B. R., & Patel, V. (2011). The integration of the treatment for common mental disorders in primary care: Experiences of health care providers in the MANAS trial in Goa, India. *International Journal of Mental Health Systems, 5*(1), 26. https://doi.org/10.1186/1752-4458-5-26

Plsek, P. E. (2003, January 27–28). *Complexity and the adoption of innovation in health care* [Paper presentation]. Accelerating Quality Improvement in Health Care Strategies to Speed the Diffusion of Evidence-Based Innovations, Washington, DC, United States.

Rao, H., Mahadevappa, H., Pillay, P., Sessay, M., Abraham, A., & Luty, J. (2009). A study of stigmatized attitudes towards people with mental health problems among health professionals. *Journal of Psychiatric and Mental Health Nursing, 16*(3), 279–284. https://doi.org/10.1111/j.1365-2850.2008.01369.x

Rössler, W. (2016). The stigma of mental disorders: A millennia-long history of social exclusion and prejudices. *EMBO Reports, 17*(9), 1250–1253. https://doi.org/10.15252/embr.201643041

Sherbourne, C. D., Wells, K. B., Duan, N., Miranda, J., Unützer, J., Jaycox, L., Schoenbaum, M., Meredith, L. S., & Rubenstein, L. V. (2001). Long-term effectiveness of disseminating quality improvement for depression in primary care. *Archives of General Psychiatry, 58*(7), 696–703. https://doi.org/10.1001/archpsyc.58.7.696

Sikorski, C., Luppa, M., König, H.-H., van den Bussche, H., & Riedel-Heller, S. G. (2012). Does GP training in depression care affect patient outcome?—A systematic review and meta-analysis. *BMC Health Services Research, 12*, 10. https://doi.org/10.1186/1472-6963-12-10

Statistics Canada. (2015). *CANSIM: Health—Mental Health and Well-Being | Country: Canada | Table: Mental Health Profile, Canadian Community Health Survey—Mental Health (CCHS)*. Data-Planet Statistical Ready Reference by Conquest Systems, Inc. http://dx.doi.org/10.6068/DP14BA889CA3A93

Stuart, H., & Sartorius, N. (2017). Opening Doors: The Global Programme to Fight Stigma and Discrimination Because of Schizophrenia. In W. Gaebel, W. Rössler, & N. Sartorius (Eds.),

The stigma of mental illness—End of the story? (pp. 227–235). Springer International. https://doi.org/10.1007/978-3-319-27839-1_13

Szeto, A., Dobson, K. S., & Knaak, S. (2019). The Road to Mental Readiness for First Responders: A meta-analysis of program outcomes. *Canadian Journal of Psychiatry. Revue canadienne de psychiatrie, 64*(1 Suppl.), 18S–29S. https://doi.org/10.1177/0706743719842562

Trautmann, S., Rehm, J., & Wittchen, H.-U. (2016). The economic costs of mental disorders: Do our societies react appropriately to the burden of mental disorders? *EMBO Reports, 17*(9), 1245–1249. https://doi.org/10.15252/embr.201642951

Turner, A., Anderson, J. K., Wallace, L. M., & Bourne, C. (2015). An evaluation of a self-management program for patients with long-term conditions. *Patient Education and Counseling, 98*(2), 213–219. https://doi.org/10.1016/j.pec.2014.08.022

Unützer, J., Schoenbaum, M., Druss, B. G., & Katon, W. J. (2006). Transforming mental health care at the interface with general medicine: Report for the Presidents Commission. *Psychiatric Services (Washington, D.C.), 57*(1), 37–47. https://doi.org/10.1176/appi.ps.57.1.37

van Schaik, D. J. F., Klijn, A. F. J., van Hout, H. P. J., van Marwijk, H. W. J., Beekman, A. T. F., de Haan, M., & van Dyck, R. (2004). Patients' preferences in the treatment of depressive disorder in primary care. *General Hospital Psychiatry, 26*(3), 184–189. https://doi.org/10.1016/j.genhosppsych.2003.12.001

Weinerman, R., Campbell, H., Miller, M., Stretch, J., Kallstrom, L., Kadlec, H., & Hollander, M. (2011). Improving mental healthcare by primary care physicians in British Columbia. *Healthcare Quarterly, 14*(1), 36–38. https://doi.org/10.12927/hcq.2011.22146

World Health Organization. (2008, January 14). *Integrating mental health into primary care: A global perspective.* https://who.int/publications/i/item/9789241563680

World Health Organization. (2017). *Depression and other common mental disorders.* https://eac.eu.com/newsletter/booklets/who%20mental%20disorders.pdf

14

Stigma Reduction for Substance Use and Opioids

Stephanie Knaak and Heather Stuart

As with many countries, Canada is facing an opioid crisis. The severity of Canada's crisis is among the worst in the world, preceded only by the United States and a few other countries, such as Libya and Russia (Global Burden of Disease Collaborative Network, 2018). The crisis has claimed the lives of over 15,393 individuals in Canada between 2016 and 2019, with 94% of apparent opioid-related fatalities believed to be accidental (Johnston, 2020). The global COVID-19 health pandemic has only exacerbated this crisis (Special Advisory Committee on the Epidemic of Opioid Overdoses, 2020). A history of high prescribing rates coupled with the introduction of synthetic opioids such as fentanyl into the illicit drug supply are two important factors that promote the crisis (Special Advisory Committee on the Epidemic of Opioid Overdoses, 2020).

As communities, first responder organizations, health authorities, and governments attempt to respond to the opioid crisis, multipillared strategies are often adopted, with attention to prevention, harm reduction, treatment, and enforcement (BC Ministry of Mental Health and Addictions, 2019; MacPherson, 2001; Mayors Task Force on the Opioid Crisis, 2017). The mobilization of harm reduction interventions is often viewed as an immediate priority, given the sheer magnitude of the crisis and death toll, but access to high-quality, evidence-based treatment services, the provision of a "safe supply" of opioids, and the criminalization of opioid use are also central to policy-related discussions (BC Ministry of Mental Health and Addictions, 2019; Mayors Task Force on the Opioid Crisis, 2017; Office of the Provincial Health Officer, 2019).

Responses to this crisis cannot be properly understood without attending to the problem of stigmatization toward people with opioid use problems (McGinty & Barry, 2020; Stuart, 2019; Volkow, 2020). This problem includes policy responses, but it also includes necessary attendance to interpersonal and individual-level stigma, such as the quality of client–provider interactions, retention in care, client satisfaction, help-seeking behaviors, and other aspects of help seeking, care delivery, and treatment (McGinty & Barry, 2020; Stuart, 2019; Volkow, 2020). There is a strong need to identify and implement interventions that effectively combat stigma in these contexts. It is also necessary to understand the qualities and characteristics of stigmatization related to opioid and other substance use problems, as well as how to disrupt these stigmatization processes, to design or identify appropriate interventions to reduce stigma in the context of providing health, safety, and social care services for people with opioid use problems and people who may be at risk of experiencing an opioid-related overdose or poisoning.

In 2019, under direction from Health Canada, the Mental Health Commission of Canada completed a national qualitative research study to understand the problem of stigma on the front lines of Canada's current opioid crisis (Knaak et al., 2019a, 2019b). The findings of this research were viewed as a guide, and the Mental Health Commission of Canada then launched a second phase of research to identify existing interventions that incorporated promising elements and approaches, with the longer term goal of evaluating the effectiveness of identified programs. This chapter reports on the main results of this qualitative research, as well as some of the early learnings from the evaluation of promising approaches and programs.

Phase 1: Qualitative Research

The objective of the qualitative research was to generate a comprehensive under-standing of stigma as it was experienced on the "front lines" of Canada's opioid crisis, particularly in the context of direct service care and response (Knaak et al., 2019a, 2019b). To support this goal, a key informant approach was adopted, and focus groups and interviews were conducted with direct service providers across the country (i.e., police officers, paramedics, firefighters, and health and social care providers). Similar work was completed with people with lived experience of an opioid use problem or who were at risk of experiencing an opioid-related poisoning or overdose. Seventy-nine individuals participated in the study through focus groups and interviews.

What Stigma Looks and Feels Like

The main results of the qualitative interviews and focus groups are highlighted in Figure 14.1. Stigma showed up in several damaging and harmful ways in the con-text of direct service care for opioid use problems and opioid-related poisoning or overdose, and stigma existed at all individual, interpersonal, and structural levels. For example, at the interpersonal level, the description of "what stigma looks and feels like" included negative judgments and stereotypes about people with substance use problems, the use of negative language and labels, and treating people with sub-stance use problems poorly in the context of direct service provision or care. Stigma was also recognized at the individual level, and many respondents spoke about the shame of addiction and how this response leads to a reluctance to seek help or sup-port for a substance use problem. Stigma at the structural level was described as being embedded within institutions and approaches to care. Perhaps the most di-rect and obvious example of structural stigma is the criminalization of many types of drug use, but this stigma can also be seen in lack of availability of services and

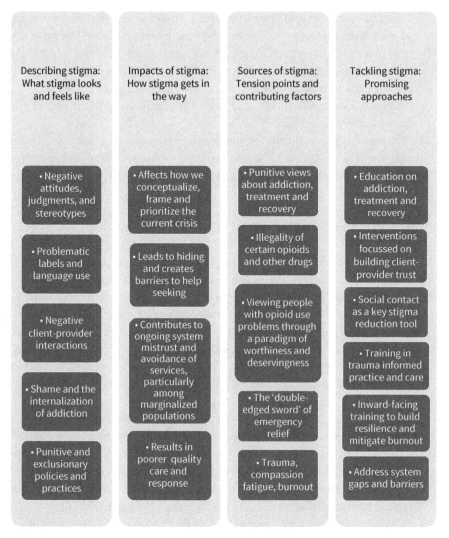

Figure 14.1 Summary of Results From Key Informant Study

stigmatizing policies and practices that exist and create additional barriers to accessing various health and social care services. The following respondent comments help to illustrate these themes:

- "Addiction is one of the only health-care problems where you're more likely to be thrown out of a hospital for showing symptoms of your illness than you are to receive care." (focus group participant)
- "I think the first assumption that people make . . . is, you're misusing. . . . And so, anybody with an addiction issue is suspect. And so, we can't treat it like a legitimate health issue." (focus group participant)

- "'If you've used drugs today, please come back tomorrow.' That seems like a perfectly reasonable thing to put on the wall. But if you use drugs every day, it's like that means I can never come to your service, even though you're a service provider and you've just been so brazenly unthinking that you would use a model like that." (focus group participant, person with lived experience of a substance use problem [PWLE])
- "Stigma is what kept us silent.... You hide a lot. There is a lot of shame." (key informant interview, PWLE)
- "They treat us like criminals . . . it shouldn't be a law issue, it's a health issue. We're sick people, it's a disease . . . let's address the problem, the real problem. Send them to rehab, they shouldn't be put . . . in jails." (focus group participant, PWLE)

How Stigma Gets in the Way

Many negative effects of stigma were identified, and stigma was described as a main force in shaping how various groups conceptualize, frame, and respond to the crisis. Stigma was also described to negatively affect the overall quality of care and response for people with opioid use problems or people at risk of experiencing an opioid-related overdose or poisoning. Another key impact of stigma was that it created barriers to help seeking. Respondents described shame and hiding from self-stigma and fear of harm and being treated poorly by service providers as the two main reasons for this response. The following comments help illustrate these themes:

- "[In a committee I sat on] they talked about ED wait time reductions and they talked about wait time reductions for key surgeries, like hip replacements and stuff. It's disappointing that they didn't talk about wait times for opioid and other types of addictions . . . but, again, that's the stigma, right?" (focus group participant)
- "My biggest factor with it—all of this opioid crisis—is the fact that we're so highly stigmatized that we do hide." (focus group participant, PWLE)
- "Stigma . . . dehumanizes people. People don't access services. People aren't taken care of when they do access services. There're assumptions made. And people use alone—because they don't want anyone to know." (key informant interview)
- "The bottom line with marginal populations is that they do not trust health care. There's huge mistrust." (Key informant interview)
- "We see a lot of our clients that we're bringing, let's say, to the hospital, and they tell us, 'no, I don't want to go there, it's degrading.'" (focus group interview)

Where Does Stigma Come From? Tension Points and Contributing Factors

The results of this study revealed both direct and indirect sources of stigma. Direct sources of stigma included punitive views about addiction, treatment and recovery, ambivalence about harm reduction and its benefits, the illegality of certain opioids and other drugs, and viewing people with opioid and other drug use problems through a paradigm of unworthiness. Some of these ideas are reflected in the following comments:

- "We're not treating addiction the same way we would treat cancer or that you have an illness. We're treating it as you have a failing." (focus group participant)
- "How can the government put money towards an anti-stigma program and expect it to work when the government itself denotes someone who is addicted to opioids a criminal? How can you fight stigma when you are labelling patients as criminals?" (key informant interview)
- "This population is seen as more difficult, hard to treat, maybe even less deserving of care." (key informant interview)

The main indirect sources of stigma were described as system inadequacies, experiences of trauma, compassion fatigue, and provider burnout. System inadequacies included the chronic underfunding of addiction treatment, understaffing and low pay in many front-line sectors, and inconsistencies in practice standards. Importantly, system inadequacies were identified as an indirect source of stigma in that they created a stressful, challenging, and ill-equipped environment in which to provide care and response to people with opioid use problems and people at risk of opioid-related poisoning. They were also recognized as examples of structural stigma toward people with substance use problems. In describing the role of trauma, compassion fatigue, and burnout and their contribution to stigma, respondents recognized that these experiences negatively affected providers' own mental health and well-being and that these problems in turn contribute to worse care, including emotional and behavioral distancing from clients. The following comments reflect the connection between system inadequacies, work-related stress, and client care:

- "Police officers, firefighters are stressed to the max because of the multiple overdose calls that they make. Emergency room workers are frustrated and of course, shelter workers, harm reduction workers, outreach workers, peer support workers are just burning themselves out like crazy trying to stick the finger in this massive hole that we have in this situation." (focus group participant)
- "In the field with the first responders . . . one of the big concerns is burnout and compassion fatigue. Because they're getting numb . . . they've just seen so much that I think they don't even have time to do self-care." (focus group participant)
- "Because of lack of treatment options and other kinds of supports it puts people who really care about their clients into a very stressful situation." (key informant interview)

The final key point that was acknowledged as an indirect source of stigma pertained to challenges responding to multiple opioid-related overdoses or poisonings.

Although respondents strongly believed that the emergency relief intervention of naloxone was an important and effective life-saving measure for people at risk of accidental overdose or poisoning, this intervention was viewed as a double-edged sword by some respondents, who thought that the availability and administration of such measures encouraged riskier drug use behaviors among some users. Respondents also articulated the emotional toll of attending to multiple overdose or poisoning emergencies and how this contributed to detachment, apathy, and burnout.

- "I can say in the last three years since the crisis has started, I had found myself and I'll admit to going, 'Why? Why this time?' Because I've seen this individual three times this week. So again, it's that ability to check in. I think the mental health of not only the patient, but of the practitioner's coincides almost exactly. The apathy just erodes confidence and you get sucked dry.'" (focus group participant)
- You start to examine your conscience. And you're like, 'This isn't why I went into nursing. What's wrong with me now that my emotion level is so blunted to this?'" (focus group participant)
- "The frustration isn't necessarily about the fact that we're attending an intervention or an overdose and administrating Narcan. It's about the fact that Narcan in and of itself sometimes feels like a double edge sword because . . . it's almost like it takes away the danger in taking something like fentanyl, which is—I mean it's just absolutely crazy." (focus group participant)

How Can Stigma Be Addressed?

The research results identified several strategies to combat opioid-related stigma and improve direct service care and response for people with opioid use problems and people at risk of an opioid-related overdose or poisoning. They are as follows.

1. Address system inadequacies that derive from structural-level stigma in health and social care systems, which underlies and contributes to ongoing individual and interpersonal-level stigma, as the following comments illustrate:
    - "We don't have a treatment system. We have a discombobulated mess of nothingness that has created where we are at today. What needs to change? First, recognition that people are going to come into contact with the system at many different touch points. Start with the touch points. Each of those touch points needs to be a way in, and people need to be directed to where they can go from there. Also, I do not think people should go to jail for substance use." (key informant interview)
    - "We need greater attention paid to structural stigma, right? I mean, you can do workshops till the cows come home, but really you need to actually be changing structures." (focus group participant)

2. Provide education and training to first responders and front-line providers that focuses on evidence-based and holistic understandings of addiction, treatment, and recovery; includes the value and importance of harm reduction as a key component of the continuum of quality care; and provides tools to improve language and behavior.
3. Provide interventions designed to build trust and understanding between providers and clients.
4. Utilize social contact-based approaches and interventions to increase human connection, understanding, and awareness and to combat feelings of apathy and helplessness. These approaches should incorporate the voices, participation, and involvement of people with lived experience of a substance or opioid use problem.
5. Provide education and training in trauma-informed care and practice.
6. Provide support and training to increase resiliency and mitigate provider burnout.

Recommendations that centered on approaches to improve the attitudes and behaviors of providers and build greater trust between clients and providers identified a need for both outward-facing approaches to improve providers' knowledge, attitudes, and behaviors toward people with opioid use problems and inward-facing approaches to improve compassion and care by attending to providers' stress resiliency and the problems of compassion fatigue, burnout, and secondary traumatic stress. The use of social contact and the meaningful inclusion of people with lived experience of opioid use emerged as a central recommendation for helping to positively shift attitudes and behaviors and improve client–provider understanding. The use of social contact was also described as a key tool to improve client–provider trust. The following comments illustrate these ideas:

- "We need to build trust with users—but how? By using people who can connect with them, whom they will trust. We are starting a program using peer navigators . . . They are getting their training upgraded as health workers." (key informant interview)
- "In a previous life I worked with men who had committed sexual offenses. You know, the best way for me to sort of get over my repugnance at their behaviour was to hear their stories. When somebody who does behavior, or exhibits behavior that people don't understand, once you hear their story you can put it all in context. It's much more difficult to be judgmental about them. That applies for anybody who's marginalized, for sure." (key informant interview)
- "I also think connection with people—peers, people with lived experiences—is so important. . . . A lot of health care providers don't really know people who are using substances, other than alcohol, they can make assumptions. Connection, bringing people together, is important. But you can't just bring anyone together, because if they're not trauma-informed, they will cause harm." (focus group participant)

Inward-facing training was identified as that which aims to help first responders and health providers develop the necessary skills and tools to build stress resiliency and improve compassion. This training included programs that provided resiliency training, compassion training, and training in trauma-informed care. The following comments illustrate:

- "We know from research that stress tolerance in the workplace through trauma exposure leads to social distance. Contemplative practices to help tolerate stress in the workplace, which keep people open and engaged and more able to deliver good care, then lessens social distance. This is what we focus on in our workshops." (key informant interview)
- "[Program on trauma-informed care] takes into account providers' own trauma. It reminds them of the way they want to show up, helps them know how to be more mindful, not just 'correct' behaviour, but see their interaction with patients as a relationship. It reminds people to be aware of the histories people carry with them—and reminds providers they don't want to inflict more harm. It reminds them of their desire to do no harm." (key informant interview)

Phase 2: Program Evaluation

The approaches that were suggested to combat stigma, as identified through the qualitative research, formed the foundation of the next major phase of this project, which was to identify promising approaches and programs and evaluate them to help establish an evidence base for effectiveness. In 2019 and early 2020, four evaluations of different training interventions targeting direct service providers were conducted (Community Addictions Peer Support Association, 2020; Knaak et al., 2021; Knaak et al., 2020; Mental Health Commission of Canada, 2020). These programs were as follows:

1. A self-directed web-based program about mental illness and substance use designed specifically for a healthcare audience. The program used social contact (including both video and in-person stories and perspectives) as a core teaching element, along with educational and action-oriented components. The course content included education and personal stories related to mental illness and substance use problems but did not address opioid use specifically. The program explained stigma in healthcare settings, described how it affected people with substance use and mental health problems, and identified ways that providers could reduce prejudice and discrimination by applying recovery-based and trauma-informed awareness in one's approach to care challenges stigma. The program also corrected common misperceptions about mental illness and addiction.
2. An in-person, half-day workshop that provided education about addiction, the effects of stigmatizing behaviors and language, and the importance of

compassion. This workshop included a combination of education and social contact components (video and in-person). The program facilitator was
a person with lived experience of a substance use problem. Core elements of
the workshop included education on the neuroscience of addiction; education
about stigma and the use of stigmatizing language; messages and personal experience stories from people with lived experience of substance use problems;
messaging around the importance of compassion, use of person-first language
and approaches, a focus on wellness as a paradigm for recovery; and action-
planning group activities on what providers can do to help reduce stigma in
their organizations and personally. This intervention was not tailored to opioid
use but was specific to substance use and substance use stigma.

3. A personal testimony–based social contact intervention delivered by a person
   with lived experience of an opioid use disorder. This 1-hour intervention was
   delivered in person to nursing students during the first lecture of a 2-week unit
   on mental health and substance use, as part of the students' regular curriculum.
   The speaker led the class in a personal narrative describing her own lived experience of opioid use disorder and recovery. She spoke about her childhood,
   how her use began, her experiences with the health system, her journey of recovery, and her current status. She also spoke about personal experiences with
   her partner, who is struggling with substance use. The course instructor participated in the session, using elements of the speaker's story to emphasize the
   importance of compassion, the role of trauma in addiction, and how addiction
   is not a choice. The instructor also connected elements of the speaker's personal
   story to the concept of internal bias, the role of the justice system in substance
   use, and the problem of diagnostic overshadowing. For this intervention, the effect of the educational component (i.e., the curricular unit on mental health and
   substance use) on students' attitudes was also assessed.

4. A 1-day, in-person trauma and resiliency–informed practice training. This was
   a mental health and resiliency training program that aimed to reduce stigmatizing behaviors by enhancing knowledge and skills related to trauma awareness, self-compassion, and compassion satisfaction. It focused on integrating
   knowledge and skills about how people are affected by trauma into workplace
   policies, procedures, and services.

The evaluation approach was outcome focused because the primary interest was
to ascertain the extent to which these interventions improved attitudes and behaviors
of service providers toward people with opioid use problems. To evaluate the programs, a pre–post design was employed, with a standardized measure that captures
stigmatizing attitudes and behaviors of service providers toward people with opioid
use problems (see Chapter 7). Some evaluations included additional measures, such
as qualitative feedback (Programs 2, 3 and 4), a measure to assess change in attitudes
toward substance use more generally (Program 2), or measures to assess improvements in resiliency, self-compassion, burnout, and compassion satisfaction (Program

4). Two programs (Programs 3 and 4) also included a follow-up assessment, in which surveys were completed again at 3 months postintervention (see Community Addictions Peer Support Association, 2020; Knaak et al., 2021; Knaak et al., 2020; Mental Health Commission of Canada, 2020, for more details).

All programs showed statistically significant improvements in attitudes and behaviors from pre- to posttraining, with improvements retained to the time of follow-up where this was measured (see Table 14.1). Some programs, however, showed stronger effect sizes than others. Based on these results, several preliminary learnings have emerged about what works to combat interpersonal-level opioid-related stigma, although more research is required.

First, similar to what has emerged to reduce stigma toward people with mental illnesses (Knaak et al., 2014; Knaak & Patten, 2016), social contact is viewed as a powerful tool to reduce substance- and opioid-related stigma, particularly at the interpersonal level. It is important to hear personal stories of substance use problems, the journey toward wellness, and experiences of both stigma and the contrast of compassionate and caring interactions with providers. Personal stories create connection between audience members and speakers. They can also disconfirm stereotypes, provide insight and understanding about substance use, and create opportunities for increased awareness, reflection, and personal change.

Second, the educational content of an intervention matters. For example, Program 3, which was the opioid-specific social contact intervention that also measured the impact of the educational content on mental illness and addiction, showed no improvement in attitudes based on the educational content alone. This result is consistent with other research that has suggested that standard curricular education focused on mental illness or substance use literacy alone does not necessarily reduce stigma (Abbey et al., 2011; Happell et al., 2104; Livingston et al., 2012; Sherwood, 2019). Educational content must be stigma informed in order to change attitudes; it must address the issue of stigma and its effect on people with substance use problems, disconfirm stereotypes and correct misinformation, use stigma-free language,

Table 14.1 Program Outcomes From Four Antistigma Programs

	n	Pre M (SD)	Post M (SD)	t test	p	Effect size (Cohen's d)
Program 1	823	2.00 (.78)	1.84 (.79)	8.63	<.001	0.20
Program 2	28	1.87 (.66)	1.69 (.64)	3.09	.005	0.27
Program 3a (social contact)	14	1.94 (.65)	1.64 (.63)	4.18	.001	0.46
Program 3b (educational content)	12	1.74 (.65)	1.74 (.69)	0.063	.951	0.01
Program 4	27	2.15 (.51)	1.94 (.44)	2.47	.020	0.44

be person centered and recovery or wellness focused, and encourage self-reflection about implicit or uninvestigated biases (Livingston et al., 2012; McGinty & Barry, 2020; Stuart, 2019).

Third, the results suggest that both in-person and web-based approaches are suitable and effective options for program delivery. Thus, web-based delivery can work if in-person delivery is not feasible or desired. However, more research is required. One important avenue for future research would be to compare the impact of the same program delivered in an in-person format and a web-based format.

Fourth, the evaluation findings suggest that general content can be used, but that tailored content is better (see also Knaak et al., 2015). The two stigma reduction programs that addressed stigma toward mental illness or substance use more generally showed improvements in opioid-specific stigma, but the improvements from these programs were not as strong as those from the opioid-specific social contact intervention. As well, the half-day workshop on substance use stigma measured pre and post attitudes related to substance use more generally, and greater improvements in attitudes were seen on this measure than on the opioid use measure (Community Addictions Peer Support Association, 2020). These results suggest that improvements likely will be greatest for the targeted domain, but that general content has "spillover" benefits to improve attitudes toward specific substances or conditions.

Last, the results suggest that inward-facing programs can have outward-facing outcomes. Program 4 taught a trauma-informed approach to care in conjunction with an equally strong focus on improving providers' self-compassion, self-care, and resiliency. Importantly, this program revealed reduced stigma from pre- to posttraining, but the results also showed a statistically significant connection between improvements in self-compassion and resiliency with these reductions in stigma.

Key Considerations and Recommendations

- Qualitative research clearly identifies stigma to be a major barrier at all individual, interpersonal, and structural levels. Stigma reduction efforts should be focused at all three levels, from legislative changes, to policy changes, to stigma interventions, to working to improve help-seeking and harm-reduction behaviors for people who use opioids.
- System-level barriers, including the ongoing issue of criminalization of certain opioids and other substances and its harms, and service and treatment gaps require prioritized attention. There is an urgent need to evaluate, understand, and address issues related to punitive or barrier-creating policies and practices, inadequate access to and quality of treatments, resource allocation, and other policy and system-level barriers to quality care and support for people with opioid use problems.
- Research provides preliminary evidence for "what works" in the design and delivery of antistigma interventions in the context of direct service provision and

care. More research is needed using a combination of education and social contact approaches, as well as training in trauma-informed care that prioritizes the health and well-being of providers.

- Antistigma interventions ought not be thought of as "one-off" interventions but as a part of a comprehensive set of tools and approaches that can be implemented as complements to each other and within a larger framework or strategy.
- Robust research and evaluation are critical to ensure that interventions meet their stated stigma reduction goals and to continue to build the evidence base for substance use stigma reduction, which is still in its relative infancy.

References

Abbey, S., Charbonneau, M., Tranulis, C., Moss, P., Baici, W., Dabby, L., Gautam, M., & Paré, M. (2011). Stigma and discrimination [Position paper] *Canadian Journal of Psychiatry*, *56*(10), 1–9.

BC Ministry of Mental Health and Addictions. (2019). *Responding to British Columbia's public health emergency progress update March—July 2019.*

Community Addictions Peer Support Association, Canadian Centre on Substance Use and Addiction, and Mental Health Commission of Canada. (2020). *Stigma ends with me: Results from the evaluation of a contact-based substance use stigma reduction intervention.* Mental Health Commission of Canada.

Global Burden of Disease Collaborative Network. (2018). *Global Burden of Disease Study 2017 (GBD 2017) Results.* Institute for Health Metrics and Evaluation. http://ghdx.healthdata.org/gbd-results-tool

Happell, B., Byrne, L., Platania-Phung, C., Harris, S., Bradshaw, J. & Davies, J. (2014). Consumer participation in nurse education. *International Journal of Mental Health Nursing, 23*, 427–434. https://doi.org/10.1111/inm.12077

Johnston, J. (2020, July 16). *June was the worst month for overdose deaths in B.C. history.* CBC News. https://www.cbc.ca/news/canada/british-columbia/overdose-deaths-b-c-june-2020-1.5652311

Knaak, S., Billet, M., Besharah, J., Karphal, K., & Patten, S. (2021). Nursing education and the value of personal story: Measuring the impact of curricular content versus social contact on substance use stigma [Manuscript submitted for publication].

Knaak, S., Christie, R., Mercer, S., & Stuart, H. (2019a) Harm reduction, stigma and recovery: Tensions on the front-lines of Canada's opioid crisis. *Journal of Mental Health and Addiction Nursing, 3*(1). https://doi.org/10.22374/jmhan.v3i1.37

Knaak, S., Christie, R., Mercer, S. & Stuart, H. (2019b). *Stigma and the opioid crisis—final report.* Mental Health Commission of Canada. https://www.mentalhealthcommission.ca/English/media/4271 24

Knaak, S., Modgill, G., & Patten, S. B. (2014). Key ingredients of anti-stigma programs for health care providers: A data synthesis of evaluative studies. *Canadian Journal of Psychiatry*, *59*(Suppl. 1), s19–s26. https://doi/10.1177/070674371405901s06

Knaak, S., & Patten, S. (2016). A grounded theory for reducing stigma in health professionals in Canada. *Acta Psychiatrica Scandinavica, 134*(Suppl. 446), 53–62. https://doi.org/10.1111/acps.12612

Knaak, S., Sandrelli, M., & Patten, S. (2020) How a shared humanity model can improve provider wellbeing and client care: An evaluation of Fraser Health's Trauma and Resiliency Informed Practice (TRIP) training program. *Healthcare Management Forum, 34*(2), 87–92https://doi.org/10.1177/0840470420970594

Knaak, S., Szeto, A., Fitch, K., Modgill, G., & Patten, S. (2015). Stigma towards borderline personality disorder: Effectiveness and generalizability of an anti-stigma program for healthcare providers using a pre–post randomized design. *Borderline Personality Disorder and Emotion Dysregulation, 2*, 9. https://doi.org/10.1186/s40479-015-0030-0

Livingston, J. D., Milne, T., Fang, M. L., & Amari, E. (2012). The effectiveness of interventions for reducing stigma related to substance use disorders: A systematic review. *Addiction, 107*(1), 39–50. https://doi.org/10.1111/j.1360-0443.2011.03601.x

MacPherson, D. (2001). *A framework for action: A four-pillar approach to drug problems in Vancouver.* City of Vancouver.

Mayors Task Force on the Opioid Crisis. (2017). *Recommendations of the Mayors' Task Force on the opioid crisis.* Federation of Canadian Municipalities. https://fcm.ca/sites/default/files/documents/resources/submission/opioid-crisis-recommendations.pdf.

McGinty, E. E., & Barry, C. L. (2020) Stigma reduction to combat the addiction crisis—developing an evidence base. *New England Journal of Medicine, 382*(14), 1291–1292. https://doi.org/10.1056/nejmp2000227

Mental Health Commission of Canada. (2020). *Understanding stigma evaluation results: Opioid-related stigma.* Mental Health Commission of Canada.

Office of the Provincial Health Officer. (2019). *Stopping the harm: Decriminalization of people who use drugs in BC. Provincial Health Officer's special report.*

Sherwood, D. A. (2019). Healthcare curriculum influences on stigma towards mental illness: Core psychiatry course impact on pharmacy, nursing and social work student attitudes. *Currents in Pharmacy Teaching & Learning, 11*(2), 198–203. https://doi.org/10.1016/j.cptl.2018.11.001

Special Advisory Committee on the Epidemic of Opioid Overdoses. (2020). *Opioid-related harms in Canada.* Public Health Agency of Canada. https://health-infobase.canada.ca/substance-related-harms/opioids

Stuart, H. (2019). Managing the stigma of opioid use. *Healthcare Management Forum, 32*(2), 78–83.

Volkow, N. D. (2020) Stigma and the toll of addiction. *New England Journal of Medicine, 382*(14), 1289–1290.

15

Media Programs

Rob Whitley

Evidence suggests that the general public uses the media as a key source of information about mental illness, including traditional media such as newspapers, as well as more modern forms of media such as social media. Surveys suggest that over three-quarters of the adult population in Canada read at least one daily newspaper each week (News Media Canada, 2019). Additionally, online news is read and shared with increasing frequency, as newspapers and other traditional media make efforts to expand their use of social media and accompanying digital platforms (Salganik, 2019).

Numerous studies from the early 2000s examined the portrayal of mental illness in the media. These include studies in the United Kingdom (Anderson, 2003; Stark et al., 2004), the United States (Corrigan et al., 2005; Wahl et al., 2002), New Zealand (Coverdale et al., 2002; Nairn & Coverdale, 2005), Australia (Francis et al., 2004; Rowe et al., 2003), and Canada (Olstead, 2002; Stuart, 2003). The results from these studies reveal a set of converging and consistent findings, regardless of time and place. Portrayals of people with a mental illness frequently revolve around negative factors such as criminality, violence, and danger. These portrayals can paint a false picture, given that research indicates that rates of crime and violence are similar between people with or without mental illness when controlling for factors such as substance use (G. Thornicroft, 2006).

Moreover, several studies indicate that media articles frequently contain stigmatizing language and rarely include more positive or hopeful stories of recovery. For example, A. Thornicroft et al. (2013) assessed over 3,000 newspaper articles about mental illness in the United Kingdom spanning a 4-year period and found that 46% of the articles were stigmatizing in content. Likewise, a Canadian analysis of articles from 2005 to 2010 found that around 40% of newspaper articles mentioning mental illness were in the context of crime and violence, while fewer than 20% mentioned recovery, treatment, or rehabilitation (Whitley & Berry, 2013a).

The preponderance of negative articles may be a consequence of editorial decision-making, or "gatekeeping," defined as the "selecting, writing, editing, positioning, scheduling, repeating and otherwise massaging information to become news" (Shoemaker & Vos, 2009, p. 73). Research on journalistic practice indicates that editors typically prefer news based on crime, conflict, or controversy, known by the saying "If it bleeds, it leads" (Harcup & O'Neill, 2017). Indeed, Shoemaker and Vos (2009) argued that editors implicitly define newsworthiness as events that are rare and out of the ordinary, especially when the event involves threats to the status quo and public order or the violation of the law or social norms. From an editor's perspective, positive and hopeful stories of recovery may be mundane and unnewsworthy, while violent events and social transgressions may be considered newsworthy "clickbait" (Chermak, 1994).

Mental health advocates have raised concerns about such patterns, because several research studies suggest that negative portrayals of people with mental illness can perpetuate stigma, suspicion, prejudice, social distance, and fear of people with mental illness. For example, Schomerus et al. (2015) examined public beliefs about mental illness after the (alleged) intentional crashing of a Germanwings aircraft by a pilot who reportedly suffered from major depressive disorder. This study revealed a significant increase in public concerns about unpredictability related to mental illness, as well as a decrease in the belief that people with mental illness are similar to the general population.

Likewise, an American study revealed an increase in negative attitudes toward people with mental illness in people who read a detailed news article about a mass shooting by an individual who suffered from mental illness. Results indicated that readers were significantly less likely to want to live near, or work with, someone with mental illness after reading the article (McGinty et al., 2013). Similarly, Australian researchers found that participants who recalled negative media coverage of mental illness were significantly more likely to believe that people with mental illness are dangerous (Reavley et al., 2016). On the contrary, one study indicated that reading a positive article about recovery reduced stigma and increased affirming attitudes among readers, meaning that the media can be a force for positive change and education (Corrigan et al., 2013).

As a whole, the mainstream media has been identified as a key factor in the perpetuation of prejudice against people with mental illness. The corpus of research indicates that media coverage can contribute to negative public attitudes, inaccurate beliefs, and erroneous stereotypes about people with mental illness, which in turn can contribute to a wider social climate that facilitates the discrimination, stigmatization, and marginalization of people with a mental illness (Crisp et al., 2000; Dinos et al., 2004). All of these forces are barriers toward service utilization, social participation, and recovery, and they worsen the situation for an already marginalized population (Rusch & Thornicroft, 2014).

Given the importance of the media as a source of potential bias, mental health advocates across the world have made strident efforts to design and implement both small-scale and large-scale interventions directed at the media in an attempt to improve media coverage of mental illness. For example, a study from Australia found that some media were featuring more hopeful and positive articles about mental illness, which was imputed to several targeted antistigma educational initiatives aimed at journalists, newsrooms, and editors (Francis et al., 2004). Another study demonstrated that reporting of mental illness in a single Jamaican newspaper was generally positive, which was attributed to informal but intense outreach to this newspaper by prominent local psychiatrists (Whitley & Hickling, 2007). In Canada, Stuart (2003) found that positive stories increased by one-third and outweighed negative stories after a targeted media intervention, again aimed at a single newspaper.

One of the most prominent large-scale recent media interventions is that organized and implemented by the Opening Minds initiative of the Mental Health Commission of Canada. This intervention will be described in depth here because it is a paradigmatic case that has become known globally as a leading example of positive and productive long-term engagement with the media. I was the principal investigator of a parallel research study that examined the tone and content of Canadian media coverage of mental health issues during this long-term intervention.

The Canadian Approach

Numerous governments have formed national mental health commissions in recent decades, including Australia, New Zealand, and Canada (Rosen et al., 2010). The precise purpose of each commission has varied, but generally involves a mandate to reduce stigma and promote recovery. The Mental Health Commission of Canada (MHCC) was formed in March 2007, with a 10-year mandate and $15 million per year in funding. This mandate was renewed in 2017 and the MHCC is still operational until further notice, on a biannual funding cycle. In 2009, the MHCC created an antistigma initiative entitled Opening Minds, described as the "largest systematic effort to reduce the stigma of mental illness in Canadian history" (Pietrus, 2013). Opening Minds involves various antistigma activities, including intense and targeted interventions with the media (Stuart et al., 2014).

The media interventions can be divided into three core activities. First, representatives from Opening Minds made contact with major journalism schools across Canada to start a conversation about the teaching of mental health issues therein. In many cases, these conversations yielded fruitful results, leading to invitations to present seminars at many of these schools, including the University of British Columbia, Carlton University (Ottawa), Ryerson University (Toronto), Mount Royal University (Calgary), and University of King's College (Halifax). These seminars used contact-based education approaches with a panel of speakers. The panel typically included (a) two local people with lived experience talking about their life with mental illness; (b) a prominent and experienced journalist talking about writing about mental illness; (c) a MHCC representative who spoke about the Opening Minds program and resources available; (d) a family member talking about the impact of mental illness and stigma on their lives; and (e) myself, talking about the ongoing results from my parallel research study. These seminars were repeated in some subsequent years and some were recorded and uploaded so that they could be shown to classes virtually. One is publicly available via YouTube, entitled "University of King's College Media Symposium." A primary aim of these sessions was to create a model and lay a foundation so that similar panels could be created independently by faculty members at the various journalism schools across Canada.

The popularity and success of the above-described seminars led the MHCC to develop a second activity, which was a free, online educational course aimed at journalism students or journalists, but freely available for anyone to take across the world. This short online course takes about 1 hour to complete and can be taken in multiple sessions. It was created with input from a variety of experts, including journalists, researchers, and people with lived experience. The course includes four modules, namely, (a) What is stigma? (b) stigma and the news media; (c) stigma, the media, and justice; and (d) the journalist's responsibilities. The MHCC has purposely disseminated this intervention to the aforementioned journalism schools, and some professors have made the online course a mandatory component of an official course (see https://www.mentalhealthcommission.ca/English/reporting-mental-health).

Third, the MHCC funded the development of a set of guidelines to help journalists better report mental illness. Known as Mindset and developed in collaboration with the Canadian Broadcasting Corporation and the Canadian Journalism Forum on Violence and Trauma, these guidelines were produced in 2014 and were made available as a short, glossy printed booklet (with English and French versions), as well as a PDF. The guidelines are available at a dedicated and regularly updated website: http://www.mindset-mediaguide.ca/. A second updated edition was released in 2017, and a third edition was released in 2020. The latest edition contains eight short chapters, with topics such as "understanding stigma," "mental illness and the law," and "mental illness and addiction." Chapters typically include a series of do's and don'ts and best practice checklists in accessible bullet-point format. Over 5,000 copies of the Mindset booklet have been sent to major newsrooms across Canada over the years, including CBC, the *Globe and Mail*, the *Toronto Star*, and a variety of other local newspapers. Copies have also been sent to major journalism schools where professors have encouraged students to download and read the guidelines as a mandatory part of courses.

These activities began with the creation of the Opening Minds initiative in 2009, and I have conducted a parallel and continuous research study examining the tone and content of news articles about mental illness from 2010 to the present. This work includes a long-term longitudinal analysis, as well as a series of substudies, with the methodology described in detail in previous papers (Whitley et al., 2015; Whitley & Berry, 2013a, 2013b; Whitley & Wang, 2017a, 2017b). In brief, we have collected news articles from print and online editions of over 20 high-circulation Canadian newspapers, as well as from selected television news from 2005 to the present using systematic retrieval software. This collection includes the retrieval of historic articles about mental illness (2005–2009), as well current articles in real time (2010–present). Articles that include key words such as "mental illness" are collected and coded daily by trained research assistants. The codes are binary responses to a series of validated questions assessing the tone and content of the articles. Abridged versions of these questions can be seen in the left-hand column of Table 15.1. Codes are entered into Excel, which is used for primary data storage, and then exported to STATA, SPSS, or R for a range of data analyses, including χ^2 and linear regression analysis.

Table 15.1 Tone and Content of News Articles Published Between January 1 and March 31, by Year

Variable	Code	2015 N = 578 (%)	2020 N = 295 (%)	χ^2	df	p value[a]
Positive or optimistic tone	Yes	136 (23.5)	213 (72.2)	190.82	1	<.001
	No	442 (76.5)	82 (27.8)			
Recovery a theme	Yes	53 (9.2)	103 (34.9)	86.467	1	<.001
	No	525 (90.8)	192 (65.1)			
Stigma in tone or content	Yes	151 (26.1)	45 (15.3)	12.64	1	<.001
	No	427 (73.9)	250 (84.7)			
Violence or crime a theme	Yes	316 (54.7)	108 (36.6)	24.79	1	<.001
	No	262 (45.3)	187 (63.4)			
Shortage of resources a theme	Yes	225 (38.9)	86 (29.2)	7.72	1	.005
	No	353 (61.1)	209 (70.8)			
Expert quoted in the text	No	422 (73.0)	193 (65.4)	68.63	3	<.001
	Yes, positive	89 (15.4)	102 (34.6)			
	Yes, negative	33 (5.7)	0 (0.0)			
	Yes, mixed	34 (5.9)	0 (0.0)			
Person with mental illness quoted in the text	No	420 (72.7)	210 (71.2)	62.11	3	<.001
	Yes, positive	57 (9.9)	75 (25.4)			
	Yes, negative	65 (11.2)	5 (1.7)			
	Yes, mixed	36 (6.2)	5 (1.7)			
Relations quoted in the text	No	499 (86.3)	246 (83.4)	28.73	3	<.001
	Yes, positive	36 (6.2)	44 (14.9)			
	Yes, negative	21 (3.6)	4 (1.4)			
	Yes, mixed	22 (3.8)	1 (0.3)			
Interventions discussed	No	367 (63.5)	242 (82.0)	32.25	3	<.001
	Yes, positive	144 (24.9)	39 (13.2)			
	Yes, negative	27 (4.7)	6 (2.0)			
	Yes, mixed	40 (6.9)	8 (2.7)			
Aetiology discussed	Not discussed	373 (64.5)	200 (67.8)	1.85	3	.60
	Biology	29 (5.0)	12 (4.1)			
	Psychosocial	152 (26.3)	75 (25.4)			
	Dual focus	24 (4.2)	8 (2.7)			

[a]Significance was set at 0.005 using a Bonferroni correction.

The results from these various analyses converge to indicate that the tone and content of media coverage of mental illness have significantly improved over the study years. For example, a regression analysis for a longitudinal series of nearly 25,000 articles between the years 2005 and 2015 revealed a significant increase over time in articles that (a) had a positive tone; (b) discussed shortage of resources; (c) quoted an expert about mental illness; (d) quoted people with mental illness; or (e) discussed mental health interventions (all at $p < .001$). Likewise, we noted a significant decreasing trend in articles that were stigmatizing in tone and content (all at $p < .001$). Analyses revealed that articles published since the formation of the MHCC were significantly more likely to be more positively oriented and less stigmatizing than earlier articles. While these results indicate significant progress in the reporting of mental illness over time, overall proportions reveal room for improvement. For example, in the last year of this study (2015), only 35% of the articles had a positive tone and only 10% had recovery as a theme, while 22% had a stigmatizing content and 51% linked mental illness to crime and violence.

Similar results were found in a study of television coverage of mental illness between 2013 and 2015. Trend analysis indicated a significant linear increase for positively oriented coverage. For example, less than 10% of clips in 2013 had a positive overall tone, whereas this figure reached over 40% by 2015. Similarly, television clips that included shortage of resources as a theme almost doubled during the same period. Moreover, articles linking mental illness to violence significantly decreased, though these remained over 50%, and again less than 10% of television clips had recovery as a theme (Whitley & Wang, 2017b). On the one hand, these analyses indicate that media coverage of mental illness in Canada has improved. On the other hand, they indicate there is more room for improvement. As such, the MHCC (with a range of other organizations) has continued their outreach work with the media, and I continue to collect data on the tone and content of media coverage.

Our most recent analysis consists of comparisons of newspaper coverage of mental illness from January to March 2015 with newspaper coverage from January to March 2020. This study used the same systematic retrieval, coding, and analysis procedures previously described. The results of this analysis can be seen in Table 15.1 and indicate further improvements in media coverage. There was a significant improvement in 8 of 10 variables between 2015 and 2020. For example, articles with a positive tone tripled, from 24% to 72%, while articles about recovery quadrupled, from 9% to 35%. Similarly, the number of articles that were stigmatizing in tone and content was halved, now making up only 15%. Recent articles are much more likely to quote people with mental illness, their family relations, and mental health experts.

The combined results from this study indicate that professional journalists in Canada have risen to the challenge and have significantly improved their coverage of mental illness. This shift could be related to the combined activities of the MHCC Opening Minds initiative, as well as to other parallel destigmatization initiatives across the country. This action-research project has prompted numerous ongoing international collaborations between myself and research teams elsewhere. For example, I received a Global Mental Health grant to visit Latin American countries, including Chile and Mexico, to present study results to researchers and Ministry of Health officials and to help launch similar action-research projects in those jurisdictions. My ideas were enthusiastically received, and I am currently collaborating with researchers to monitor and transform media coverage of mental illness in Latin America.

Moreover, we have supplemented the broad approach of analyzing general patterns and trends with a more stratified approach examining differential media coverage according to the sociodemographic characteristics of the people portrayed. For example, we recently conducted an analysis that examined three types of newspaper articles: those that focus on (a) mental illness generically, (b) a woman with mental illness, and (c) a man with mental illness. The findings revealed that generic articles were more positive than articles about individuals. These articles were significantly more likely to quote mental health experts and have recovery, inadequate resources, and etiology as themes. In contrast, articles that depicted men were significantly more likely to have stigmatizing content and violence as themes, while articles depicting women were significantly more likely to quote mental health experts, discuss mental health interventions, and have recovery and inadequate resources as themes (Whitley et al., 2015). The results from this study indicate a new frontier in research on media coverage of mental illness, which is to examine differential coverage according to sociodemographic factors. This type of research could point to specific areas in need of intervention.

Citizen Journalism

While these results should be considered good news, the study period overlaps with massive changes in the media industry, with social media progressively usurping the traditional media as a go-to source of news and information. This brings new challenges as well as opportunities, and researchers are still grappling with methodological and ethical issues regarding the systematic examination of social media, not least issues of retrieval, analysis, and intervention. This has prompted small-scale yet innovative projects to help develop and assess new social media resources in a grassroots fashion. Much of this has been built around the concept of "citizen journalism." This emerging practice offers an opportunity for people with mental illness to produce alternative bottom-up, locally grounded portrayals suitable for social media that may dispel common myths and erroneous stereotypes and further inform the public about life with a mental illness.

Citizen journalism involves ordinary community members producing media pieces about topics and issues that affect them and their communities. These items can include videos, podcasts, and blogs suitable for social media dissemination. Citizen journalists are not formally trained in journalism and are not employed by mainstream media outlets. Instead, they are concerned citizens generating their own content, often aiming to inform and educate the general public about a misunderstood issue (Carpenter, 2010). By nature, citizen journalism approaches are truly a grass-roots, bottom-up approach with the potential for a wide reach, in part because they bypass the editorial "gatekeepers" who guard access to the mainstream media.

While there has been little action or research specifically related to citizen journalism and mental health, related research suggests that citizen journalism may have the potential to diversify media coverage of marginalized communities and provide educational counternarratives to negative mainstream media representations (Wall, 2015). For example, marginalized communities such as indigenous groups and ethnic minorities have used citizen journalism to obtain a public voice and offer alternative (typically, more positive and nuanced) representations that differ from those frequently found in the mainstream media (Farinosi & Treré, 2014; Luce et al., 2017). In other instances, citizen journalists have brought attention to human rights abuses or aspects of human suffering (and resilience) that have been overlooked by the mainstream media (Allan et al., 2007).

But citizen journalism has its challenges. Some research indicates that citizen journalism is often perceived as less credible than traditional journalism (Swasy et al., 2015) and that it can be harmful if it contributes to the distribution of misinformation or an exaggerated sense of risk and threat in certain situations (Mythen, 2010). Citizen journalism is also often prompted by a desire to promulgate a specific idea or perspective, and so the distinction between reporting and advocacy may become blurred. In short, citizen journalism has strengths and weaknesses that have not been sufficiently studied in the mental health context.

One citizen journalism approach that is particularly suitable for the social media age is known as participatory video (PV). PV is a collaborative, grass-roots, bottom-up approach that involves three core steps. First, participants with a shared experience are recruited into a workgroup, which considers issues faced by their demographic through discussion and analysis. Second, video cameras are given to the workgroup, who receive technical training in videography, scripting, and editing in regular sessions. Third, the workgroup deploys these new skills to produce locally grounded educational videos, which can be shared online (and shown at organized screenings) to raise awareness and catalyze change (Parr, 2007; Sitter, 2012). The videos are rooted in a local context, and the workgroup has complete editorial control over content and themes. Such videos can be based on a unifying topic in a documentary-style format or on the experience of a single individual. This latter approach is known as *digital storytelling*, with an individual sharing "their story" on camera, often focusing on overcoming challenges and strategies of resilience. Of note, PV is always a group activity and works best in preexisting homogenous groups where people face the same societal problems. In sum, participants in a PV project become grass-roots community educators, aiming to raise awareness and reframe discussions from their perspective (Mitchell, 2008).

These visual and digital methods have much potential to reduce mental illness stigma because much social science research indicates that we now live in a "digital age" with increasing numbers of people obtaining information via online videos embedded in social media on mobile phones, tablets, and home computers (Salganik, 2019). Indeed, the whole PV approach proceeds on the well-grounded knowledge that videos can educate, challenge, and change public attitudes and behaviors (Parr,

2007; White, 2003). Moreover, PV can create a form of "virtual contact," with the potential to confront stereotypes and illuminate day-to-day "behind the scenes" realities of recovery, in a manner similar to contact-based education. Such virtual contact may be especially important during COVID-19, where legislation is discouraging in-person, contact-based sessions. It may prove to be important in the post-COVID-19 era as well, because institutions may continue to prefer virtual education and sessions to in-person activity.

Given the potential of digital PV, I recently completed an action-research project that involved developing a new citizen journalism/PV intervention aimed at people with mental illness, with parallel research to assess (a) feasibility of the intervention; (b) impact on viewer beliefs and stigma; (c) impact on the recovery of workgroup members; and (d) tone and content of the resultant videos. The project involved multiple steps. To start, three workgroups of between 4 and 10 core members with mental illness were gathered in different Canadian cities (Montreal, Toronto, Halifax). This involved collaboration with a local psychosocial rehabilitation center in each city to recruit participants and help conduct the project. Second, we hired a professional videographer-facilitator at each site to conduct classroom instruction in video scripting, filming, and editing. This instruction occurred twice weekly at the rehabilitation centers during the first few months of the project. Third, the workgroups were tasked with creating a series of documentary-style or digital storytelling videos about mental illness using their newly learned skills, with assistance from the group videographer-facilitator over an 18-month period. Each workgroup was given complete editorial control over the content, themes, segmentation, and length of videos. Fourth, the workgroups made efforts to disseminate the videos on social media and organize a series of in-person screenings of the videos to target groups, including (a) tertiary students and young adults, (b) health and social-service providers, and (c) the general public. To encourage engagement and create a recognizable brand, we entitled the project and its activities Recovery Advocacy Documentary Action Research. The videos and other information are available at https://www.radarmentalhealth.com.

Study results indicated that the citizen journalism/PV approach is a feasible and potentially effective antistigma intervention (Whitley et al., 2020). Over the course of 18 months, the workgroups produced 26 videos (7 in Halifax, 10 in Toronto, and 9 in Montreal), with a median length of 10 minutes. The workgroups also organized 49 screenings (13 in Halifax, 18 in Montreal, 18 in Toronto), which reached more than 1,500 people. Audience members ($N = 1,104$, 72% response rate) completed a postscreening questionnaire assessing impact on knowledge, beliefs, and attitudes. Aggregated responses indicate a positive impact of the videos on viewers, because they overwhelmingly agreed that the videos had increased their understanding of stigma and recovery and changed their attitudes toward people with mental illness for the better. The questionnaire data were augmented by six focus groups with viewers ($N = 30$), which also indicated that the videos had a positive impact on viewers. Four clear themes emerged from the analysis of focus group data, indicating that viewers typically found the videos: (a) educational and informative; (b) real and relatable; (c) attention grabbing; and (d) change inducing.

All videos were uploaded to a dedicated YouTube channel. The most popular video (about homelessness) has over 9,000 views, while two other videos (one about stigma and one digital storytelling video about recovery) have over 3,000 views. A conscious effort was made to share videos on other social media platforms, and some videos were embedded in articles on popular websites, including *Psychology Today* and the *Huffington Post*, thus extending their reach.

Another aim of the project was to assess the impact of project involvement on workgroup members, in particular on recovery and self-stigma. This work was done through qualitative interviews ($n = 20$). Participants reported that regular involvement in this project fostered their recovery and reduced their self-stigma in a variety of ways, imparting multiple psychosocial benefits, which are summarized in five themes: (a) skill-acquisition, (b) platform and voice, (c) connectedness, (d) a meaningful focus, and (e) personal development (Whitley et al., in press).

A final aim of this project was to compare the tone and content of the 26 project videos with the tone and content of mainstream television portrayals of mental illness. To meet this aim, we randomly selected 26 television clips mentioning mental illness from CBC Toronto, one of Canada's most popular television channels, and conducted a comparative analysis between the two sets of videos. The analysis indicated that the participatory videos produced by the citizen journalists tended to be much more positive and hopeful than the videos produced by the CBC professional journalists. For example, over 60% of the citizen journalism videos focused on recovery compared to 27% of the television clips. Conversely, over 40% of the television clips focused on crime, violence, or legal issues, in comparison to only 23% of the citizen journalism videos. The citizen journalism videos were also more likely to highlight social issues experienced by people with mental illness, especially the problem of stigma (Carmichael et al, 2019). In sum, this project offers preliminary evidence that participatory video is a feasible and potentially effective antistigma intervention with broad potential use.

Recommendations

The literature described in this chapter implies that a multipronged approach is necessary to tackle stigma in the media, pointing to three specific recommendations. First, carefully crafted long-term interventions targeted at professional journalists and the mainstream media can be successful in improving coverage and reducing stigma. Such interventions may be most effective when supported and implemented by well-organized and well-funded national-level organizations such as the MHCC. These interventions are more of a top-down type of initiative, because they typically involve collaboration between professionals including researchers, journalists, and program managers. Indeed, co-creation of such interventions with journalists should be considered essential to ensure that the interventions are relevant, accessible, and feasible. Like any attempt to change embedded practice, a long-term approach is necessary, and incremental progress in the short term can lead to significant progress in the long term.

Second, top-down national or regional-level initiatives can be complemented by more bottom-up, locally grounded, grass-roots approaches that harness the power of social media. Indeed, the research reviewed in this chapter indicates that citizen journalism and participatory video are powerful group interventions that can produce content to educate viewers and reduce public stigma, while positively benefiting workgroup participants in terms of recovery and self-stigma. As such, psychiatric rehabilitation centers and other mental health advocacy organizations should consider initiating similar citizen journalism projects in their own locales. Such endeavors may be especially important in the COVID-19 era, as more and more events occur virtually and social media has become increasingly prominent.

Third, research indicates the importance of a stratified approach that attends to differential media coverage according to factors such as age, gender, disorder, ethnocultural status, and other important sociodemographic factors. As stated, my own analyses indicated that articles that focused on a man with a mental illness were significantly more negative and stigmatizing than the articles that focused on a woman, which were more likely to be compassionate and sympathetic (Whitley et al., 2015). More recently, I have been commissioned by Veteran's Affairs Canada to conduct a 2-year study (2020–2022) to examine the tone and content of media coverage of veteran's mental health and suicide, given the elevated rates of suicide and mental illness in this population. An aim of this research is to produce educational material (including guidelines) to help journalists report about Canadian veterans in a fair, balanced, and responsible manner and to move beyond stigmatizing stereotypes. Similar analyses are encouraged elsewhere to identify subgroups of people with mental health issues that may be particularly misrepresented in the media and to develop relevant interventions accordingly.

Conclusion

Since the beginning of the 21st century, a rich and diverse literature has emerged to examine media coverage of mental illness. These studies have spurred numerous top-down interventions and programs designed to reduce stigma and stereotypes in the mainstream media and promote more positive, balanced, and accurate coverage. In parallel, numerous bottom-up and locally grounded interventions have emerged attempting to promote positive and hopeful content about mental illness in social media. This multipronged approach appears to have success in the struggle against stigma, and it is hoped that such interventions will be intensified, implemented, and evaluated elsewhere.

Key Recommendations

- It is necessary to take a multipronged approach to tackle stigma in the media, combining top-down and bottom-up activity to reach both traditional media and social media.
- Like any attempt to change embedded practice, a long-term approach is necessary, and incremental progress in the short term can lead to significant progress in the long term.
- This should involve the development and implementation of educational resources aimed at the mainstream media, co-created with input from researchers, journalists, and others.
- Such resources can include the development of (a) reporting guidelines; (b) in-person trainings for journalists and journalism students; and (c) online courses.
- This should be complemented by bottom-up citizen journalism approaches, which can result in sharable content for social media that can educate viewers and reduce stigma.
- Participatory video may be a particularly effective intervention because we now live in a "digital age" with increasing numbers of people obtaining information via videos.
- Psychiatric rehabilitation centers and other mental health advocacy organizations should consider initiating locally grounded citizen journalism or participatory video projects.
- All interventions with the mainstream media should be evaluated by systematic research examining the tone and content of media coverage before and after interventions.
- All citizen journalism and participatory video interventions should be evaluated by systematic research assessing user engagement and impact on media consumers.
- A stratified approach can identify subgroups of people with mental health issues that may be particularly misrepresented in the media, leading to targeted intervention.

References

Allan, S., Sonwalkar, P., & Carter, C. (2007). Bearing witness: Citizen journalism and human rights issues. *Globalisation, Societies and Education, 5*(3), 373–389.

Anderson, M. (2003). "One flew over the psychiatric unit": Mental illness and the media. *Journal of Psychiatric and Mental Health Nursing, 10*(3), 297–306.

Carmichael, V., Adamson, G., Sitter, K. C., & Whitley, R. (2019). Media coverage of mental illness: A comparison of citizen journalism vs. professional journalism portrayals. *Journal of Mental Health, 28*(5), 520–526.

Carpenter, S. (2010). A study of content diversity in online citizen journalism and online newspaper articles. *New Media & Society, 12*(7), 1064–1084.

Chermak, S. (1994). Crime in the news media: A refined understanding of how crimes become news. In G. Barak (Ed.), *Media, process, and the social construction of crime: Studies in newsmaking criminology* (pp. 95–129). Garland.

Corrigan, P. W., Powell, K. J., & Michaels, P. J. (2013). The effects of news stories on the stigma of mental illness. *Journal of Nervous and Mental Disease, 201*(3), 179–182.

Corrigan, P. W., Watson, A. C., Gracia, G., Slopen, N., Rasinski, K., & Hall, L. L. (2005). Newspaper stories as measures of structural stigma. *Psychiatric Services, 56*(5), 551–556.

Coverdale, J., Nairn, R., & Claasen, D. (2002). Depictions of mental illness in print media: A prospective national sample. *Australian and New Zealand Journal of Psychiatry, 36*(5), 697–700.

Crisp, A. H., Gelder, M. G., Rix, S., Meltzer, H. I., & Rowlands, O. J. (2000). Stigmatisation of people with mental illnesses. *British Journal of Psychiatry, 177*, 4–7.

Dinos, S., Stevens, S., Serfaty, M., Weich, S., & King, M. (2004). Stigma: The feelings and experiences of 46 people with mental illness. Qualitative study. *British Journal of Psychiatry, 184*(2), 176–181.

Farinosi, M., & Treré, E. (2014). Challenging mainstream media, documenting real life and sharing with the community: An analysis of the motivations for producing citizen journalism in a post-disaster city. *Global Media and Communication, 10*(1), 73–92.

Francis, C., Pirkis, J., Blood, R. W., Dunt, D., Burgess, P., Morley, B., Stewart, A., & Putnis, P. (2004). The portrayal of mental health and illness in Australian non-fiction media. *The Australian and New Zealand Journal of Psychiatry, 38*(7), 541–546.

Harcup, T., & O'Neill, D. (2017). What is news? News values revisited (again). *Journalism Studies, 18*(12), 1470–1488.

Luce, A., Jackson, D., & Thorsen, E. (2017). Citizen journalism at the margins. *Journalism Practice, 11*(2-3), 266–284.

McGinty, E. E., Webster, D. W., & Barry, C. L. (2013). Effects of news media messages about mass shootings on attitudes toward persons with serious mental illness and public support for gun control policies. *American Journal of Psychiatry, 170*(5), 494–501.

Mitchell, C. (2008). Taking the picture, changing the picture: Visual methodologies in educational research in South Africa. *South African Journal of Educational Research, 28*(3), 365–383.

Mythen, G. (2010). Reframing risk? Citizen journalism and the transformation of news. *Journal of Risk Research, 13*(1), 45–58.

Nairn, R. G., & Coverdale, J. H. (2005). People never see us living well: An appraisal of the personal stories about mental illness in a prospective print media sample. *The Australian and New Zealand Journal of Psychiatry, 39*(4), 281–287.

News Media Canada. (2019, November 28). Newspaper *readership remains strong*. https://nmc-mic.ca/2019/11/28/newspaper-readership-remains-strong/

Olstead, R. (2002). Contesting the text: Canadian media depictions of the conflation of mental illness and criminality. *Sociology of Health & Illness, 24*(5), 621–643.

Parr, H. (2007). Collaborative video-making as process, method and text in mental health research. *Cultural Geographies, 14*(1), 114–138.

Pietrus, M. (2013). *Opening Minds interim report*. Mental Health Commission of Canada.

Reavley, N. J., Jorm, A. F., & Morgan, A. J. (2016). Beliefs about dangerousness of people with mental health problems: The role of media reports and personal exposure to threat or harm. *Social Psychiatry and Psychiatric Epidemiology, 51*(9), 1257–1264.

Rosen, A., Goldbloom, D., & McGeorge, P. (2010). Mental Health Commissions: Making the critical difference to development and reform of mental health services. *Current Opinion in Psychiatry, 23*(6), 593–603.

Rowe, R., Tilbury, F., Rapley, M., & O'Ferrall, I. (2003). "About a year before the breakdown I was having symptoms": Sadness, pathology and the Australian newspaper media. *Sociology of Health & Illness, 25*(6), 680–696.

Rusch, N., & Thornicroft, G. (2014). Does stigma impair prevention of mental disorders? *British Journal of Psychiatry, 204*, 249–251.

Salganik, M. J. (2019). *Bit by bit: Social research in the digital age*. Princeton University Press.

Schomerus, G., Stolzenburg, S., & Angermeyer, M. C. (2015). Impact of the Germanwings plane crash on mental illness stigma: Results from two population surveys in Germany before and after the incident. *World Psychiatry, 14*(3), 362–363.

Shoemaker, P. J., & Vos, T. P. (2009). *Gatekeeping theory*. Routledge.

Sitter, K. C. (2012). Participatory video: Toward a method, advocacy and voice (MAV) framework. *Intercultural Education, 23*(6), 541–554.

Stark, C., Paterson, B., & Devlin, B. (2004). Newspaper coverage of a violent assault by a mentally ill person. *Journal of Psychiatric and Mental Health Nursing, 11*(6), 635–643.

Stuart, H. (2003). Stigma and the daily news: Evaluation of a newspaper intervention. *The Canadian Journal of Psychiatry, 48*(10), 651–656.

Stuart, H., Chen, S. P., Christie, R., Dobson, K., Kirsh, B., Knaak, S., Koller, M., Krupa, T., Lauria-Horner, B., Luong, D., Modgill, G., Patten, S. B., Pietrus, M., Szeto, A., & Whitley, R. (2014). Opening minds in Canada: Targeting change. *The Canadian Journal of Psychiatry, 59*(10, Suppl. 1), S13–S18.

Swasy, A., Tandoc, E., Bhandari, M., & Davis, R. (2015). Traditional reporting more credible than citizen news. *Newspaper Research Journal, 36*(2), 225–236.

Thornicroft, A., Goulden, R., Shefer, G., Rhydderch, D., Rose, D., Williams, P., Thornicroft, G., & Henderson, C. (2013). Newspaper coverage of mental illness in England 2008–2011. *The British Journal of Psychiatry, 202*(s55), s64–s69.

Thornicroft, G. (2006). *Shunned*. Oxford University Press.

Wahl, O. F., Wood, A., & Richards, R. (2002). Newspaper coverage of mental illness: Is it changing? *Psychiatric Rehabilitation Skills, 6*(1), 9–31.

Wall, M. (2015). Citizen journalism: A retrospective on what we know, an agenda for what we don't. *Digital Journalism, 3*(6), 797–813.

White, S. A. (2003). *Participatory video: Images that transform and empower*. Sage.

Whitley, R., Adeponle, A., & Miller, A. R. (2015). Comparing gendered and generic representation of mental illness in Canadian newspapers: An exploration of the chivalry hypothesis. *Social Psychiatry and Psychiatric Epidemiology, 50*(2), 325–333.

Whitley, R., & Berry, S. (2013a). Trends in newspaper coverage of mental illness in Canada: 2005–2010. *The Canadian Journal of Psychiatry, 58*(2), 107–112.

Whitley, R., & Berry, S. (2013b). Analyzing media representations of mental illness: Lessons learnt from a national project. *Journal of Mental Health, 22*(3), 246–253.

Whitley, R., & Hickling, F. (2007). Open papers, Open Minds? Media representations of psychiatric deinstitutionalization in Jamaica. *Transcultural Psychiatry, 44*(4), 659–671.

Whitley, R., Sitter, K. C., Adamson, G., & Carmichael, V. (2020). Can participatory video reduce mental illness stigma? Results from a Canadian action-research study of feasibility and impact. *BMC Psychiatry, 20*(1), 16.

Whitley, R., & Wang, J. (2017a). Good news? A longitudinal analysis of newspaper portrayals of mental illness in Canada 2005 to 2015. *The Canadian Journal of Psychiatry, 62*(4), 278–285.

Whitley, R., & Wang, J. (2017b). Television coverage of mental illness in Canada: 2013–2015. *Social Psychiatry and Psychiatric Epidemiology, 52*(2), 241–244.

16

Dissemination and Implementation Science in Stigma Programs

Keith S. Dobson and Heather Stuart

As the earlier chapters in this volume attest, there has been a remarkable amount of research conducted over the past decade to develop, validate, and use stigma assessment tools and stigma reduction programs related to mental illnesses. While the focus of the Opening Minds program within the Mental Health Commission of Canada was originally youth, healthcare providers, the workplace, and the media (see other chapters in this volume), recent developments have included student populations, including both postsecondary and high school levels. Programs in other parts of the world have emphasized broad-based social marketing education and stigma interventions for the public at large (Henderson & Thornicroft, 2009, 2013; Thornicroft et al., 2013) and for targeted mental disorders in others (Jorm et al., 2006). Most of these programs are situated in a specific national and cultural context, and although the evaluation of stigma reduction programs has certainly increased in recent years, there are many programs that are still developed and used without strong theoretical or logic models, relatively poorly defined outcomes, and limited evaluation.

We believe that the field of antistigma programming is on the threshold of a large step forward. Early work helped to define the parameters of stigma, which are now generally agreed to involve social stigma, self-stigma, and structural stigma (see Chapter 1), and tools to measure these various dimensions (see Yang & Link, 2015; other chapters in this volume). Although structural stigma is a construct that has been known for some time, the field is only now starting to distinguish the various attitudes, emotions, and discriminatory behaviors that can be monitored within organizations and at the structural levels of healthcare and other systems, to both recognize the elements of structural stigma in the first instance and then (hopefully) document their decrease over time.

The reliable and valid measurement of constructs such as social stigma, self-stigma, and structural stigma is a relatively simple task, certainly as compared to the development and validation of programs to modify these constructs. The design of a specific intervention, even within a specific context or for a specific target group, is itself a challenging process, not to mention its implementation and evaluation. In this chapter we will discuss some of the more salient issues related to design and evaluation, which are hopefully followed by the dissemination and implementation of evidence-based programs to reduce various forms of stigma. In doing so, we differentiate among the ideas of development and evaluation, dissemination, and implementation, so these terms are briefly defined.

Development and evaluation of a particular intervention usually occurs within a defined context (place, population) and a particular time, as well as with intended outcomes. For example, a public information campaign might be launched in a specific country with the goal of improving knowledge about the frequency of occurrence of mental illnesses in the entire population. The development of this program requires a theory of change or logic model: statements about the proposed program elements that will modify certain mechanisms to achieve the desired outcomes. The logic model requires a defined target audience and defined outcomes that can be measured to know if the program "succeeded." Assuming the logic model is sensible, it may be possible to move ahead to a study that provides "proof of concept": that the program might work in the original context, as designed.

Even with this simple example, multiple questions must be addressed and there are many problems to solve. Will the information campaign be targeted toward the entire population or only selected sectors? If the latter, how will these sectors be chosen, and why? Who is the target audience? What medium for information will be used: television, print, social media, live productions, all of the above? What specific information is to be provided to the public? Who will produce the public information content, and how? What is the putative mechanism of action for program success, and how might it be evaluated? Are the mechanisms of action themselves based on evidence, or are they unique? Who will ensure that the program is delivered as intended? What is the baseline level of knowledge about the issue being discussed? How much of a change would be considered a program success? How will the outcome be measured? Is there a validated assessment tool, or does one need to be developed? What type of sampling will be used to evaluate the program's outcomes? Would the developers be happy with strong media presence but weak outcomes on the designated measure? How long might the potential outcome last; how long will it be measured? Is the hypothetical outcome something that can be quantified and analyzed statistically, or does the program need a qualitative evaluation, or both? Who will conduct the evaluation, with what measures, when, and with what reporting mechanism? How much will it cost to achieve an effect? How often does it need to be delivered to maintain its effect? Is it sustainable?

Even a simple idea such as a public information campaign entails a myriad of specific questions. Every decision represents increased specificity, but also limits the results to that unique design, implementation, and evaluation. Put otherwise, the generalizability of any given program is delimited by the number of specific decisions made for a unique program instantiation. The issues associated with research design, methods to evaluate outcomes, and the meanings attached to statistical versus clinical/social significance of study results are well known in the field of clinical science and field research (Brownson et al., 2012; McHugh & Barlow, 2012) and remain hot topics of debate.

Imagine, however, that a program is developed, evaluated using a mixed method design, and found to have merit. Perhaps a public information campaign in a certain country has increased public awareness of the prevalence of mental illnesses by 20%, and this increased awareness surpasses the expected outcome. Then imagine that this campaign's results last for 6 months, which is longer than anticipated. How, then, is this program to be used? Can it be taken to another country and simply used as it was first developed? What language, cultural, or other changes are required? How acceptable will the messages embedded in the information campaign be in the new country? Can its outcomes be replicated? These are the issues associated with dissemination.

Program Dissemination

Dissemination is the practice of taking a validated program more or less in its original form into a new context for re-evaluation. A formal definition is that "dissemination is an active approach of spreading evidence-based interventions to the target audience via determined channels using planned strategies" (Rabin & Brownson, 2012, p. 26). This type of work is critical for a number of reasons. At a very basic level, the replication of an initial result is important to document that the initial result was not a statistical anomaly. Conventional statistics are typically declared significant if the probability of error is 5% or less. A 5% error rate is not particularly critical if the outcome being assessed is benign, such as reducing stigma. However, if it turns out that a national media campaign is very expensive (as it is), then an erroneous claim of success can be an expensive problem, especially if another country elects to adopt the same program based on the evidence. In this situation, it is critical to evaluate if the program can be successfully disseminated and validated in a second setting. From a purely statistical perspective, although the chance of a given error may be 5% or .05, the probability of the same error being made twice is $.05 \times .05$, or .0025, which is slight. Put otherwise, the replication of a successful program is an essential requirement to ensure program outcomes and to validate the program.

Even assuming that a program can achieve statistically significant change twice, and so is unlikely to yield spurious outcomes, the issue of dissemination is important from the perspective of generalizability. For example, can a public information campaign developed and validated in one country simply be taken and implemented without change in another country? Is it reasonable to expect the same results in the new context? What necessary modifications must be made? Can the program be delivered with the same fidelity as in the original project? Does the target audience in the new context mirror the original? To the extent that the second context is a direct reflection of the first, then the dissemination is likely to move uneventfully, and replication can be assessed. To the extent that the second context differs, then the second instantiation of the program is a test of the program's generalizability to a new setting, audience, mode of delivery, etc., and the identification of whatever parameters require adjustment.

One of the clear advantages of a replication setting that is similar in most respects to the original is that the results from the second evaluation process can be more or less directly compared to the original (assuming that the same outcomes have been assessed). This process of "benchmarking" the results of the second study against the original are clear (Spilka & Dobson, 2015), and even if the second setting is different in some definable ways, the benchmark set by the original study can be used to see if the results are equivalent or different. Indeed, if there are multiple replications that vary in known ways, it may be possible to discern which variations are associated with reduced replication (or possible enhancement!) of the original results.

A number of factors affect dissemination (Colditz, 2012). As shown in Table 16.1, these factors center around issues related to the available quality and type of information that exists about a given program or intervention; the clarity of its contents; the values, preferences, and beliefs of the group or organization that is considering if they will disseminate the program; and the context for dissemination. Note that all of these factors can be either facilitative or preventative of dissemination, depending on how they are structured.

Assuming that a group or organization chooses to engage in dissemination of an existing program, a host of considerations emerge. A major issue is whether adaption is required. This issue is sometimes framed as a question of fidelity: Can the program be delivered in the dissemination project in the same manner as in the original? Are the same methods available? Can the people who deliver the program be trained to a

Table 16.1 Factors That Affect Dissemination

Category	Factor
Information	• Scientific basis; knowledge about causality • Source (professional, governmental, media, social) • Format and framing
Clarity of contents	• Perceived validity • Perceived relevance • Perceived strength of the message • Intervention cost
Values, preferences, beliefs	• Role of the decision-maker • Background (education, economic, personal experience) • Political affiliation • Willingness to adopt innovations (readiness for change) • Willingness to accept uncertainty • Willingness to accept risk • Ethical decision-making
Context	• Culture • Political opportunities and constraints • Timing • Media attention • Financial factors

Adapted from Bero et al. (1998), Anderson et al. (2005), and Colditz (2012).

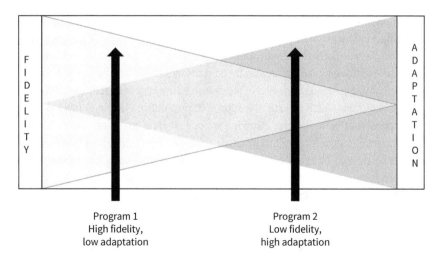

Figure 16.1 A Conceptual Framework to Consider Fidelity and Adaption for Dissemination

high standard, to match the original program? Are the same outcome measures available? To the extent that the answer to this series of question is yes, then the results should, in theory, be similar to the original. Such a situation would be represented by Program 1 in Figure 16.1, which would represent a dissemination project with higher fidelity and lower levels of adaptation. In contrast, to the extent that adaptation or "fit" to the new context is required, results may vary. Such adaptations may include more straightforward issues such as language translation, but may also involve a host of other issues such as the people who are trained, the quality of training, the settings in which the program is offered, and much more. Program 2 in Figure 16.1 represents a program wherein there has been more adaptation to novel circumstances in the dissemination site.

Dissemination can be haphazard, in the sense that a second group or organization may learn about an outcome in the original setting and simply choose to study the program within their context. This type of dissemination project may lead to no lasting change and largely serve as a stand-alone research project. Dissemination can also be purposeful and employ strategically chosen parameters to test the generalizability of an original program to new subgroups, cultural groups, languages groups, or countries. The latter process is more likely when an organization develops the original program and is motivated to test the value of the program in new settings, which can also be considered new markets.

Implementation and Implementation Science

In contrast to dissemination work, implementation science (IS) is a somewhat newer and broader concept (Bauer & Kirchner, 2020; Damschroder et al., 2009). According to Rabin and Brownson (2012), implementation is "the process of putting to use or integrating evidence-based interventions within a setting" (p. 26). In this sense, IS predicated on preexisting evidence, as can be gleaned from both basic and dissemination research. Indeed, it would generally be somewhat risky to attempt to implement a program based on a single project or study and without at least replicating the benefits of the program within a particular setting or population. Implementation is also a broader construct than dissemination in the sense that its goal is typically a sustained or long-term change in policy and practice, whereas a dissemination study may have a shorter term goal of examining the generalizability of a program or project as a proof of concept, with no intention of longer term sustainability.

Different models of IS exist (Gaglio & Glasgow, 2012). The PRECEDE–PROCEED model (Green & Kreuter, 2005) defines two broad aspects of implementation. In the PRECEDE part of the model are considerations most relevant to basic and dissemination research: predisposing, reinforcing and enabling constructs in educational/environmental diagnosis, and evaluation. These aspects deal with issues already discussed in this chapter relevant to both the conduct of foundational program research and its generalization to novel settings and contexts. The PROCEED aspect of the model relates to a broader implementation, because the acronym speaks to policy, regulatory, and organizational constructs in educational and environmental development. These factors were added after than the original PRECEDE dimensions, but directly reference the need to consider the nature of the organization in which an intervention or program is being implemented and the ways in which policy, regulatory, and organizational factors can either help or hinder the adoption and maintenance of that program (see http://www.lgreen.net/precede.htm) .

An alternative IS framework, and one that has become increasing popular, is the RE-AIM model (see https://www.re-aim.org). RE-AIM stands for research, effectiveness, adoption, implementation, and maintenance. The model is founded on the idea of foundational and dissemination research, and in terms of effectiveness it also considers issues related to the demonstrable measure of intended outcomes (including both positive intended outcomes and minimal or no negative outcomes). The latter three aspects of the RE-AIM framework explicitly reference the utilization of programs in broader settings. Thus, adoption considerations include whether the program can be generalized to real-world settings. Will the program have broad acceptability, for example, in both the service providers and the recipients of the program? Is the program politically acceptable and likely to be adopted? Implementation deals with further study of the program in its novel setting. Considerations here include adaptations of the program for the new context, the ability to deliver the program with fidelity, the training costs and benefits, and any potential unforeseen difficulties in the delivery of the program. Finally, maintenance is related to considerations such as funding policies, economic costs and offsets of the program, the sustainability of the program as intended, and the "political capital" that a program can engender, which may make it more difficult to terminate. A key consideration in the maintenance of a program is its acceptability to providers, recipients, agencies, and funders. In order to sustain a program, there is a high probability that the evaluation process needs to include key participants, including the public. Ideally, it will also be possible to document not only the direct costs of providing a program (to show that the funding is sustainable), but also that the program engenders cost savings or offsets. Although the formal computation of a "return on investment" is often difficult to document in the field of mental health, it can be critical, if and when it is possible.

In addition to the PRECEDE–PROCEED and RE-AIM models, there are now a growing number of models and systems for implementation study and research. Moore and colleagues (2014, 2015) have developed a process framework to evaluate the design and implementation of programs and projects across their development and field evaluation. The World Health Organization has developed an Implementation Research Toolkit (World Health Organization, 2014) to help groups and organization design and evaluate real-world programs. In addition to the issues already discussed in this chapter, their framework references the need for program implementation work to be systematic, multidisciplinary, contextual, and complex in its formulation (see Table 16.2).

Table 16.2 Key Characteristics of Implementation Research

Characteristic	Description
Systematic	• The systematic study of how evidence-based public health interventions are integrated and provided in specific settings and how resulting health outcomes vary across communities • Balances relevance to real-life situations with rigor, strictly adhering to norms of scientific inquiry
Multidisciplinary	• Analysis of biological, social, economic, political, system, and environmental factors that impact implementation of specific health interventions • Interdisciplinary collaborations between behavioral and social scientists, clinicians, epidemiologists, statisticians, engineers, business analysts, policy makers, and key stakeholders
Contextual	• Demand driven; framing of research questions is based on needs identified by implementers in the health system • Research is relevant to local specifics and needs and aims to improve healthcare delivery in a given context • Generates generalizable knowledge and insights that can be applied across various settings • Mindful of cultural and community-based influences
Complex	• Dynamic and adaptive • Multiscale: occurs at multiple levels of health systems and communities • Analyses multicomponent program and policies • Nonlinear, iterative, evolving process

From World Health Organization, 2014.

Dissemination and IS Research in the Field of Stigma

As documented in this book and elsewhere (Arboleda-Flórez & Sartorius, 2008; Stuart et al., 2012), there are many models to identify, mitigate, reduce, or eliminate stigma related to mental illnesses. Some models have a sound logic to them, use established and validated metrics, and are evaluated using established research methodologies, including mixed methods research. Unfortunately, such models are the exception rather than the rule. More commonly, stigma approaches are developed at a local level based on a common-sense logic or belief and with poorly articulated processes of change and limited evaluation. Some well-intentioned mental health campaigns may have the paradoxical effect of increasing stigma if they are not well conceptualized and conducted (Corrigan, 2018).

The methods of dissemination research and implementation science are not a panacea to poorly conducted investigations. Further, the development and evaluation of a given project or program must take place within a historical, contextual, and practical set of circumstances. Nonetheless, it is our firm conviction that developers should review the issues seen in Tables 16.1 and 16.2 prior to embarking on any novel program or project in the area of mental illness stigma. In this context, several key considerations emerge.

Individuals or groups that wish to promote stigma reduction programs must have a logic model (Gasper, 1997; Kellogg Foundation, 2006; Knowlton & Philips, 2013). A logic model is the framework that describes the relationships among factors such as the required resources for a program, the intended activities, and the expected outcomes. Often a logic model is graphically presented, but it forms a blueprint for the organization, planning, implementation, and evaluation of a program. A logic model compels the organizer to consider the proposed mechanisms of action for the program and the linkage between the program's activities and the expected outcomes. These considerations can expose flaws in the logic; for example, a simple educational program about the nature of mental illnesses is unlikely to shift discriminatory behaviors in healthcare because there is no clear logical linkage between education or information alone and behavior change—something that many intervention programs naively assume.

The development of a logic model should encourage program developers to consider validated theories or best practices, as have been established in prior research, and further contemplate if these theories and practices should be incorporated into the current program. As noted earlier in this chapter, there are a series of factors to consider in the adoption of prior knowledge, including whether the existing theory and research apply in the context for the new or innovative application. To the extent that the current program area is similar to past research, we would argue that dissemination methods can be applied. In such instances, there should be efforts to obtain prior materials and to use them with minimal modification but higher fidelity to the original program and the same or very similar outcome measurement to ascertain if the results can be replicated in the new context. In contrast, to the extent that the novel setting or application is different from the locations or contexts where the development work was conducted, then the principles of IS (Damschroder et al., 2009; Peters et al., 2013) should be adopted, and enhanced modification and revalidation of expected outcomes will be necessary. In this instance, it will be important to evaluate not just stigma reduction outcomes, but also the acceptability of the programs in the novel context and their potential sustainability as secondary outcomes.

As the field of antistigma research and programs develops, we can expect that more new measures will emerge. This volume documents a wide variety of measures that assess aspects of public stigma and self-stigma, particularly with an emphasis on either attitudinal or emotional aspects of stigma. Measures of discriminatory behavior have been relatively underdeveloped, as have measures of structural stigma, so enhanced measurement in those domains are recommended areas for future development. The field has also seen a dramatic increase in recent years of field-tested stigma reduction programs in areas as diverse as public information, educational settings, healthcare, the workplace, and media outlets. The chapters in this volume document the creativity of researchers and the range of outcomes that have already been established. These outcomes represent critical reference points for future theory and program development and are recommended as benchmarks for future stigma reduction programming.

The continued use of evolving theory and research will no doubt yield innovations in models and methods to conceptualize and measure aspects of stigma and to develop and validate models and methods to reduce the stigma of mental illnesses. The frameworks that exist within dissemination research and IS are strongly recommended as the way in which the field will develop and grow to reduce stigma and promote the health and well-being of the hundreds of millions of individuals who experience mental illnesses globally. Bridging the science-to-action gap will be essential to creating a world where people with mental and substance use disorders can live their lives as full and effective members of their communities.

Key Considerations

- The optimal methods for the design and delivery of stigma reduction tools and programs rest on a sound logic model, established outcome measures, and replication procedures.
- Dissemination science methods can be used to determine whether a program that was developed in one context can be implemented successfully elsewhere, with a novel target audience, or focused on a specific aspect of stigma.
- For broader study of the ability to translate and broadly implement methods that have initial success, IS methods can be utilized to encourage the development of programs that are systemic, multidisciplinary, contextual, and complex in nature.

References

Anderson, L. M., Brownson, R. C., Fullilove, M. T., Teutsch, S. M., Novick, L. F., Fielding, J., & Land, G. H. (2005). Evidence-based public policy and practice: Promises and limits. *American Journal of Preventative Medicine, 28* (5 Suppl.), 226–230.

Arboleda-Flórez, J., & Sartorius, N. (Eds.). (2008). *Understanding the stigma of mental illness: Theory and interventions.* J. Wiley & Sons.

Bauer, M. S., & Kirchner, J. (2020). Implementation science: What is it and why should I care? *Psychiatry Research, 283,* 112376. https://doi.org/10.1016/j.psychres.2019.04.025

Bero, L., Grillr, R., Grimshaw, J., Harvey, E., Oxman, A. D., & Thompson, M. (1998). Closing the gap between research and practice: An overview of systematic reviews of interventions to promote the implementation of research findings. *British Medical Journal, 317,* 465–468.

Brownson, R. C., Colditz, G. A., & Proctor, E. K. (Eds.). (2012). *Dissemination and implementation research in health: Translating science to practice.* Oxford University Press.

Colditz, G. A. (2012). The promise and challenges of dissemination and implementation research. In R. C. Brownson, G. A. Colditz, & E. K. Proctor (Eds.), *Dissemination and implementation research in health: Translating science to practice* (pp. 3–22). Oxford University Press.

Corrigan, P. W. (2018). *The stigma effect: Unintended consequences of mental health campaigns.* Columbia University Press.

Damschroder, L. J., Aron, D. C., Keith, R. E., Kirsh, S. R., Alexander, J. A., & Lowery, J. A. (2009). Fostering implementation of health services research findings into practice: A consolidated framework for advancing implementation science. *Implementation Science, 4,* 50. https://doi.org/10.1186/1748-5908-4-50

Gaglio, B., & Glasgow, R. E. (2012). Evaluation approaches for dissemination and implementation research. In R. C. Brownson, G. A. Colditz, & E. K. Proctor (Eds.), *Dissemination and implementation research in health: Translating science to practice* (pp. 327–356). Oxford University Press.

Gasper, D. R. (1997). *"Logical frameworks," a critical assessment: Managerial theory, pluralistic practice.* ISS Working Papers, General Series 19007. International Institute of Social Studies of Erasmus University Rotterdam.

Green, L. W., & Kreuter, M. W. (2005). *Health Program Planning: An Educational and Ecological Approach.* 4th edition. NY: McGraw-Hill Higher Education.

Henderson, C., & Thornicroft, G. (2009) Stigma and discrimination in mental illness: Time to change. *Lancet, 373,* 1928–1930.

Henderson, C., & Thornicroft, G. (2013) Evaluation of the Time to Change programme in England 2008–2011. *British Journal of Psychiatry, 55,* s45–s48.

Jorm, A. F., Christensen, H., & Griffiths, K. M. (2006). Changes in depression awareness and attitudes in Australia: The impact of beyondblue: The national depression initiative. *Australian and New Zealand Journal of Psychiatry, 40,* 42–46.

Kellogg Foundation. (2006). *Logic model development guide.* http://www.wkkf.org/resource-directory/resource/2006/02/wk-kellogg-foundation-logic-model-development-guide

Knowlton, W. L., & Philips, C. C. (2013). *The logic model guidebook: Better strategies for great results* (2nd ed.). Sage.

McHugh, R. K., & Barlow, D. H. (Eds.). (2012). *Dissemination and implementation of evidence-based psychological interventions.* Oxford University Press.

Moore, G., Audrey, S., Barker, M., Bond, L., Bonell, C., Hardeman, W., Moore, L., O'Cathain, A., Tinati, T., Wight, D., & Baird, J. (2015). Process evaluation of complex interventions: Medical

Research Council guidance. *British Medical Journal, 350,* h1258. http://www.bmj.com/content/350/bmj.h1258.long

Moore, G., Barker, M., Bond, L., Bonell, C., Hardeman, W., Moore, L., O'Cathain, A., Tinati, T., Wight, D., & Baird, J. (2014). *Process evaluation of complex interventions: Medical Research Council guidance.* MRC Population Health Science Research Network. http://www.populationhealthsciences.org/MRC-PHSRN-Process-evaluation-guidance-final-2-.pdf

Peters, D. H., Tran, N. T., & Adam, T. (2013) *Implementation research in heath: A practical guide.* World Health Organization. https://www.who.int/iris/bitstream/10665/91758/1/9789241506212_eng.pdf

Rabin, B. A., & Brownson, R. C. (2012). Developing the terminology for dissemination and implementation research. In R. C. Brownson, G. A. Colditz, & E. K. Proctor (Eds.), *Dissemination and implementation research in health: Translating science to practice* (pp. 23–51). Oxford University Press.

Spilka, M. J., & Dobson, K. S. (2015). Promoting the internationalization of evidence-based practice: Benchmarking as a strategy to evaluate culturally transported psychological treatments. *Clinical Psychology: Science and Practice, 22,* 58–75.

Stuart, H., Arboleda-Flórez, J., & Sartorius, N. (2012). *Paradigms lost: Fighting stigma and the lessons learned.* Oxford University Press.

Thornicroft, C., Wyllie, A., Thornicroft, G., & Mehta, G. (2013). Impact of the "Like Minds, Like Mine" anti-stigma and discrimination campaign in New Zealand on anticipated and experienced discrimination. *Australian & New Zealand Journal of Psychiatry, 48* (4), 360–370. https://doi.org/10.1177/0004867413512687

World Health Organization. (2014). *Implementation Research Toolkit Workbook.* WHO Document Production Services. https://www.who.int/tdr/publications/topics/ir-toolkit/en/

Yang, L. H., & Link, B. G. (2015). Measurement of attitudes, beliefs and behaviors of mental Health and mental Illness. Unpublished manuscript, Columbia University, USA. Retrieved June 24, 2021 from https://sites.nationalacademies.org › dbasse_170048

17

Future Directions of Stigma Reduction

Lessons Learned

Heather Stuart and Keith S. Dobson

The Goal Is to Make a Meaningful Difference in the Lives of People With Mental Illnesses

Almost anyone can show their program is effective if they carefully pick the right outcomes and use a broad definition of stigma that includes literacy and mental health awareness. It is relatively easy to show noteworthy increases in knowledge or awareness, even after a brief intervention, but it is much more difficult to show improvements in social inclusion or reductions in structural inequities. We have learned that improving mental health literacy or reducing negative and stereotypic attitudes will not necessarily lead to improved social outcomes for people with mental illnesses. Targeting behavioral outcomes—at both the individual and the organizational level—is necessary to promote full and effective social participation as envisioned by the UN Declaration on the Rights of Persons With Disabilities (United Nations General Assembly, 2006).

Public attitude surveys are a favored method for examining changes in stigma at the population level. However, public attitude surveys are susceptible to social responsibility bias, particularly in areas where active antistigma programming has been operating. Members of the public may mask their true feelings to provide a socially desirable response. Even though public surveys may report fewer negative attitudes and greater compassion, respondents may not be practicing more inclusive behaviors. Thus, changes in public expressions of stereotypical attitudes may be a poor yardstick to measure success in antistigma programming because it is impossible to know if they signify meaningful changes in the day-to-day lives of people with a mental illness (Stuart et al., 2012).

To begin to address this problem, all of the instruments developed by the Opening Minds research team included a measure of social distance that is a proxy (albeit an imperfect one) for behavior change. It measures behavioral intentions under a series of hypothetical circumstances, such as in employment circumstances, housing, friendships, or romantic relationships. The social distance measures were considered the key benchmarks for success.

Targeted Interventions Have a Better Chance of Succeeding

Although the cognitive and social mechanisms underlying the nature and nurture of stigma are similar (we might even say universal), the way in which they play out is determined by the local context. To maximize success, interventions must be targeted and take account of cultural nuances and cultural dynamics (Yang et al., 2007). What we want a family physician to do with respect to someone who has an opioid addiction, for example, is not what we want a police officer to do when dealing with someone who is suicidal. Similarly, the cultural dynamic in an emergency room is not the same as the cultural dynamic of an inpatient psychiatric unit or community mental health program; and the nature of stigma in a large, urban, multicultural setting is not the same as that in a rural or indigenous community. While stigma may be present in all of these places, the remedies that will have local traction will differ. Although early antistigma efforts tended to be global in nature, such as large social marketing campaigns, it is now clear that one size does not fit all.

Opening Minds researchers learned this lesson early on, after pilot testing a large public education campaign. The campaign used various media sources to transmit messages emphasizing the effectiveness of treatment and the possibilities of recovery (Stuart et al., 2014c). Following best practice principles, first-person accounts were featured as a key ingredient for change. Ads were included in major newspapers, prime-time television commercials, and social networking sites. A marketing firm was enlisted to conduct pretest and posttest surveys of 2,000 media-engaged Canadians, defined as those who regularly used media, because they would have been the most likely to have seen or heard the campaign's messages (83.9% return). Despite this, there were no appreciable improvements in any of the survey items. For example, only about one-third of the sample agreed that people with a mental illness could make a complete recovery—one of the central messages of the campaign—and this increased by only 1.1% on the posttest. Given the costs associated with mounting and sustaining large media campaigns and the lackluster results of the pilot, Opening Minds reoriented its approach to more intensive and targeted interventions.

Initially, the targeted approach was met with skepticism in some quarters, given that large campaigns tended to be the go-to method for marketing health messages in Canada and elsewhere and were emerging as a prominent feature of several antistigma initiatives worldwide. In England, for example, a series of large social marketing campaigns were undertaken as the centerpiece to the Time to Change program. They targeted men and women in their mid-20s to mid-40s. Each year there were two main bursts of marketing activity, including national television, print, radio, cinema, outdoor advertisements, and online advertisements. Pretest and posttest surveys conducted by an external marketing firm showed no significant longitudinal improvement in knowledge or intended behavior over the six bursts of media activity, despite the fact that modest levels of campaign awareness were achieved, ranging from 30% to 59% of the sample, depending on the burst (Evans-Lacko et al., 2013). In Sweden, mass media social marketing campaigns were used alongside more targeted initiatives, with some overall positive change. However, it is not possible to disentangle the different influences of these components, making it unclear what were the discrete effects of the population marketing campaign versus the more targeted interventions (Henderson et al., 2016). Even if well-conducted social marketing campaigns could improve knowledge about mental illnesses or change attitudes, it is unlikely that they would be potent enough to alleviate many of the most disturbing consequences of stigma, such as social marginalization or social inequity (Stuart et al., 2012).

Antistigma Interventions Must Be Based on Best Practices and Principles

When the Mental Health Commission of Canada was first funded and it became known that part of the funding would be used to support antistigma initiatives, programs from all over Canada solicited Opening Minds for financial support. A decision was made not to "reinvent the wheel" if there were strong, evidence-based programs that could be scaled up. However, virtually no program had evaluation data supporting its effectiveness. Some had satisfaction data. Many had collected pre- and posttest attitudinal and social distance data but had used unstructured scales and had not had the resources to conduct quantitative analyses. Because different measures were used across programs, data could not be compared to identify the most promising practices. A complete description of the Opening Minds approach is contained elsewhere (Stuart et al., 2014a, 2014b).

Two target groups were chosen to begin work, youth and healthcare workers. A formal request for interest was circulated to a broad array of stakeholders in these groups asking if they would be willing to become pilot evaluation sites. To do this, they had to agree to work with a coordinating team to develop and conduct evaluations, provide a description of the structure and processes needed to mount their respective programs, participate in the development of a theory of change outlining how program resources were supposed to bring about change, and quantify program outputs using a standardized collection strategy. On the advice of an international review panel, programs using contact-based education that directly or indirectly involved people with lived experience to tell recovery stories and encourage active learning were prioritized for evaluation support. Formal partnership agreements were established (Stuart et al., 2014a).

Though the process of soliciting requests for interest did not fit well with the other two target groups subsequently identified (workplaces and media), it did cement an underlying principle that all partnering programs contributed to data collection and evidence building. Only those programs that appeared to be effective (or efficacious) were identified as promising or best practices and became candidates for wider distribution. Individual programs received analytic support from university-based researchers (who received and analyzed the data) and were provided with technical reports outlining their performance. Researchers took considerable time and effort to present findings to program staff in ways that would be understandable to them, provide opportunities for discussion and reflection, and promote better practice alternatives. Programs used these findings to fine-tune their approach. In several cases, programs that were demonstrated to be ineffective independently took the decision to wind down rather than reformulate. Working with teams of university researchers, the emphasis was on reporting anonymized results in the academic literature where they could become part of best practice policy reviews. The technical reports and academic publications were also used by programs to engage funders and solicit more sustainable resources.

While it is difficult to quarrel with evidence-based approaches, the production of evidence in the stigma and broader mental health fields has been subject to resource inequities. The current evidence-based paradigm in medicine largely ignores the social and cultural forces that influence both the production of evidence and the distribution of research and evaluation resources. With fewer prospects for funding, researchers who may have contributed to antistigma evaluations migrate to other areas. Therefore, developing a strong evidence base to support antistigma programming was viewed as an important advocacy tool (Stuart, 2008).

In addition to the Opening Minds program, other large national programs have made a point of building formal ties with university researchers to conduct third-party evaluations. For example, the Time to Change program in the United Kingdom partnered with university researchers from the Institute of Psychiatry at King's College in London. Together they crafted an extensive evaluation plan and produced evidence-based reviews of their activities that have been published in the academic literature (e.g., Evans-Lacko et al., 2013). New Zealand's Like Minds Like Mine antistigma program worked with researchers from the United Kingdom to evaluate the most common stigma experiences reported by service users—information that is vital to correctly targeting programs. These partnerships are exemplary of a new model of research in the stigma field that includes a broad array of program stakeholders as equal partners, particularly those with lived experience of a mental illness.

Understanding Why a Program Works Is Key to Scaling Up

It is one thing to know that a program works and quite another to understand why it works—information that is vital in order to scale programs up to achieve population-level change. All programs have a theory of change or internal logic that outlines how the various components fit together to create a specific outcome. Sometimes these are explicit, logical, and evidence informed. Most of the time in the antistigma field, they are implicit, poorly articulated, illogical, and inconsistent with best practices.

For example, the belief that one needs to change negative and prejudicial attitudes in order to reduce discrimination (a centerpiece of many programs) is not borne out in the social-psychological literature. A meta-analytic review of 60 studies published between 1930 and 1993 showed that prejudice was only rarely predictive of discrimination (Schütz & Six, 1996). Less than 10% of the variation in measures of discriminatory behaviors could be accounted for by prejudicial attitudes. Other research has demonstrated that the relationship between attitudes in general (not necessarily prejudice) and behaviors is weak and sometimes negligible, though some of this work has been criticized for attempting to predict too specific an act from too general a measure (Duckitt, 1992). Given the potential complexity of the relationship between attitudes and behaviors, it is best not to naively assume that upstream changes in stigmatizing attitudes will ipso facto result in the downstream nondiscriminatory behavioral outcomes desired. Greater focus on the behaviors and their specific determinants is needed with the goal of articulating specific theories of change to guide antistigma programming. From a public health perspective, this means identifying the principles and procedures involved in successful antistigma programming in such a way that they can be meaningfully tested using a variety of research methods and, if found to be effective, widely disseminated. It does the field little good to know that gifted antistigma advocates can achieve local successes when what is critical is that these interventions can be clearly specified and taught (Stuart, 2008).

Two of the Opening Minds research teams have grappled with this problem by attempting to identify the key ingredients needed to make a program effective. Knaak and colleagues (2014) identified the program characteristics across 22 programs targeting healthcare providers that were most predictive of positive outcomes. Each program was qualitatively reviewed and coded for the presence or absence of six potential key ingredients or intervention elements that were considered particularly important for improving attitudes and behavioral intentions, as follows: the program should contain social contact in the form of personal testimony from a trained speaker with lived experience of a mental illness; the program should employ multiple points of social contact through, for example, presentations from a live speaker, video presentations, and multiple first-person speakers; the program should focus on behavioral change by teaching skills that could help healthcare workers know what to say and do; the program should engage in myth-busting; the program should use an enthusiastic facilitator or instructor who models a person-centered approach to set the tone for messaging; and the program should emphasize and demonstrate recovery as a key part of the messaging. Programs containing all six ingredients performed significantly better. Two particularly potent ingredients were the inclusion of multiple forms of social contact and an emphasis on recovery.

Similarly, Chen and colleagues (2016) evaluated 18 Canadian antistigma programs that targeted youth aged 12–18 and were affiliated with the Opening Minds initiative. All programs offered some form of contact-based education in the classroom. Using purposive sampling, key stakeholders and program staff were interviewed to determine what components were considered key in mounting a successful program and bringing about the desired change. Site visits were also conducted in 7 programs. Several key constructs were developed from this broad array of information. The first pertained to the speakers. Speakers had to be in recovery, living well with their illness, ready to share their personal stories, and able to engage with students in an open, genuine, and confident way. Speakers had to be equipped with the public speaking skills and knowledge needed to deliver the program. Speaker training was an important part of program success. Finally, speakers had to act as role models for recovery. Second, the program had to correct misperceptions and myths. One important misconception that was widely addressed was the dangerousness attribution—the idea that people with a mental illness are generally dangerous and a public risk. Third, connecting students with resources was considered a key ingredient. This included disseminating information through booklets, handouts, and websites. Finally, authentic and intensive interaction between speakers and students was key to transformative learning. This could be achieved through question-and-answer sessions with students in small classroom groups (e.g., as opposed to large theater-style presentations). An important focus of the interaction was empowerment: empowering students to access resources and empowering students to make positive changes in their schools and wider communities to reduce stigma.

Future Challenges

Although research has demonstrated that stigma is universal, it plays out in different ways in different local contexts. The experience of someone with a mental illness in the United States will be different than the experience of someone in a low- or middle-income country, where mental health systems may be rudimentary or lacking altogether, human rights infractions are frequent, research on best practices is lacking, and local advocacy structures are nonexistent. Similarly, the experience of someone in a large, multicultural urban setting will be different than that of someone in a rural or indigenous community. Programs that hold providers to rigorous fidelity criteria may be too inflexible to meet the needs of people in various settings. Understanding why programs work will be key to adapting and disseminating them on a broader scale.

Future research that examines stigma across cultural settings is scarce, but beginning to grow (e.g., Lasalvia et al., 2015; Pescosolido et al., 2008). Much more research is needed to understand how unique social and cultural factors might influence the nature of stigma and the feasibility and acceptability of antistigma interventions. For example, the World Psychiatric Association, through the Open the Doors program, has successfully mounted antistigma interventions in low-, middle-, and high-income countries. Important to the success of these initiatives has been setting broad principles, building on the activities of local community groups and volunteers, ensuring activities address problems that are locally important, and allowing for flexibility in the way programs are implemented so that they can be adapted to local contexts (Sartorius & Schulze, 2005). As we move forward, it will be important to develop processes that can be used to support local advocates to create cultural adaptations of programs and evaluate their effects.

A second challenge is embedding mental health awareness and antistigma programming into school curricula at all levels of the educational system, from kindergarten to graduate school. While contact-based education programs targeting high school students have been the norm and have been demonstrated to be effective (see other chapters in this book), they have remained an add-on to the curriculum and are included largely at the pleasure of individual teachers, rather than embedded into the fabric of the educational system. (Indeed, much the same could be said for stigma intervention programs in workplaces and healthcare settings and those targeting the media.) Currently, contact-based programs are largely one size fits all. A speaker joins a class at the invitation of the teacher, provides an engaging personal story of recovery and hope, and then answers students' questions. While this model has been widely used with high school students, teachers have been reticent to involve younger children. Taking a life course perspective, it is important to begin early with children and ensure that messages are appropriately targeted to their level of cognitive and emotional development and that they evolve as children grow and develop. Thus far, no systematic attempt has been made to consider how antistigma messages could be tailored to specific grades or how they would build on each other and evolve to give comprehensive knowledge and skills.

A third challenge is to continue to build an evidence base to support antistigma advocacy and practice (Stuart, 2008). One of the major claims of the evidence-based approach is that it provides objective data about the effectiveness of interventions. It eliminates possibilities for subjective decision-making and volunteer bias. The promise of evidence-based practice is that it will result in greater fairness and reduce inequities. Although it is difficult to quarrel with this premise, a closer look at the nature of the evidence required and the methods currently favored to generate it yields several significant challenges for those who would view evidence-based practice as an antistigma tool. This is largely because the evidence-based paradigm ignores the social and cultural forces that influence both the production of evidence and the distribution of resources. It fails to recognize that these processes are themselves subject to significant bias. A recent report produced by the International Alliance of Mental Health Research Funders highlights a number of funding inequities, including that research into mental health is underfunded compared to research for other physical diseases that often account for a smaller proportion of the global disease burden. They also note that the majority of mental health research funding is spent on basic research, rather than applied, health services, or clinical research (Woelbert et al., 2020).

A second problem with the evidence-based paradigm that is particularly relevant for antistigma programming is that the production of "evidence" favors interventions that can be studied using double-blind, randomized controlled trials and summarized using systematic reviews and meta-analyses. While experimental studies and meta-analyses are possible (see Corrigan et al., 2012), many stigma interventions are not oriented to individual-level treatments, with the result that they are not amenable to classical experimental designs. As antistigma efforts increasingly address structural stigma through mechanisms such as legislative change, policy reform, or advocacy, a broader and more eclectic approach to the production of evidence will be required. Notwithstanding the difficulties of combining studies that have used diverse designs, nonexperimental approaches will be disadvantaged in policy reviews because they are currently deemed to provide evidence of a lower quality. As we move forward, it will be important to embrace broader interpretations of "evidence" (Stuart, 2008).

A fourth challenge moving forward will be in developing theories of change for complex, community-based antistigma programs. This will be a daunting task because there is currently little empirical evidence on which to draw to support causal pathways or set plausible thresholds for success. Often antistigma programs are complex and work across several systems or sectors to bring about cultural or community-level change. A major assumption underlying these efforts is that changes at the level of the community (such as legislative or policy reform) will improve the lives of people with a mental illness, through some unspecified trickle-down effect (Stuart, 2008). Nowhere are the difficulties with assumption more evident than in the context of disability legislation. Disability legislation is one component of a larger and complex regulatory framework focusing on human rights and nondiscrimination—one that imposes specific duties on employers to accommodate disabled employees. Despite the duty to accommodate, many employers express concerns about the potential costs of accommodations and show a reluctance to hire disabled people. In the United States, for example, employers have strongly opposed their obligations to make reasonable accommodations and have fought strenuously to legally restrict the definition of disability to exclude many chronic but intermittent conditions such as mental disorders (Stuart, 2007). As this example illustrates, little is known about the components of the wider community that are amenable to change or the specific pathways through which structural or community-level changes result in improvements in individual-level outcomes.

Ultimately, building better practices in antistigma programming will require research and practitioner communities to work together in strategic alliances to develop plausible interventions, evaluate their effects, and ensure that results are used to inform policy and programming. A push to ensure that results are published in the academic literature will enlarge the evidence available to inform policy and practice. In turn, this will make it increasingly difficult for policy makers and funders to be swayed by negative and prejudicial public opinions and overlook the importance of creating sustainable funding options in support of antistigma programming.

Key Considerations

As awareness of the hidden burden of stigma has grown, so have antistigma activities. While a number of national programs have developed, the typical antistigma program is locally developed by enthusiastic advocates, often volunteers, and exists on a shoestring budget. Funding is precarious and there is little opportunity for critical reflection or program evaluation. Many lay theories of stigma reduction, which are based on local wisdom and experience, never make it into the published scientific literature where they can be used to inform policy. The development and evaluation work conducted by the Mental Health Commission of Canada's Opening Minds antistigma initiative made a concerted attempt to harness local wisdom and conduct systematic evaluations of these programs using comparable methods and measures. In so doing, a number of key considerations and lessons have emerged.

- The primary goal is to make meaningful changes in the lives of people with mental and substance use disorders so that they are full and effective members of society. There is no evidence to suggest that changes in knowledge or attitudes can automatically reduce prejudicial beliefs or structural barriers to promote inequities.
- Targeted interventions to key community groups, such as youth, healthcare providers, media, or workers, using contact-based education are more likely to show noteworthy change compared to population-level educational campaigns, which are costlier and more difficult to sustain, or programs focusing on mental health literacy.
- Antistigma programs must continually strive to use best practice evidence to create plausible theories of change that can be systematically tested and, if found to be effective, more broadly disseminated. Charisma and enthusiasm are not scalable or sustainable.

References

Chen, S. P., Koller, M., Krupa, T., & Stuart, H. (2016). Contact in the classroom: Developing a program model for youth mental health contact-based anti-stigma education. *Community Mental Health Journal, 52*(3), 281–293. https://doi.org/10.1007/s10597-015-9944-7

Corrigan, P. W., Morris, S. B., Michaels, P. J., Rafacz, J. D., & Rusch, N. (2012). Challenging the public stigma of mental illness: A meta-analysis of outcome studies. *Psychiatric Services, 63*(10), 963–973. https://doi.org/10.1176/appi.ps.005292011

Duckitt, J. (1992). Prejudice and behavior: A review. *Current Psychology, 11*(4), 291–307. https://doi.org/10.1007/BF02686787

Evans-Lacko, S., Malcolm, E., West, K., Rose, D., London, J., Rüsch, N., Little, K., Henderson, C., & Thornicroft, G. (2013). Influence of Time to Change's social marketing interventions on stigma in England 2009–2011. *British Journal of Psychiatry, 202*(Suppl. 55), 77–88. https://doi.org/10.1192/bjp.bp.113.126672

Henderson, C., Stuart, H., & Hansson, L. (2016). Lessons from the results of three national antistigma programmes. *Acta Psychiatrica Scandinavica, 134.* https://doi.org/10.1111/acps.12605

Knaak, S., Modgill, G., & Patten, S. B. (2014). Key ingredients of anti-stigma programs for health care providers: A data synthesis of evaluative studies. *Canadian Journal of Psychiatry. Revue canadienne de psychiatrie, 59*(10), S19–S26. https://doi.org/10.1177/070674371405901s06

Lasalvia, A., Van Bortel, T., Bonetto, C., Jayaram, G., Van Weeghel, J., Zoppei, S., Knifton, L., Quinn, N., Wahlbeck, K., Cristofalo, D., Lanfredi, M., Sartorius, N., & Thorncroft, G. (2015). Cross-national variations in reported discrimination among people treated for major depression worldwide: The ASPEN/INDIGO international study. *British Journal of Psychiatry, 207*, 507–514. https://doi.org/10.1192/bjp.bp.114.156992

Patten, S. B., Williams, J. V. A., Lavorato, D. H., Bulloch, A. G. M., Charbonneau, M., Gautam, M., Moss, P., Abbey, S., & Stuart, H. (2016). Perceived stigma among recipients of mental health care in the general Canadian population. *Canadian Journal of Psychiatry, 61*(8). https://doi.org/10.1177/0706743716639928

Pescosolido, B. A., Olafsdottir, S., Martin, J. K., & Long, J. S. (2008). Cross-cultural aspects of the stigma of mental illness. *Understanding the Stigma of Mental Illness: Theory and Interventions, 19–35.* https://doi.org/10.1002/9780470997642.ch2

Sartorius, N., & Schulze, H. (2005). *Reducing the stigma of mental illness.* Cambridge University Press.

Schütz, H., & Six, B. (1996). How strong is the relationship between prejudice and discrimination? A meta-analytic answer. *International Journal of Intercultural Relations, 20*(3–4), 441–462. https://doi.org/10.1016/0147-1767(96)00028-4

Stuart, H. (2008). Building an evidence base for anti-stigma programming. In J. Arboleda-Flórez & N. Sartorius (Eds.), *Understanding the stigma of mental illness: Theory and interventions* (pp. 135–145). John Wiley & Sons. https://doi.org/10.1002/9780470997642.ch8

Stuart, H., Arboleda-Flórez, J., & Sartorius, N. (2012). *Paradigms lost: Fighting stigma and the lessons learned.* Oxford University Press.

Stuart, H., Chen, S.-P., Christie, R., Dobson, K., Kirsh, B., Knaak, S., Koller, M., Krupa, T., Lauria-Horner, B., Luong, D., Modgill, G., Patten, S. B., Pietrus, M., Szeto, A., & Whitley, R. (2014a). Opening Minds in Canada: Background and rationale. *Canadian Journal of Psychiatry. Revue canadienne de psychiatrie, 59*(10, Suppl. 1), S8–S12.

Stuart, H., Chen, S.-P., Christie, R., Dobson, K., Kirsh, B., Knaak, S., Koller, M., Krupa, T., Lauria-Horner, B., Luong, D., Modgill, G., Patten, S. B., Pietrus, M., Szeto, A., & Whitley, R. (2014b). Opening minds in Canada: Targeting change. *Canadian Journal of Psychiatry. Revue canadienne de psychiatrie, 59*(10, Suppl. 1), S13–S18.

Stuart, H. (2007). Employment equity and mental disability. *Current Opinion in Psychiatry, 20*(5), 486–490. https://doi.org/10.1097/YCO.0b013e32826fb356

Stuart, H., Patten, S. B., Koller, M., Modgill, G., & Liinamaa, T. (2014). Stigma in Canada: Results from a rapid response survey. *Canadian Journal of Psychiatry. Revue canadienne de psychiatrie, 59*(10), S27–S33. https://doi.org/10.1177/070674371405901s07

United Nations General Assembly. (2006). *Convention on the rights of persons with disabilities (CRPD).* http://www.un.org/disabilities/convention/conventionfull.shtml

Woelbert, E., White, R., Lundell-Smith, K., Grant, J., & Kemmer, D. (2020). *The inequities of mental health research funding.* International Alliance of Mental Health Research Funders. https://www.drugsandalcohol.ie/33429/1/The_Inequities_of_Mental_Health_Research.pdf

Yang, L. H., Kleinman, A., Link, B. G., Phelan, J. C., Lee, S., & Good, B. (2007). Culture and stigma: Adding moral experience to stigma theory. *Social Science and Medicine, 64*(7), 1524–1535. https://doi.org/10.1016/j.socscimed.2006.11.013

Appendices

Appendices are listed in the order they appear throughout the volume and are numbered to correspond to their respective chapter. Thus, the first two appendices of Chapter 5 are numbered 5.1 and 5.2, respectively.

Appendix 5.1

The Opening Minds Scale–Workplace Attitudes

The Opening Minds Scale–Workplace Attitudes (OMS-WA) is a 23-item measure that examines attitudes, stereotypes, and beliefs toward people with mental illnesses. This measure is composed of five subscales: avoidance/social distance (Items 1, 3, 4, 8, 12, 14), danger/unpredictability (Items 10, 13, 15, 19, 23), work-related beliefs/competency (Items 2, 6, 7, 11, 17), helping behaviors (Items 16, 18, 20, 22), and perceptions of responsibility (Items 5, 9, 21). All items from the helping behavior subscale (Items 16, 18, 20, 22) should be reverse coded.

Because of the different number of times within each subscale, we recommend that the mean score be used. As such, subscale mean scores should be calculated by adding all subscale items together and dividing by the number of subscale items. When calculating the mean scale score for the OMS-WA, all items should be summed together and divided by 23. Note that Item 12 may not be appropriate in the workplace setting because feedback from some participants has indicated that agreement with the item may arise as a result of workplace dating policies or personal beliefs that one should not date someone from work, not because of having more stigmatizing attitudes.

Opening Minds Survey for Workplace Attitudes

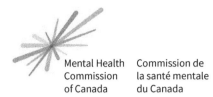

Mental Health Commission de
Commission la santé mentale
of Canada du Canada

This survey was developed as part of the Opening Minds initiative of the Mental Health Commission of Canada to assess opinions in the workplace toward co-workers who may have a mental illness. There are no right or wrong answers to these questions, as everyone will have different attitudes and opinions, based on their own experiences in life.

Please read each of the following statements carefully and decide how much you agree or disagree with each statement. Place an "X" in the correct column for each statement to indicate your response.

	Strongly Disagree	Disagree	Neither Agree nor Disagree	Agree	Strongly Agree
1. I would be upset if a co-worker with a mental illness always sat next to me at work.	☐	☐	☐	☐	☐
2. Most employees with a mental illness are too disabled to work.	☐	☐	☐	☐	☐
3. I would not want to be supervised by someone who had been treated for a mental illness.	☐	☐	☐	☐	☐
4. I would not be close friends with a co-worker who I knew had a mental illness.	☐	☐	☐	☐	☐
5. Employees with a mental illness tend to bring it on themselves.	☐	☐	☐	☐	☐
6. The quality of the work performed by employees with a mental illness is unlikely to meet the expectations of the job.	☐	☐	☐	☐	☐
7. Jobs with tight deadlines and high demands are harmful to employees with mental illnesses.	☐	☐	☐	☐	☐
8. I would try to avoid a co-worker with a mental illness.	☐	☐	☐	☐	☐
9. Employees with a mental illness could snap out of it if they wanted to.	☐	☐	☐	☐	☐
10. Employees with a mental illness are often more dangerous than the average employee.	☐	☐	☐	☐	☐
11. It would be better for employees with mental illnesses to participate in work activities that are outside of the paid labor force.	☐	☐	☐	☐	☐
12. If I knew a co-worker who had a mental illness, I would not date them.	☐	☐	☐	☐	☐
13. Employees with a mental illness often become violent if not treated.	☐	☐	☐	☐	☐
14. I would not want to work with a co-worker who had been treated for a mental illness.	☐	☐	☐	☐	☐

	Strongly Disagree	Disagree	Neither Agree nor Disagree	Agree	Strongly Agree
15. Most violent crimes in the workplace are committed by employees with mental illness.	☐	☐	☐	☐	☐
16. I would tell my supervisor if a co-worker was being bullied because of their mental illness.	☐	☐	☐	☐	☐
17. You can't rely on an employee with a mental illness.	☐	☐	☐	☐	☐
18. I would stick up for a co-worker who had a mental illness if they were being teased.	☐	☐	☐	☐	☐
19. You can never know what an employee with a mental illness is going to do.	☐	☐	☐	☐	☐
20. I would help a co-worker who got behind in their work because of their mental illness.	☐	☐	☐	☐	☐
21. Most employees with a mental illness get what they deserve.	☐	☐	☐	☐	☐
22. I would volunteer my time to work in a program for people with mental illnesses.	☐	☐	☐	☐	☐
23. Employees with serious mental illnesses need to be locked away.	☐	☐	☐	☐	☐

Appendix 5.2

Health and Work Performance Questionnaire Core Questions

1. How many hours does your employer expect you to work in a typical 7-day week? If it varies, estimate the average. If you are self-employed, estimate the number of hours you would consider a full work week. If you have more than one job, combine the total number of hours for all jobs.

_____ NUMBER OF HOURS

2. Now please think of your work experiences over the past 7 days. In the spaces provided below, write the number of days you spent in each of the following work situations.

In the past 7 days, how many days did you . . .   NUMBER OF DAYS

a. . . . miss an **entire** work day because of problems with your
   physical or mental health?   _____
b. . . . miss an **entire** work day for any other reason (including vacation)?   _____
c. . . . miss **part** of a work day because of problems with your physical
   or mental health?   _____
d. . . . miss **part** of a work day for any other reason (including vacation)?   _____
e. . . . come in early, go home late, or work on your day off?   _____

3. About how many hours altogether did you work in the past 7 days? (See examples below.) If you have more than one job, report the combined total number of hours for all jobs. If you did not work at all in the past 7 days, enter "0" and skip to question B1.

_____ NUMBER OF HOURS

Examples for Calculating Hours Worked in the Past 7 Days
8 hours per day for 5 days = 40 hours
7 hours per day for 5 days = 35 hours
8 hours per day for 4 days plus 4 hours per day for 1 day = 36 hours
7 hours per day for 3 days plus 4 hours per day for 2 days = 29 hours

---

3. Did you have any of the following experiences at work in the past 7 days?

	Yes	No
a. Any special work success or achievement?	1	2
b. Any special work failure?	1	2
c. An accident that caused either damage, work delay, a near miss, or a safety risk?	1	2

d. If you answered "Yes" to any of the above questions, please describe what happened.

_____

_____

_____

5. The next questions are about the time you spent during your hours at work in the past 7 days. Circle the one number from each question that comes closest to your experience.

	All of the time	Most of the time	Some of the time	A little of the time	None of the time
a. How often was your performance **higher** than most workers on your job?	1	2	3	4	5
b. How often was your performance **lower** than most workers on your job?	1	2	3	4	5
c. How often did you do not work at times when you were supposed to be working?	1	2	3	4	5
d. How often did you find yourself not working as **carefully** as you should?	1	2	3	4	5
e. How often was the **quality** of your work lower than it should have been?	1	2	3	4	5
f. How often did you not concentrate enough on your work?	1	2	3	4	5
g. How often did health problems limit the kind or amount of work you could do?	1	2	3	4	5

6. On a scale from 0 to 10 where 0 is the worst job performance anyone could have at your job and 10 is the performance of a top worker, how would you rate the usual performance of most workers in a job similar to yours? *(Circle the number)*

Worst Performance										Top Performance
0	1	2	3	4	5	6	7	8	9	10

7. Using the same 0-to-10 scale, how would you rate your usual job performance over the past year or two? *(Circle the number)*

Worst Performance										Top Performance
0	1	2	3	4	5	6	7	8	9	10

8. Using the same 0-to-10 scale, how would you rate your overall performance on the days you worked during the past 7 days? *(Circle the number)*

Worst Performance										Top Performance
0	1	2	3	4	5	6	7	8	9	10

9. How would you compare your overall job performance on the days you worked during *the past 7 days* with the performance of most other workers who have a similar type of job? *(Circle the number)*

1. You were **a lot better** than other workers
2. You were **somewhat better** than other workers
3. You were **a little better** than other workers
4. You were about **average**
5. You were **a little worse** than other workers
6. You were **somewhat worse** than other workers
7. You were **a lot worse** than other workers

Scoring Rules for the HQP 7-Day Version

Scoring Absenteeism

Absolute absenteeism:	$4^* Q1 - 4^* Q3$
Relative absenteeism:	$(4^* Q1 - 4^* Q3) / (4^* Q1)$
Relative hours of work:	$Q3/Q1$

Scoring Presenteeism

Absolute presenteeism:	$10^* Q8$
Relative presenteeism:	$Q8/Q6$

For additional information on the HPQ go to: http://www.hcp.med.harvard.edu/hpq/info.php

Appendix 5.3

The Internalized Stigma of Mental Illness Inventory

We are going to use the term "mental illness" in the rest of this questionnaire, but please think of it as whatever you feel is the best term for it. For each question, please mark whether you strongly disagree (1), disagree (2), agree (3), or strongly agree (4).

	Strongly Disagree	Disagree	Agree	Strongly Agree
1. I feel out of place in the world because I have a mental illness.	1	2	3	4
2. Mentally ill people tend to be violent.	1	2	3	4
3. People discriminate against me because I have a mental illness.	1	2	3	4
4. I avoid getting close to people who don't have a mental illness to avoid rejection.	1	2	3	4
5. I am embarrassed or ashamed that I have a mental illness.	1	2	3	4
6. Mentally ill people shouldn't get married.	1	2	3	4
7. People with mental illness make important contributions to society.	1	2	3	4
8. I feel inferior to others who don't have a mental illness.	1	2	3	4
9. I don't socialize as much as I used to because my mental illness might make me look or behave "weird."	1	2	3	4
10. People with mental illness cannot live a good, rewarding life.	1	2	3	4
11. I don't talk about myself much because I don't want to burden others with my mental illness.	1	2	3	4
12. Negative stereotypes about mental illness keep me isolated from the "normal" world.	1	2	3	4
13. Being around people who don't have a mental illness makes me feel out of place or inadequate.	1	2	3	4
14. I feel comfortable being seen in public with an obviously mentally ill person.	1	2	3	4
115. People often patronize me, or treat me like a child, just because I have a mental illness.	1	2	3	4
16. I am disappointed in myself for having a mental illness.	1	2	3	4
17. Having a mental illness has spoiled my life.	1	2	3	4

	Strongly Disagree	Disagree	Agree	Strongly Agree
18. People can tell that I have a mental illness by the way I look.	1	2	3	4
19. Because I have a mental illness, I need others to make most decisions for me.	1	2	3	4
20. I stay away from social situations in order to protect my family or friends from embarrassment.	1	2	3	4
21. People without mental illness could not possibly understand me.	1	2	3	4
22. People ignore me or take me less seriously just because I have a mental illness.	1	2	3	4
23. I can't contribute anything to society because I have a mental illness.	1	2	3	4
24. Living with mental illness has made me a tough survivor.	1	2	3	4
25. Nobody would be interested in getting close to me because I have a mental illness.	1	2	3	4
26. In general, I am able to live my life the way I want to.	1	2	3	4
27. I can have a good, fulfilling life, despite my mental illness.	1	2	3	4
28. Others think that I can't achieve much in life because I have a mental illness.	1	2	3	4
29. Stereotypes about the mentally ill apply to me.	1	2	3	4

Appendix 6.1

Opening Minds Provider Attitudes Towards Opioid Use Scale

This survey asks for your opinions on a series of statements about people with opioid use problems. Examples of opioids include medications such as Percocet, Vicodin, morphine, and oxycodone. It also includes heroin, fentanyl, and carfentanil. By "opioid use problem" we mean a pattern of use that leads to serious harms, impairment, or distress. Please answer the questions according to your own beliefs, feelings, and experiences.

Please indicate the extent to which you agree or disagree with each of the following statements.	Strongly Disagree	Disagree	Neutral	Agree	Strongly Agree
1. I have little hope that people with opioid use problems will recover.	☐	☐	☐	☐	☐
2. People with opioid use problems are weak willed.	☐	☐	☐	☐	☐
3. People with opioid use problems are to blame for their problems.	☐	☐	☐	☐	☐
4. I tend to use negative terms to talk about people with opioid use problems.	☐	☐	☐	☐	☐
5. People with opioid use problems cost the system too much money.	☐	☐	☐	☐	☐
6. I would see myself as weak if I had an opioid use problem.	☐	☐	☐	☐	☐
7. I tend to act more negatively toward people with opioid use problems than other people I help.	☐	☐	☐	☐	☐
8. People with opioid use problems can't be trusted.	☐	☐	☐	☐	☐
9. People with opioid use problems who take drug therapies like methadone are replacing one addiction with another.	☐	☐	☐	☐	☐
10. I tend to be less patient toward people with opioid use problems than other people I help.	☐	☐	☐	☐	☐
11. People with opioid use problems only care about getting their next dose of drugs.	☐	☐	☐	☐	☐
12. When people with opioid use problems ask for help with something, I have a hard time believing they are sincere.	☐	☐	☐	☐	☐
13. People with opioid use problems should be cut off from services if they don't try to help themselves.	☐	☐	☐	☐	☐

Please indicate the extent to which you agree or disagree with each of the following statements.	Strongly Disagree	Disagree	Neutral	Agree	Strongly Agree
14. I tend to negatively judge people with opioid use problems.	☐	☐	☐	☐	☐
15. People with opioid use problems who relapse while trying to recover aren't trying hard enough to get better.	☐	☐	☐	☐	☐
16. I tend to speak down to people with opioid use problems.	☐	☐	☐	☐	☐
17. Most people with opioid use problems engage in crime to support their addiction.	☐	☐	☐	☐	☐
18. If a co-worker says something negative about people with opioid use problems, I would be more likely to speak negatively when discussing them myself.	☐	☐	☐	☐	☐
19. I tend to think poorly about people with opioid use problems.	☐	☐	☐	☐	☐

Appendix 7.1

The Youth Opinion Survey

Now that you have heard our presentation, we are going to ask you a few questions about mental illnesses. This will help us in further developing our class materials and allow us to meet your learning needs.

Some General Info About You:

Year of birth: _____ Month of birth: _____ Day of birth: _____

Female ( )   Male ( )   Other ( )   What grade are you in? _____

What words or phrases come to your mind to describe someone with a mental illness?

1. _____ 2. _____ 3. _____

The next few questions ask you to agree or disagree with a series of statements. Please check the box that best fits your opinion.

	Strongly Disagree	Disagree	Unsure	Agree	Strongly Agree
Most people with a mental illness are too disabled to work.	O	O	O	O	O
People with a mental illness tend to bring it on themselves.	O	O	O	O	O
People with mental illnesses often don't try hard enough to get better.	O	O	O	O	O
People with a mental illness could snap out of it if they wanted to.	O	O	O	O	O
People with a mental illness are often more dangerous than the average person.	O	O	O	O	O
People with a mental illness often become violent if not treated.	O	O	O	O	O
Most violent crimes are committed by people with a mental illness.	O	O	O	O	O
You can't rely on someone with a mental illness.	O	O	O	O	O
You can never know what someone with a mental illness is going to do.	O	O	O	O	O
Most people with a mental illness get what they deserve.	O	O	O	O	O
People with serious mental illnesses need to be locked away.	O	O	O	O	O

Please tell us what you think you would do in these different circumstances.

	Strongly Disagree	Disagree	Unsure	Agree	Strongly Agree
I would be upset if someone with a mental illness always sat next to me in class.	O	O	O	O	O
I would not be close friends with someone I knew had a mental illness.	O	O	O	O	O
I would visit a classmate in hospital if they had a mental illness.	O	O	O	O	O
I would not try to avoid someone with a mental illness.	O	O	O	O	O
I would not mind it if someone with a mental illness lived next door to me.	O	O	O	O	O
If I knew someone had a mental illness I would still date them.	O	O	O	O	O
I would mind being taught by a teacher who had been treated for a mental illness.	O	O	O	O	O
I would tell a teacher if a student was being bullied because of their mental illness.	O	O	O	O	O
I would stick up for someone who had a mental illness if they were being teased.	O	O	O	O	O
I would tutor a classmate who got behind in their studies because of their mental illness.	O	O	O	O	O
I would volunteer my time to work in a program for people with a mental illness.	O	O	O	O	O

Do you, or does someone you know, have a mental illness?

- o No
- o Uncertain
- o Yes, a close friend
- o Yes, a close family member
- o Yes, someone other than a close friend or family member
- o Yes, I do

Thank you for completing this questionnaire!
In additional to all the above questions the posttest also included the following:

These questions ask you about how you felt about the presentation.

	Strongly Disagree	Disagree	Unsure	Agree	Strongly Agree
I enjoyed learning about mental illnesses.	O	O	O	O	O
Now I think about mental illnesses in a new way.	O	O	O	O	O
I would like to have more presentations like this.	O	O	O	O	O
More class time should be spent learning from people with mental illnesses.	O	O	O	O	O

What did you like?

_____

_____

_____

_____

What didn't you like?

_____

_____

_____

_____

What did you learn about mental illnesses?

_____

_____

_____

_____

Thank you for completing this questionnaire!

Appendix 8.1

The Opening Minds Scale for Health Care Providers

These questions ask you to agree or disagree with a series of statements about mental illness. There is no correct answer. Please mark the box that best fits your opinion.

	Strongly Disagree	Disagree	Neither Agree nor Disagree	Agree	Strongly Agree
1. I am more comfortable helping a person who has a physical illness than I am helping a person who has a mental illness.	☐	☐	☐	☐	☐
2. If a colleague with whom I work told me they had a mental illness, I would be just as willing to work with him/her.	☐	☐	☐	☐	☐
3. If I were under treatment for a mental illness I would not disclose this to any of my colleagues.	☐	☐	☐	☐	☐
4. I would see myself as weak if I had a mental illness and could not fix it myself.	☐	☐	☐	☐	☐
5. I would be reluctant to seek help if I had a mental illness.	☐	☐	☐	☐	☐
6. Employers should hire a person with a managed mental illness if he/she is the best person for the job.	☐	☐	☐	☐	☐
7. I would still go to a physician if I knew that the physician had been treated for a mental illness.	☐	☐	☐	☐	☐
8. If I had a mental illness, I would tell my friends.	☐	☐	☐	☐	☐
9. Despite my professional beliefs, I have negative reactions towards people who have mental illness.	☐	☐	☐	☐	☐
10. There is little I can do to help people with mental illness.	☐	☐	☐	☐	☐
11. More than half of people with mental illness don't try hard enough to get better.	☐	☐	☐	☐	☐
12. I would not want a person with a mental illness, even if it were appropriately managed, to work with children.	☐	☐	☐	☐	☐
13. Healthcare providers do not need to be advocates for people with mental illness.	☐	☐	☐	☐	☐
14. I would not mind if a person with a mental illness lived next door to me.	☐	☐	☐	☐	☐
15. I struggle to feel compassion for a person with mental illness.	☐	☐	☐	☐	☐

Appendix 11.1

The Opening Minds Scale for Supervisor Workplace Attitudes

Read the following statements, and decide how much you to agree or disagree with that statement. Place an "X" in the correct column for each item to indicate your response.

	Strongly Disagree	Disagree	Unsure	Agree	Strongly Agree
1. It is in the interest of employers to support people with mental health difficulties so as to retain their skills and experience.					
2. You would employ someone who you knew had a history of mental health difficulties.					
3. People with mental health difficulties are less reliable than other employees.					
4. Employees who have been off work with a mental health difficulty for more than a few weeks are unlikely ever to return.					
5. Organizations take a significant risk when employing people with mental health difficulties.					
6. Negative attitudes from co-workers are a major barrier to employing people with mental health difficulties.					
7. Employers should make a special effort to accommodate the particular needs of employees with mental health difficulties in the workplace.					
8. If one of your employees had a mental health difficulty, you would want him/her to tell you.					
9. If you knew that an employee had a mental health difficulty, you would be likely to reduce the responsibility given to them.					
10. If you knew that an employee had a mental health difficulty, you would be unlikely to consider them for a promotion.					
11. You would feel comfortable talking about a mental health difficulty at work.					

Appendix 11.2

A Checklist to Engage Organizations in Antistigma Implementation and Evaluation Work

"Champion"/workplace liaison engaged ☐	• Managerial-level within organization • Pre-existing understanding of importance and impact of mental health and mental illness in the workplace • In person meetings, if possible
Senior leadership/executive level engaged ☐	• Pre-existing understanding of importance and impact of mental health and mental illness in the workplace OR • Provide supporting information on importance of mental health in the workplace and benefits of anti-stigma initiatives • Receive all levels of approval
Program for implementation ☐	• Present program options for organizations • Address barriers/concerns to implementation (e.g. cost, logistics) • Receive endorsement for program from senior leadership/executives
Commitment to evaluation component ☐	• Provide rationale for importance of evaluation • Address barriers/concerns to commitment (e.g. time constraints)
Organizational clearance/REB for evaluation component ☐	• What REB clearances are required from the researchers end and/or the organization's end in order to conduct the evaluation?
Other factors to consider ☐	• Account for timing throughout process (e.g. summer months, holidays) • Account for organizational turnover and engage new stakeholders as needed

Appendix 11.3

An Evaluation Framework to Be Designed Collaboratively Among Employers, Programs, and Researchers

Evaluation objectives: List the various objectives of your evaluation

Main evaluation question: What is your main evaluation question?

Framework for evaluation of changes resulting from the program

Assumed impact on:	Components of program addressing this:

What components of the program will impact what?

Evaluation tool	What does it evaluate	When will it be administered

What are your evaluation tools/ outcome measures? What component of the program or impact of the program does it evaluate? When will they be administered?

Program implementation: What is the structure of the program implementation process?

Evaluation procedures: What are your evaluation procedures? Who and how is data being collected? How long will the measures take to be completed? How will you link surveys over time? Etc.

Anticipated outputs: What type of reports will be provided?

Appendix 13.1

PSP Pre Learning Module Questionnaire

Module to be Conducted in the _____ DISTRICT HEALTH AUTHORITY

PART 1. Socio-Demographic and Context Questions for Physicians Who Will Complete the Module

We would like to have a better understanding about you and the context in which you work. Please answer the following questions:

1. Date you will attend the Mental Health Module: _____/_____
    Month/Year

2. What is your gender? ☐ Male ☐ Female

3. Which age group applies to you?
    20–29 years
    30–39 years
    40–49 years
    50–59 years
    60–69 years
    70 years of age or older

4. How long have you been practicing family medicine? _____ ☐ Not Applicable

5. What is your pattern of work?
    ☐ Full time
    ☐ Part-time
    ☐ Other-Specify_____

6. What is the nature of the practice in which you work most of the time?
    ☐ Solo practice
    ☐ Two physician practice
    ☐ Small group practice (4 or fewer physicians)
    ☐ Large group practice (5 or more physicians)

7. How many unique patients are seen in your practice in a year?
    ☐ Fewer than 1,000
    ☐ 1,000 to 1,999
    ☐ 2,000 to 2,999
    ☐ 3,000 or more
    ☐ Primarily work in a drop in clinic
    ☐ Other (hospitalist, work as a locum etc.)

Approximately what percentage of patients in your practice have mental health concerns?

8. Are you currently, or have you in the past, attended any other practice support modules?

    ☐ Yes   ☐ No   If YES, which one(s)?

    _____

PART 2: Your Current Practice and Experiences With Mental Health Care

In this set of questions, we ask about your current practices regarding depression and your **overall, general level of confidence** in your skills in dealing with mental health issues, and the impact that the learning module may have had on these aspects of your practice.

1. Approximately what percentage of patients do you screen for depression? _____%

    If you do screen for depression:
    a. Do you use formal screening instruments?   ☐ Yes   ☐ No
       If YES, which one(s)? _____

       _____

       _____

    b. If you suspect that a patient is depressed, based on your screening, do you follow a specific interview protocol to screen for other mental health and addictions conditions?
                          ☐ Yes   ☐ No

       If YES, please describe what you do. _____

       _____

       _____

2. Does the Diagnostic Assessment Interview help you identify any mental health conditions other than depression?
                          ☐ Yes   ☐ No

    a. If YES, what was the most commonly identified mental health condition other than depression?

       _____

    b. If YES, does the Family Physician Guide provide adequate information and assistance for further treatment and follow-up?
                          ☐ Yes   ☐ No

    c. Please provide any comments or suggestions about the Diagnostic Assessment

3. Please rate your current level of confidence in your ability to:	Very Confident	Somewhat Confident	Not Very Confident	Not at all Confident
(a) Diagnose depression				
(b) Screen for addictions				
(c) Screen for other mental health conditions				
(d) Treat depression				
(e) Treat other mental health disorders				

3. Please rate your current level of confidence in your ability to:	Very Confident	Somewhat Confident	Not Very Confident	Not at all Confident
(f) Prescribe medications for mental health conditions				
(g) Assess patients' problems and strengths				
(h) Develop systematized care plans for patients where the Mental Health Care plan is not appropriate				
(i) Create a Mental Health Care plan fitting the MSP guidelines				
(j) Engage mental health patients in a range of interventions (e.g., Cognitive Behavioural Interpersonal Skills training).x				
(k) Offer and coach the Antidepressant Skills Workbook.				
(l) Access the Mental Health Coaching Program materials and services for your patients.				
(m) In general, how confident are you in the quality of mental health care you provide to your patients?				

4. Please rate your current level of confidence in your knowledge/ awareness of:	Very Confident	Somewhat Confident	Not Very Confident	Not at all Confident
(a) Non-pharmacological interventions (cognitive behavioral skills such as activation, relaxation, negative thinking).				
(b) Regional mental health resources for mental health patients.				

PART 3. New Tools and Skills for Mental Health Care

Please reflect on your familiarity with the tool or skill *prior to* the Learning Module, your *current* levels of confidence in and comfort with using the tool or skill, and your perceptions of how your patients who require mental health care responded to it (if applicable).

Note: Part 3 consisted of 17 items, all asked in the same format. For the sake of space the first item is shown completely below, and then the complete list of items is provided.

Item	Your FAMILIARITY with the tool/ skill <u>now</u>	Your CONFIDENCE in the tool/ skill <u>now</u>	Your COMFORT with using the tool/ skill <u>now</u>	Your PATIENTS' responses to the tool/ activity
1. PHQ9 & PHQ2	☐ very high ☐ high ☐ moderate ☐ low ☐ very low ☐ not at all ☐ not applicable	☐ very high ☐ high ☐ moderate ☐ low ☐ very low ☐ not at all ☐ not applicable	☐ very high ☐ high ☐ moderate ☐ low ☐ very low ☐ not at all ☐ not applicable	☐ very positive ☐ positive ☐ neutral ☐ negative ☐ very negative ☐ not used ☐ not applicable

All items:

1. PHQ9 & PHQ2
2. AUDIT (Alcohol Use Disorders Identification Test)
3. SMMSE (Standardized Mini-Mental State Exam)
4. MOCA (Montreal Cognitive Assessment)
5. GAF (Global Assessment of Functioning)
6. GAD-7 (Generalized Anxiety Disorder)
7. The Family Physician Guide
8. CBIS Manual (binder or e-version)
9. Electronic hyperlinked mental health algorithm
10. Add Mental Health Coaching Program name
11. Referrals for Add Mental Health Coaching Program name
12. Antidepressant Skills Workbook & coaching skills
13. Diagnostic assessment interview skills
14. Problem List Action Plan
15. CBIS Resource List
16. CBIS skills handouts
17. Medication algorithm

Index

Tables, figures, and boxes are indicated by an italic t, f, and b following the page number.

Printed in the USA
CPSIA information can be obtained
at www.ICGtesting.com
CBHW062317050324
5012CB00004B/84

9 780197 572597